SOUTH SIDE HITMEN

THE STORY OF THE 1977 CHICAGO WHITE SOX

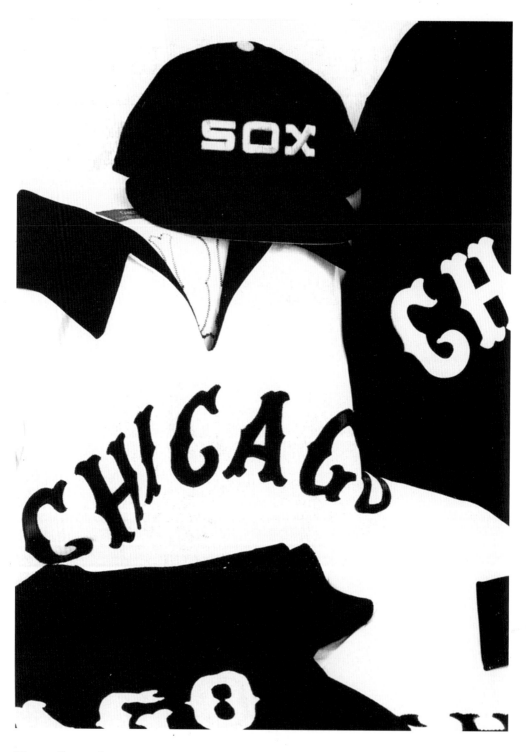

This collage of 1977 South Side Hitmen uniforms, ball, and hat comes from the Gerry Bilek memorabilia collection. (Photo by Mark Flectcher.)

SOUTH SIDE HITMEN

THE STORY OF THE 1977 CHICAGO WHITE SOX

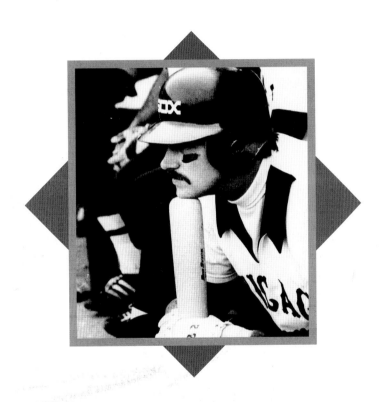

Dan Helpingstine,
with photographs from Leo Bauby

ARCADIA

Published by Arcadia Publishing
Charleston SC, Chicago IL, Portsmouth NH, San Francisco CA

Printed in Great Britain

Library of Congress Catalog Card Number: 2005931665

For all general information contact Arcadia Publishing at:
Telephone 843-853-2070
Fax 843-853-0044
E-mail sales@arcadiapublishing.com
For customer service and orders:
Toll-Free 1-888-313-2665

Visit us on the Internet at www.arcadiapublishing.com

This book is dedicated to Nancy Puhr-Morris.

Thanks for the friendship and professionalism.

One day I will pay you back fully.

CONTENTS

ACKNOWLEDGMENTS

The first thing I would like to do is thank three individuals who helped me with this book and who also assisted on my first book published by Arcadia, *The Chicago White Sox: 1959 and Beyond.* These three gentlemen provided the book's photographs, and they also provided technical expertise, memories, and historical perspective.

The overwhelming majority of the photographs in this book come from the Leo Bauby collection. Bauby's collection spans most of the 20th century and neatly captures the storied history of the White Sox. The pictures can be viewed at http://www.chicago-baseball-photos. com, a collection that brings back powerful memories in images. His collection of White Sox photos is staggering.

Gerry Bilek's basement recreation room looks like a small White Sox museum. He has a turnstile from old Comiskey and other relics that would take a Sox fan down a true nostalgic trip to the past. His recollections and photograph contributions are an essential part of this book.

Mark Fletcher is a photographer as well as a collector. His expert photography has helped restore past feelings about the White Sox. He took photographs of some of Bilek's memorabilia to bring back the flavor of 1977.

I would also like to thank Vivian Jones of the Chicago White Sox Media Relations office for helping me secure the interviews with former White Sox.

I am also appreciative to White Sox fan and historian Mark Liptak. Liptak still follows the team religiously from his home in Idaho, where he claims to be one of the few Sox fans in that part of the country. (He is probably right.) I am more than grateful for all his ongoing help.

Keith Scherer was gracious enough to allow me to use an online ESPN article of his in which he gave a great analysis of what derailed the White Sox in August 1977. Scherer's well-written article appeared in 2003 and illustrated the staying power the South Side Hitmen.

The author used his own memories, newspaper accounts from the *Chicago Sun-Times*, and *Chicago Tribune*, and interviews with the people listed in the following introduction. One of the handiest resources was *The White Sox Encyclopedia* by Rich Lindberg with photographic history from Mark Fletcher.

I would like to thank Arcadia editor Jeff Ruetsche for his ongoing confidence in me. Ruetsche allowed me the creative freedom to put my spin on this little slice of Chicago White Sox history.

The year 1977 was very special for me personally, as I got married that September. My wife Delia has been very supportive of me in my writing throughout all these years and that is something I do not take for granted. She also helped with the editing of this book, cleaning up my sometimes awkward phrasing.

INTRODUCTION

Baseball was still young in 1977. Yes, the sport had its problems—as it always has—but the seven-day-a-week, 24-hour-a-day hype wasn't over-exposing the industry. If a fan wanted to know what was happening with his team and couldn't watch or listen to the game, he picked up the paper in the morning. There is something simple and gratifying about reading about it in the newspaper. Today's glut of cable TV and radio talk shows is simply too loud. I am happy to include some of the memories of sportswriters who covered the South Side Hitmen.

Long time columnist Bill Gleason, now retired, has often been considered the city's number one White Sox fan. When he lived in Chicago, the last four digits of his home phone were 1959. During the second half of the 20th century, he covered Bill Veeck, the Allyns, and Jerry Reinsdorf. Gleason helped form the panel on the radio show, the Sportswriters, which aired Sundays from 4:00 to 6:00 p.m. on WGN-AM, 720. Former boxing promoter Ben Bentley, *Chicago Tribune* sports editor George Langford, and *Chicago Tribune* sports reporter Bill Jauss discussed with him the state of Chicago and national sports. The Sportswriters did not take calls from listeners. However, Gleason and other panelists often read listener letters and actually treated listener opinions with respect. I learned a great deal about the White Sox from Gleason and I am pleased to have several of his observations in this book.

Bill Jauss covered two key series in the 1977 South Side Hitmen season. He was at rollicking Comiskey for both the July 4 holiday weekend four-game set against Minnesota and the four-game series against Kansas City that ended the month. A few of his keen observations are also quoted in the book. Jauss has always been a fan advocate, and it was great talking to him about the 1977 season.

One of the hardest things for any reporter to do is to write some tough things about people he knows and associates with on a daily basis. I am grateful to former *Chicago Sun-Times* reporter Joe Goddard for recalling a story he did on Sox manager Paul Richards in 1976. It was still somewhat painful for Goddard to remember his story about a man who otherwise had a great baseball career. Maybe Goddard should write a book about the White Sox someday. He knows a great deal about the team and has an excellent memory for detail.

Gary Peters is profiled in chapter 1. Peters was one of the toughest left-handers in the American League during the mid-1960s. I am grateful for the time he gave me recalling his White Sox career. This included memories of the 1967 White Sox, a team that came very close to a World Series, but has been almost forgotten in the fog of baseball history.

Eric Soderholm also gave his time. His comeback season in 1977 had a profound impact on him. His return, his career year, and his bonding with Sox fans have been a great story. Soderholm was somewhat surprised that a book about the 1977 Sox was being written. He shouldn't have been surprised; 1977 was a historic season for the team in many ways.

Steve Stone is now a large part of Chicago baseball history. He has won over many Cub fans for his candor in the broadcast booth. As a student of the game, I enjoyed my conversation with him. I never would mind Steve Stone disagreeing with me. I would gain from the experience of listening to someone who knows the game. His comments to me about 1977 were as honest as anything that has been said on the air.

Rich "Goose" Gossage was a large part of the 1977 White Sox since he was packaged in the trade that brought Richie Zisk to Chicago. But no fan with vivid memories of the 1970s will forget Gossage's windmill motion and a fast ball most hitters couldn't see. His recollections about Bill Veeck and the 1976 season help put a perspective on the state of the franchise during the mid-1970s.

I remember sitting at a bar enjoying a beer and watching Oscar Gamble golf one deep into the right field upper deck for a three-run homer. Gamble made Sox history in 1977 even though he had expected to play for the Yankees that year. I appreciated the time Gamble gave me as he recalled the "offensive balance" of the 1977 team and dreamed of what would have been if the team had been kept together until more pitching arrived.

Nancy Faust will be forever connected to the South Side Hitmen. Picking up on the frenzy and emotion of the most exciting days of the summer of 1977, musician Faust played a song that remains a rallying cry for the team. Faust understands that entertaining fans largely comes from spontaneity. Are you listening, Major League Baseball?

History doesn't occur in a vacuum. This book is not just a recollection of an emotional and memorable season. The author has attempted to put the team in its proper place in Chicago White Sox history. To say that 1977 was a breakthrough season is an understatement. It is also safe to say that the South Side Hitmen helped keep the team in Chicago. It is hard to imagine the future of the White Sox had they gone through another 90-loss season in 1977. Instead, the team had its best attendance since 1960, the year after it went to its last World Series of the 20th century. More importantly, it gave fans their greatest memories of the 1970s that have lasted into the 21st century.

1967

END OF THE NO-HIT ERA

The seeds of the exciting, 1977 slugging South Side Hit Men were actually sown exactly 10 years earlier by a White Sox team that couldn't hit a beach ball into Lake Michigan while standing on the sand. In one of the last years of one divisional play, the 1967 team was not eliminated from the pennant chase until the 160th game of the season. Although it competed gamely in a race with the Twins, Red Sox, and Tigers, where there was a strong possibility of a four-way tie for first, the 1967 White Sox are rarely talked about in the same breath as other great Sox teams. They put together a 10-game winning streak in early May and were in first place from June 10 until August 13. Yet, the contending White Sox had to fight off criticism that they were a boring team that relied too much on pitching while lulling their fans to sleep with a small-ball offense. Even Manager Eddie Stanky, a staunch defender of his club, thought they were boring, calling them the "dullest ball club I have ever seen."

Getting anywhere near the World Series was not expected when the 1967 season began. The consensus of experts predicted a fourth place finish. From 1951 through 1967, the Sox had sported winning records, one of the most successful such runs by any Major League Baseball franchise. There was the pennant year of 1959 and six 90-win seasons. They had three straight second place finishes in the then one ten-team division from 1963 to 1965, winning 94, 98, and 95 games, respectively. But in 1966, their record slipped to 83-79, and they needed a strong finish to again land on the sunny side of .500.

Starting with the second game of a doubleheader against Cleveland on April 30, the Pale Hose went on their 10-game winning streak. Except for a 13-1 blowout of Baltimore, the wins were low scoring affairs which included two 1-0 triumphs, one of which was in 10 innings. The streak ended when Chicago was shut out 1-0 by Minnesota's Dean Chance. The White Sox were perched in first place at the All-Star break, but they were not running away with anything. They led second place Detroit by two, and third place Minnesota by two and a half games. To shore up their low scoring attack, Chicago picked up two aging sluggers in late July: Ken Boyer from the Mets and Rocky Colavito from the Indians.

Boyer and Colavito made only occasional contributions and may have disrupted team chemistry. As the season progressed, cynics were ready to bury the White Sox any time they lost, especially when their weak offense failed to support their excellent pitching. Manager Eddie Stanky lashed out at the naysayers on September 9, when his club blew a 3-0 ninth inning lead and lost to co-contender Detroit 7-3 in a nationally televised game.

"They discount the guts of this club," Stanky said, defending his often maligned but winning team. "All year long this team had guts."

The Sox somewhat vindicated Stanky the next day with a doubleheader sweep by shutting out the heavy hitting Tigers in both games. In game one, righty and Cy Young Award candidate Joe Horlen delivered a brilliant performance when he pitched a no-hitter, beating Detroit 6-0 for one of his 19 wins that year.

By the end of September, the White Sox were in excellent shape and ready to prove their detractors wrong once and for all. With five games remaining in the season, the second place Sox were but one game behind first place Minnesota. The remaining Sox schedule looked easy as they faced the last place Kansas City Athletics twice in Kansas City, and the seventh place Washington Senators three times to close out the year at Comiskey Park.

A rain out in Kansas City forced a Wednesday night doubleheader. That September 27, 1967, became known as "Black Wednesday" as Chicago sent out their ace pitchers Gary Peters and Joe Horlen and still lost 5-2 and 4-0. They barely avoided a double shut out by scoring two in the ninth in game one. The South Siders went from being on the verge of the World Series to getting eliminated unless they swept the lowlife Senators.

Tommy John started the Friday night game at Comiskey and gave up an unearned run in the first. So desperate for any kind of offense, the Sox lifted John for a pinch hitter in the fifth even though they trailed only 1-0. There was no designated hitter back then, and the Sox could have used one.

Phil Ortega, on the mound for the Senators, hadn't won a game in nearly two months. After giving up two singles in the first, Ortega surrendered only two more hits for the remainder of a complete game performance. Facing the virtual end of their season in the ninth when they trailed 1-0, the Hitless Wonders couldn't put the ball into fair territory. Ken Boyer struck out, Ron Hansen fouled out to the catcher, and J. C. Martin struck out. Ortega pitched one of the best games of his 46-62 career, and the banjo hitting White Sox proved their critics right by getting shut out in a must-win game. Elimination came on that 160th game of the season even though a great pitching staff had thrown eight shut outs during the stretch month of September. And after losing the last two games of the season, the White Sox actually finished in fourth, three games behind pennant winning Boston.

In many ways, Gary Peters—a 1960s Chicago White Sox icon—symbolized the South Side ball club during that decade. From 1963 to 1967, he was one of the toughest left-handed pitchers in the American League. Though 1967 wasn't his winningest year, in many ways it was a career year for Peters and his last great season with the White Sox. He made his only All-Star appearance in Anaheim, pitching three perfect innings. In the process he fanned Willie Mays, Orlando Cepeda, Dick Allen, and Roberto Clemente. Peters finished the year with 215 strikeouts, and, with Tom Bradley and Ed Walsh, was one of three White Sox pitchers to record 200 or more strikeouts in two or more seasons. Yet Peters was not concerned with piling up strikeouts or pitch counts.

"I didn't consider myself a power pitcher," Peters told the author in 2005. "I threw my fast ball high and inside. I never left it out over the plate. I had a sinker and slider and in one complete game I only threw 70 pitches."

In the middle of that wild pennant race in 1967, Peters was involved in a somewhat typical and yet amazing type hitless-wonder win.

On September 13, the White Sox beat the Cleveland Indians 1-0 in a 17-inning night game. Peters started the game and walked 10 batters in 11 innings. He gave up a second inning triple to catcher Joe Azcue and nothing more. Peters ended up throwing nine and two-thirds innings of hitless ball only to get a no-decision. Reliever Don McMahon picked up the win by pitching a scoreless 17th inning. The Sox finally won with the help of a passed ball.

"We had guys who knew how to pitch," Peters recalled. "We didn't have many seven run leads. We couldn't just let them hit it. We could never afford that mentality."

As a result, Peters said, this philosophy (of not giving in to hitters) was reflected in the staff's low earned run average of 2.45 in 1967. But the shortage of offense finally caught up with the White Sox during the September 27 doubleheader against Kansas City. Peters, however, doesn't hold any grudges against his offense. He takes the responsibility for one of the most significant losses for the White Sox during the 1960s.

"Kansas City was in a good position where they could play the spoiler," Peters remembered, "but I didn't pitch that well. I gave up too many runs. That's just the way I look at it."

Peters also thinks the 1967 White Sox should be remembered as a good team, and that their boring persona was overblown.

"I came up in the fall of 1959," Peters said. (Peters made two appearances and pitched one inning.) "Everybody thought that team was exciting. It [the 1967 team] was the same kind of club but in '59 we had more guys who could steal. I never heard that we weren't exciting. We weren't playing to be exciting. We were playing to win."

The collapse during the final week of the 1967 season actually helped set the stage for the fan euphoria of 1977. After seeing their team average a little over three runs a game in 1967 and sleep walking through decades of low scoring games, White Sox fans were ready to leave the legacy of the Go-Go White Sox behind them. The 1-0 wins and the 3-2 losses had grown old and stale. How about a team that could just hit the cover off the ball? Bill Melton won the American League home run championship on the last day of 1971, and Dick Allen had his MVP year in 1972. The Sox even led the American League in homers in 1974. But the first truly exciting offensive club to come along to thrill fans didn't appear on the scene until a decade after a great World Series opportunity was lost due to an anemic offense that had a hard time getting the ball out of the infield.

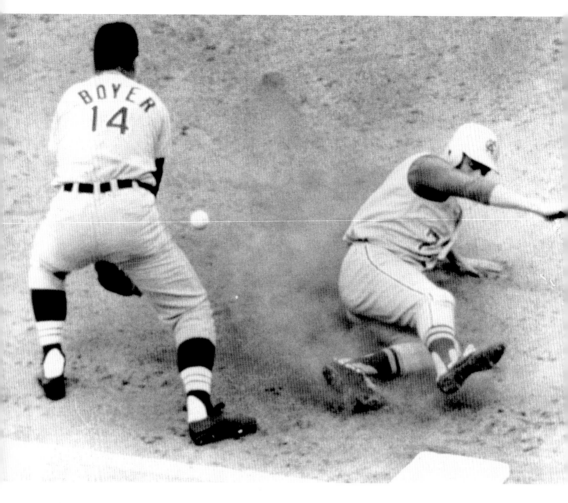

Boyer and Bando were two great third baseman. Sal Bando slides into third while Ken Boyer appears to have a sinking, helpless feeling. Boyer won the National League Most Valuable Player Award in 1964 while leading St. Louis to a World Championship. Bando played on the World Champion A's of 1972–1974. This play occurred on Black Wednesday, September 27, 1967, when Kansas City swept the Sox in a mid-week doubleheader and virtually ended Chicago's season. (Leo Bauby collection.)

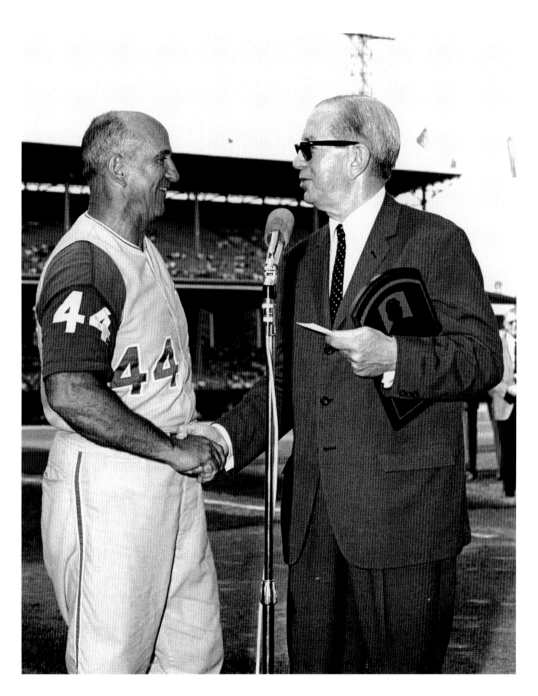

Ex-White Sox great Luke Appling takes part in pre-game ceremony with long-time Sox radio play-by-play announcer Bob Elson. Ironically, Appling was the interim manager of the Kansas City A's on Black Wednesday. Appling finished his career with 2,749 career hits, a .310 lifetime batting average, and he set the single season record for batting average for the White Sox with a .388 mark in 1936. (Gerry Bilek collection.)

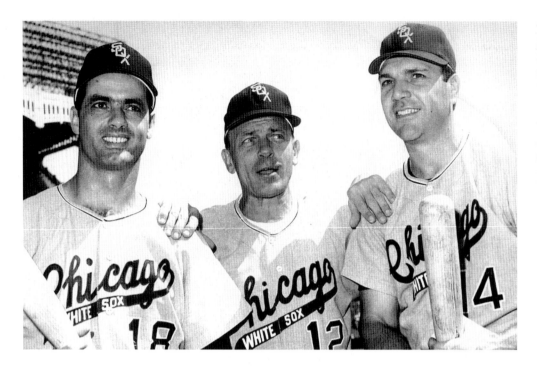

Manager Eddie Stanky stands in between sluggers Rocky Colavito (left) and Ken Boyer. The two hit a combined 656 home runs in their careers and a total of seven in the last half of 1967 after they were acquired in mid-season trades. It would have been great if the Sox had picked them up in 1964 when each was still in his prime.

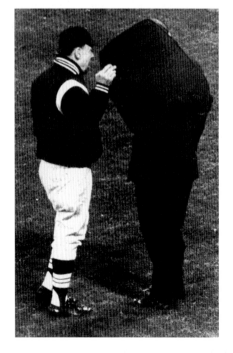

In this picture, it appears that the umpire is hiding from Eddie Stanky. Stanky was not shy about arguing with umpires—or anyone else. Even though he admitted his 1967 team was as dull as it could be, Stanky took high offense at anyone who suggested the same. Richard Nixon had a better relationship with the media. (Gerry Bilek collection.)

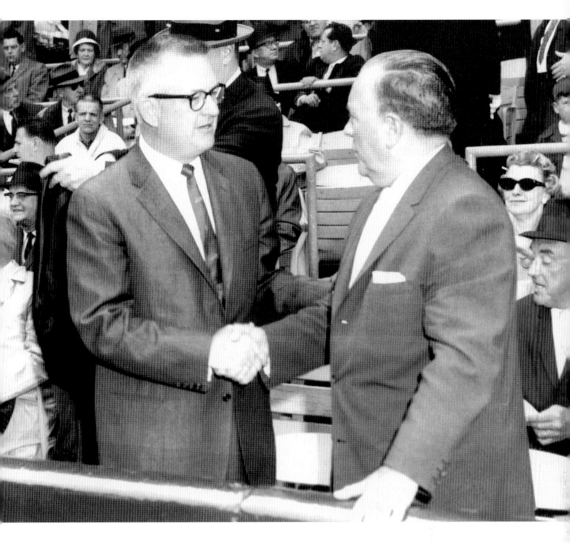

Arthur Allyn and Richard J. Daley were the two biggest White Sox fans during the 1960s. Allyn owned the Sox from June 1961 until September 1969. Daley was "His Honor," the mayor of Chicago, a position he held from 1955 through his death in December 1976. (Gerry Bilek collection.)

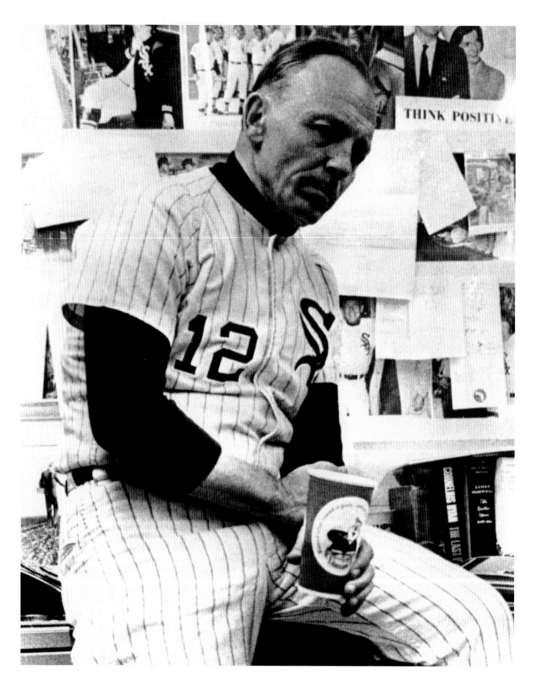

Eddie Stanky is seen here after the White Sox were officially eliminated from the 1967 pennant race by the Washington Senators. Washington shut out the Sox 1-0. The crusty manager, who defended his team time and again during the grueling last month of the race, ended up leaving the room in tears. White Sox fans cried right along with him. (Leo Bauby collection.)

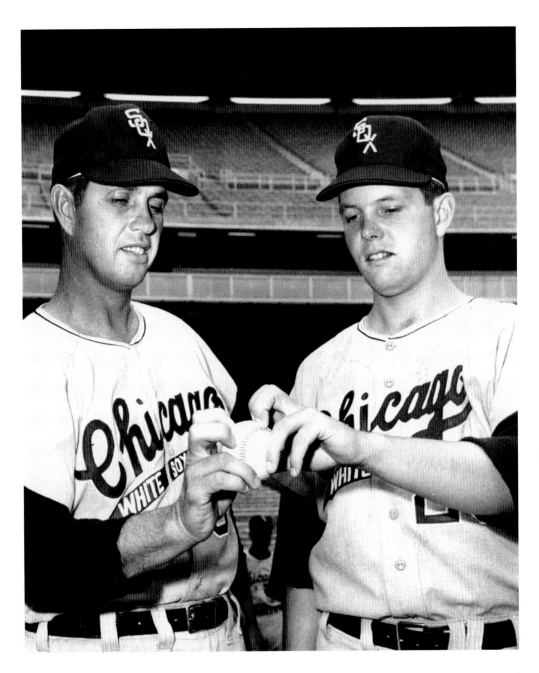

Wilbur Wood and Hoyt Wilhelm were the lefty-righty knuckle ball combination coming out of the bullpen for the Sox. According to Roland Hemond, Wood was not crazy about the shift to a role as a starting pitcher in 1971, as Wood thought he had found himself as a reliever. In his career, Wilhelm appeared in 1,070 games. The two men were a combined 12-5 in the tragic year of 1967. (Leo Bauby collection.)

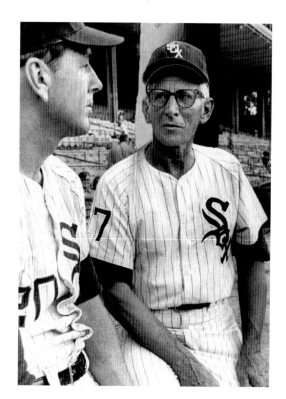

Nineteen-game winner Joe Horlen is pictured with mentor and pitching coach, Ray Berres, in 1968. It is funny how there so few sore arms on the Sox staff when Berres was coach. (Leo Bauby collection.)

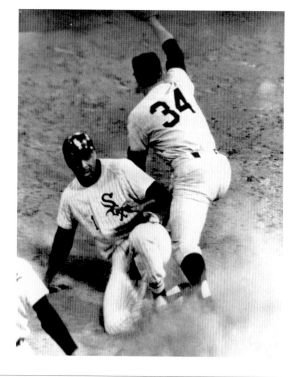

Center fielder Tommie Agee disappointed Sox fans when his averaged dipped to .234. He was traded to the Mets after the season and starred in the 1969 World Series. No White Sox player played in a World Series until 2005, unless they did it for other teams. (Gerry Bilek collection.)

Considered a great clutch hitter, shortstop Ron Hansen grounded out to third to end a White Sox rally (at least by 1967 standards) and finish off the first game of the doubleheader against the Kansas City A's on Black Wednesday. The bases were loaded at the time, and a grand slam would have put the Sox ahead by one. He is shown here in 1964, a year in which he hit 20 homers. (Leo Bauby collection.)

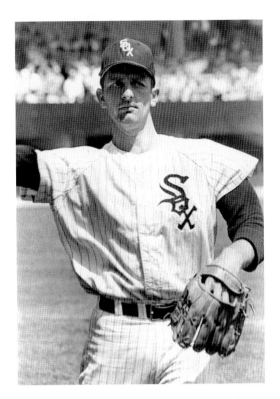

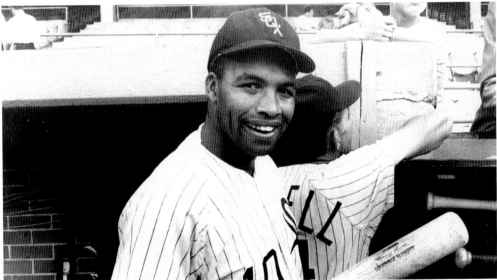

Tommy Davis looks awfully happy here, but looks are truly deceiving. Acquired in an after-season trade between the 1967 and 1968 campaigns, the two-time National League batting champion was looked as the offensive savior for the White Sox in 1968. He was nothing of the kind. His batting average dropped 34 points and he had 50 lonely RBIs. (Gerry Bilek collection.)

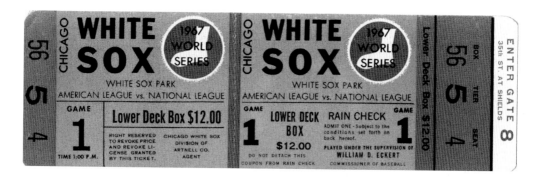

This 1967 World Series ticket was never used. The 1967 season was over-achieving and ended in a nightmare. The 1977 South Side Hitmen, who never really came close to winning anything, overshadow this club in many ways. Regardless, it would have been an interesting had the hitless 1967 wonders played in the World Series against the Cardinals. (Leo Bauby collection.)

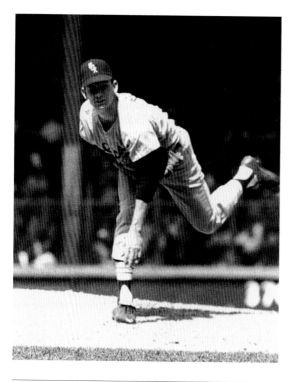

Gary Peters shows the form that made him one of the great left-handed pitchers in the American League during the mid-1960s. He won 16 in 1967. He would have won more with a better hitting team, which is a real understatement. (Leo Bauby collection.)

1967: END OF THE NO-HIT ERA

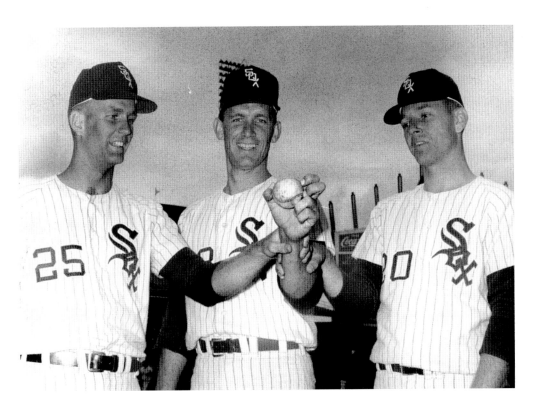

Tommy John (left), Gary Peters (middle), and Joe Horlen were the top three pitchers for the White Sox in 1967. The three threw a combined 15 shutouts that year. (Leo Bauby collection.)

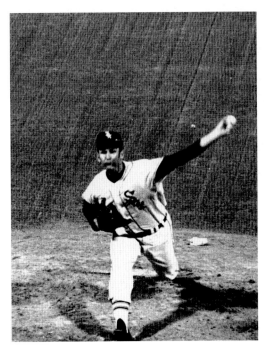

Tommy John is shown here during the disastrous 106-loss 1970 season. John started and lost the pennant-race eliminating game against the Washington Senators in 1967, even though he gave up only one unearned run in five innings. The run was scored in part because Senator Fred Valentine got new life when his foul ball landed in a camera well set up for a hoped for World Series. There was no World Series. You can't win when you can't score. (Leo Bauby collection.)

SOUTH SIDE HITMEN

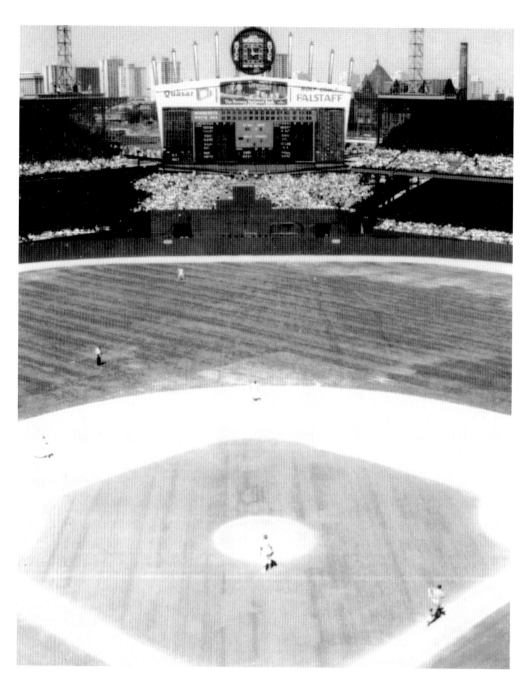

In 1969, much to the dismay of the pitching staff, the White Sox installed Astroturf in the infield to help their ground balls sneak out to the outfield. According to Gary Peters, the turf helped the opposition more because the Sox staff was full of low-ball, sinker throwing pitchers. Additionally, it made the infield look like a pool table and ruined the natural beauty of Comiskey Park. (Leo Bauby collection.)

2

1976

BARELY HANGING ON

At the start of the 1976 season, the Chicago White Sox were still a franchise at a crossroads. In late 1975, it appeared that the charter member of the American League was on its way out of Chicago. Financially strapped owner John Allyn had just seen his team draw barely over 770,000, a drop of almost a quarter of a million from 1974. One-time budding stars Bill Melton and Carlos May neared the end of their careers. After putting together four straight 20-win seasons, Wilbur Wood slumped to 16-20 with an ERA of over four for the first time in his career. No one from the Sox farm system showed any real promise of reviving the team. And after winning only 75 games and finishing 22 ½ games out of first place, the club had little talent to offer in the way of trades.

As the winter meetings approached in late 1975, Seattle loomed as the new home for the White Sox. The Sox had been losing money every year since 1970. By the end of 1975, the franchise had lost $8 million. That was a lot of money in those days.

"Poor John Allyn is broke," one American League owner said of the Sox boss. "If he doesn't get rid of the club soon, he won't have a dime left."

Finally, Bill Veeck, the last owner to take a White Sox team to a World Series, at that time, stepped in with an investment group to purchase the club when no other local businessman or entities were interested in risking money on the sagging franchise.

Bill Veeck was not your stereotypical owner. After wrestling control of the White Sox from the Comiskey family, he constructed "the Monster" in center field at Comiskey Park. "The Monster" was the huge fireworks-erupting scoreboard that celebrated rare White Sox home runs, delighting Chicago fans and infuriating opponents and the baseball establishment. He was the first owner to put names on the backs of uniforms, a move that drew intense criticism. Veeck took the Sox to the World Series in 1959, but some fans thought he sold the future of the team away by trading young promising players for veterans in an attempt to repeat the next year. Fans also felt deserted and betrayed when Veeck sold the team to Arthur Allyn in June 1961.

No matter how his baseball legacy would be judged, the American League wasn't impressed with Veeck's offer to purchase the White Sox in 1975. (A majority of owners must approve the sale of any franchise.) In addition to some owners not wanting the renegade Veeck back in major league baseball, the powers that be didn't think Veeck had enough financial backing and resources to make the purchase. So they gave him a chance to restructure his deal. If he failed to deliver, however, the franchise's 75-year old connection to Chicago and the Midwest would end.

Fans, with the prompting of WBBM/Channel 2 TV sportscaster, Johnny Morris, offered to send in donations to keep the team in the city. However, Illinois State law prevented Veeck from having more than 50 investors in his group. Legally, Veeck could not form a partnership with the fans to keep the White Sox in Chicago.

"There are people who say they have only a couple of bucks, but they're pulling for me," Veeck said, touched by fan sentiment. "Those are the ones who get to you."

On December 10, 1975, Veeck presented his new financial package to the owners. Whether they wanted him in their exclusive little group or not, the American League owners approved the sale by a 10-2 vote. The White Sox stayed in Chicago.

In a move to revive memories of the "Go-Go" Sox of the 1950s, Veeck brought back 67-year-old Paul Richards to manage the club. During his first tenure as Sox manager, Richards had averaged 88 wins from 1951 to 1954 with a 154-game schedule, even though Richards left the club on September 10, 1954, due to a salary dispute.

A new optimism greeted the Sox in the Bicentennial year of 1976. The media was behind Veeck, even praising the new paint job Comiskey Park had received. An hour or two before the home opener, Veeck made his way through the stands and was greeted by fans grateful for his keeping the Sox in the city. A crowd engulfed him, patting him on the back and shaking his hand as he walked through the lower deck on the third base side. Along with this newborn optimism, the sweet smell of marijuana was in the air. The 40,318 fans, hopefully more high on the occasion, attended the successful season home opener in which Wilbur Wood threw a 4-0 whitewashing of the Kansas City Royals. Nothing could spoil the day, not even the scoreboard firing a dud after a Jim Spencer two-run homer to right.

Later in the season, Veeck dressed his team up in shorts to get publicity and have fun. The Sox won one game largely because a Texas outfielder couldn't find a fly ball in the early June fog. Attendance climbed back over the 900,000 mark—not great but quite an improvement after the apathetic 1975 campaign nearly drove the team out of the city.

The year 1976, however, was not good for the White Sox. On May 9, Wood took a line drive on the knee off the bat of Tiger outfielder Ron LeFlore in Detroit. Wood was only 4-3 at the time but had an ERA of 2.25. His absence for the remainder of the season didn't help an already thin pitching staff. The short pants stunt drew derision as well as laughter. By the end of August, the *Chicago Sun-Times* depicted manager Paul Richards as a lonely man who had taken a job that wasn't right for him at that time in his life. More than one player complained to reporter Joe Goddard about Richards.

"He'd fall asleep during games," Goddard recalled in 2005. "He was late for games, not that he would be late for the actual start, but he would show only a half hour before. One time he gave a lineup card to third baseman Bill Stein to run out to the umpires. Stein noticed there were four outfielders but no third baseman. When Stein went back, Richards asked Stein where he usually batted. Stein said third and Richards said, 'put yourself down for third.'"

"His heart just wasn't in it," Goddard concluded.

According to Goddard, almost everybody connected with the White Sox organization didn't appreciate the story. Bill Veeck told Goddard that he "should have let the team be sold to Seattle." Veeck's son, Mike, angrily told Goddard that it "took a lot of guts" for Goddard to show up the day after the story ran. Harry Caray lit into Goddard claiming that Richards had taken the managerial job for one year as a favor to Veeck, an arrangement that Goddard said he knew nothing about. Goddard said he actually felt bad writing a story about an otherwise good baseball man.

Meanwhile—as Richards dismissed the article and showed enough class to co-exist with Goddard—Jim Spencer and Jorge Orta went on to lead the team in the home run department with 14 each, a puny number, hardly enough to entertain fans. In the last half of September, the team mailed their season in, failing in their last 15 of 16 games. The squad, labeled as quitters, finished with a last place record of 64-97, their second worst season in 25 years.

"It was a three ring circus, and we were the third act." This Rich Gossage quote easily described the 1976 Chicago White Sox season. Equipped with little pitching, defense, or hitting, the team's biggest accomplishment was staying in Chicago after the near move to Seattle at the end of 1975. However, Gossage wasn't referring to the team's performance where they barely missed losing 100 games.

Throughout his career, Bill Veeck was criticized for denigrating the sport by doing just about anything to draw attention and fans. Pinch hitting little people, martians landing in the middle of the Comiskey Park, and the exploding scoreboard offended many. Gossage holds Veeck in high regard, but he had little use for the many similar Veeckian brainstorms in 1976.

For almost his entire career, Gossage was a relief pitcher. The nickname of "Goose" was in reference to the number of zeros he placed on the scoreboard. He had a Hall of Fame type career notching 310 saves. But in 1976, he was slotted into the starting rotation for the pitching-poor White Sox. His changed routine of warming up before games, instead of in the middle as a reliever, was constantly interrupted by some eye-catching promotion.

"There were cattle, elephants, and dancing girls," Gossage said in 2005, still not amused. "Many times I didn't get a chance to warm up. It's hard to pitch the first inning when you haven't thrown. But the umpires wouldn't delay the game."

"He was a great promoter," Gossage said of Veeck. "But it got old."

Gossage also had few fond memories of the 1976 Sox, the team Veeck worked so hard to promote. He remembered leaving games with leads that weren't protected and a team defense that did little to reassure a pitcher.

"Bart Johnson [Sox right-hander] was on the mound and Paul Richards went out to talk to him," Gossage recalled. "He told Johnson to pitch around the next hitter. Johnson pointed to the Sox outfield and asked, 'How do I pitch around them?' Richards said, 'Young man, you have a point.'"

Needless to say, Johnson didn't pitch around the next hitter.

A little more than two months after the 1976 season mercifully ended, Gossage was traded to the Pirates along with Terry Forster in exchange for Richie Zisk and pitcher Silvio Martinez. Despite spending his formative major league years with the White Sox, Gossage said he was "happy to get out of that situation," not only because he was departing from a bad team, but because he was able to rejoin former Sox manager, Chuck Tanner, who was now managing Pittsburgh.

"It was a good trade for both teams," said Gossage, who wasn't surprised by the success of the South Side Hitmen. "Getting Zisk was good for the White Sox. They really needed the hitting."

Free agency was in its infancy in 1977. Other teams, even those that would be considered small market teams today, began signing star players to expensive, long-term contracts. Bill Veeck, the one-time players' advocate, had little means to seriously compete in this market. Yet, to improve attendance he couldn't field a team as boring as the 1976 edition. He might have been looked upon as a savior in late 1975, but White Sox fans had had enough of losing teams contending for last place.

So what did the White Sox do? They began by trading two of their hardest throwing pitchers—Rich Gossage and Terry Forster—to the Pirates for right fielder Richie Zisk. They also signed free-agent third baseman Eric Soderholm. Soderholm had injured his knee in a freakish, off the field accident in September 1975 and spent 1976 rehabbing. Finally, two days before the season was to begin, the White Sox sent shortstop Bucky Dent to the New York Yankees for pitchers LaMarr Hoyt and Bob Polinksy, and outfielder Oscar Gamble.

Zisk, Gamble, and Soderholm would end up leading the Sox to an incredible year. White Sox fans, so used to watching dull teams scratch for runs and then lose, fell in love with a club that could just plain hit. Huge Comiskey Park rocked with large crowds singing good-bye songs to vanquished opponents and demanding players come out of the dugout to acknowledge curtain calls after dramatic home runs. Many of the players, once considered outcasts, fed off the energy and emotion to have career years. Baseball was not merely revived on the South Side of Chicago; the enthusiasm from a once dormant fan base attracted national attention.

The 1977 White Sox became known as the South Side Hitmen, a name they more than lived up to. They didn't win the World Series or even a division championship, but they posted their best record in 12 years and set a White Sox attendance record. Their 192 home runs set another team record. They thrilled home crowds with long homers, come-from behind victories, and an offensive barrage that left opponents dazed and defeated. Two years earlier, many were ready to see the team leave for the great Northwest. Now they bonded with their favorite baseball club in a way that hasn't been matched since.

The 1977 South Side Hitmen. Just the name stirs memories of excitement and hope that had abandoned Chicago during the late 1970s. They are arguably one of the most loved teams in franchise history. Too bad they didn't have more pitching. Or more defense. Or the luck that always seemed to elude Chicago baseball teams. But in 1977, when baseball was still young, the South Side Hit Men were what the sport should be all about.

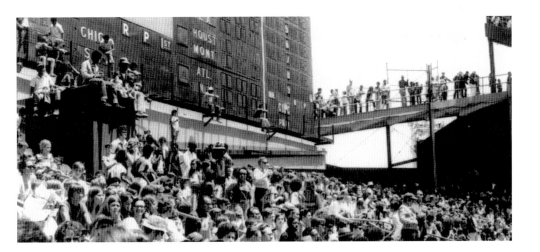

The White Sox had their problems with attendance during the late 1960s and mid-1970s. This was not the case on May 20, 1973. In those days, there was a great deal of general admission seating at Comiskey. Many fans ended up not seeing the game because there was no place for them to stand or sit. (They received refunds for the tickets.) Many sat in the aisles or, as in this photograph, stood on the scoreboard catwalk. The emotion at the ballpark was at near 1977 levels when Bill Melton and Carlos May homered in the first game, which the Sox won 9-3. (Leo Bauby collection.)

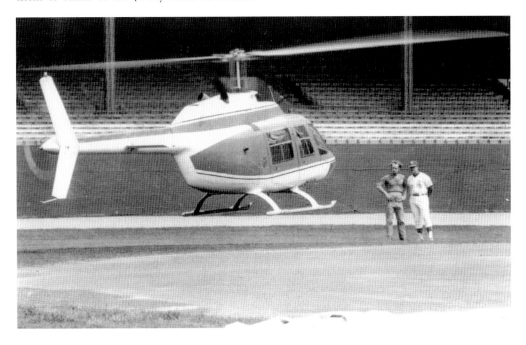

No, this was not some Bill Veeck–type stunt like bringing martians to Comiskey. Early Chicago springs are often cold and wet putting a damper on everything. In 1973, a helicopter was brought into Comiskey to dry the wet turf. (Leo Bauby collection.)

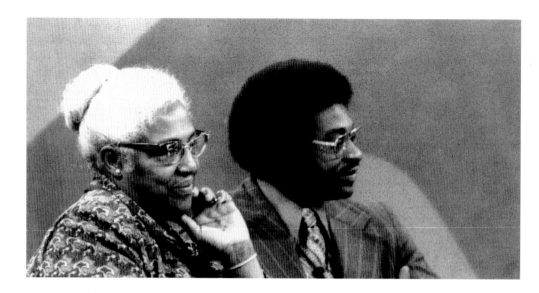

Dick Allen was the rage when he had his MVP season in 1972. Here he is shown with his mother on his TV show. Allen "retired" in the early part of September 1974 and then returned to play for his once hated Phillies. The White Sox tinkered with the idea of bringing him back in 1977 but thought better of it. It turned out to be a very wise decision. (Leo Bauby collection.)

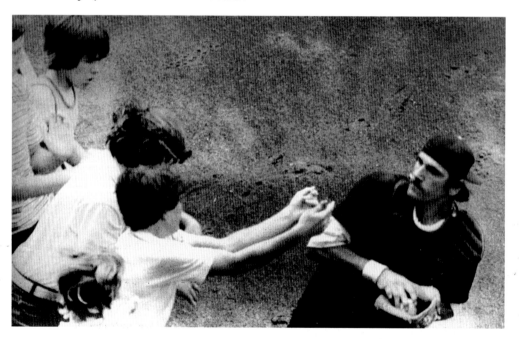

Jim Essian fights with a fan for foul ball in 1976. Essian ended up being the main compensation to the Sox when they traded Dick Allen after the disappointing 1974 season and would have a nice year for the 1977 South Side Hitmen. (Leo Bauby collection.)

Flame-throwing Terry Forster mows them down and looks great while doing it. It was short pants day at Comiskey on August 8, 1976. It was actually a kind of brisk day for August, never getting out of the 1970s. Yet the Sox were dressed for a day at the beach. They won the game but never were that fashionable again. (Leo Bauby collection.)

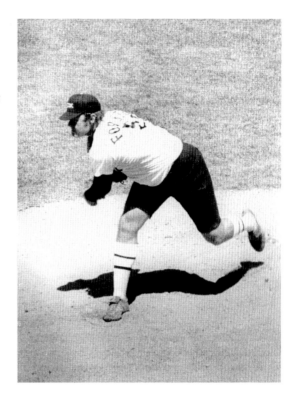

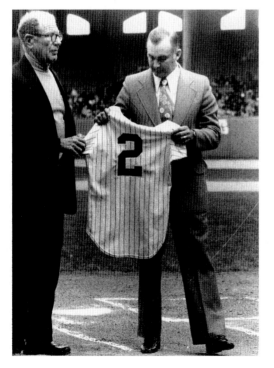

The number of Nelson Fox is retired. The second baseman was one the most memorable players from the Go-Go era, and won the American League Most Valuable Player Award in the 1959 pennant-winning season. Fox was a throwback player, never worrying about getting hit by a pitch, and more than willing to use his body to block a ground ball. He was also an excellent bunter. Fox died on December 1, 1975, and a well-organized campaign helped get him elected to the Hall of Fame in 1997. His uniform was retired during this 1976 ceremony. (Leo Bauby collection.)

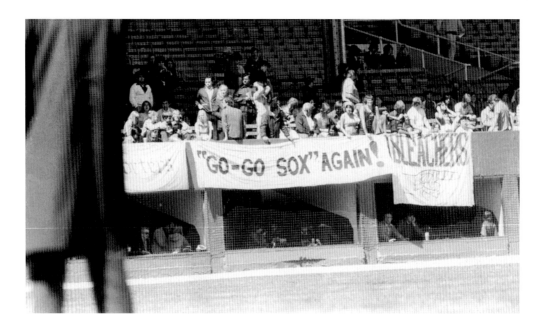

Banners in the left field seats celebrate what some fans thought was the reincarnation of the winning teams of the 1950s. Not quite in 1976, although the Sox did show some speed running after the ball after they missed it. (Leo Bauby collection.)

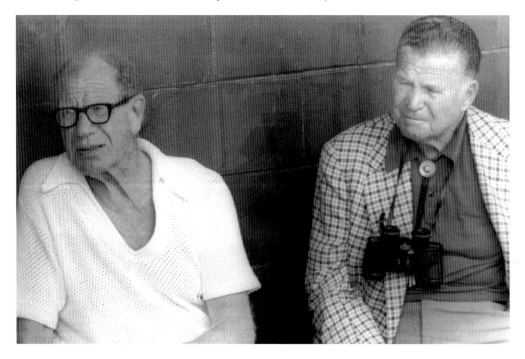

Another blast from the Go-Go past—Bill Veeck poses with former GM Frank Lane. (Leo Bauby collection.)

1976: BARELY HANGING ON

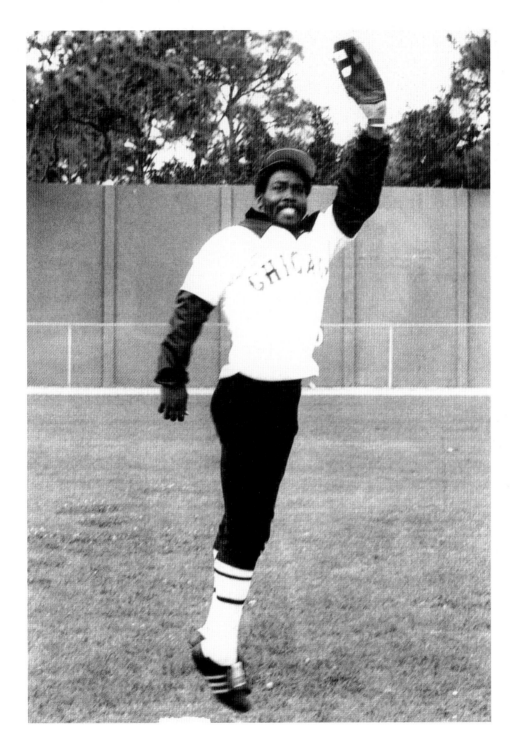

Chet Lemon is pictured just before he started his first full season with the White Sox in 1976. The ball club was a little uncertain where it wanted to play him—third base or center field. Lemon ended up in center, which turned out to be a good choice. (Leo Bauby collection.)

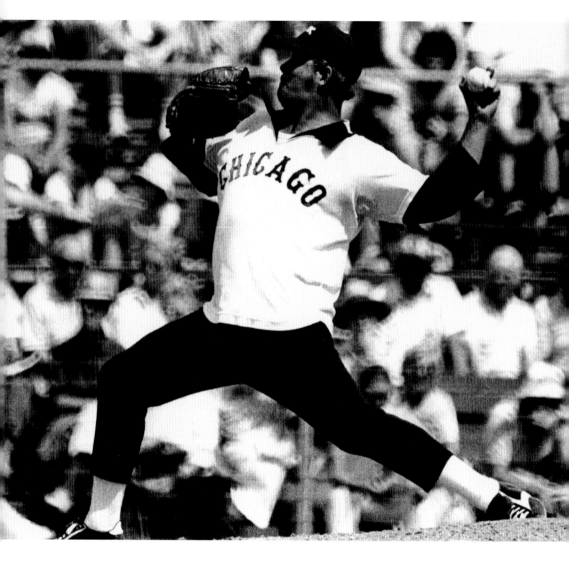

Wilbur Wood gets in tune during spring training, 1976. Despite losing 20 games in 1975, Wood was still considered the number one pitcher on the staff as the White Sox headed into the 1976 season. Even with the 20-loss season, Wood was one of the amazing stories in baseball during the first half of the 1970s. (Leo Bauby collection.)

1976: BARELY HANGING ON

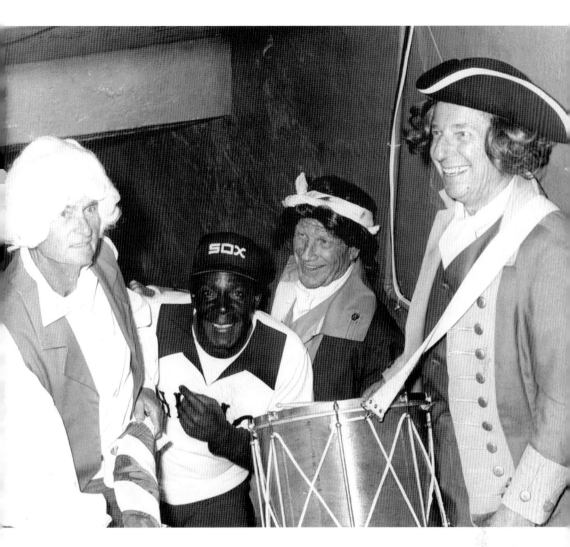

If nothing else, Bill Veeck was a great showman. On Opening Day at Comiskey during the bicentennial year, Veeck and company marched out on the field in 1776 wear. Veeck looked like a natural with his peg leg. It was a great day for the White Sox as fans were grateful that the team had been saved from a move to Seattle. The Sox won 4-0 on a sunny day that was basked in a new optimism. (Leo Bauby collection.)

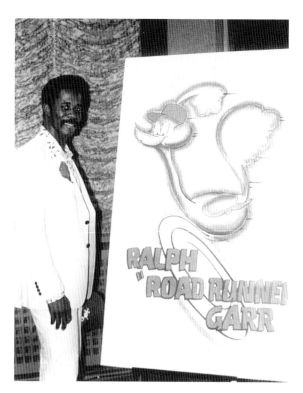

The spirit of 1976 was also wedded to the spirit of the Go-Go 1950s. Ralph Garr was obtained from Atlanta in an effort to put speed on the basepaths. Here Garr is shown beaming next to a poster of the roadrunner. Garr led the White Sox in hitting with an even-steven .300 average. (Leo Bauby collection.)

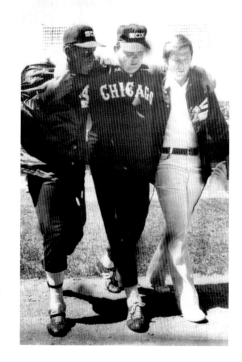

The end of the 1976 season came on May 9. Here, Wilbur Wood is being helped off the field after a line drive hit by Detroit's Ron LeFlore ripped into his knee. There was no way the Sox could recover from this bad break. They had no one else on the staff that could start between 40 and 50 games and log in well over 300 innings. Wood tried to make a comeback in 1977 and 1978, but the knuckleballer was never the same again. (Leo Bauby collection.)

1976: BARELY HANGING ON

Wilbur Wood recovers in the hospital after his injury. Doesn't look good, does it? In this case, looks were not deceiving. (Leo Bauby collection.)

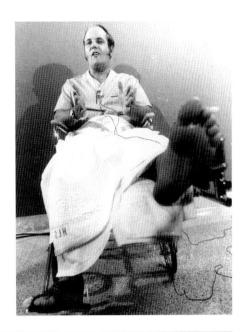

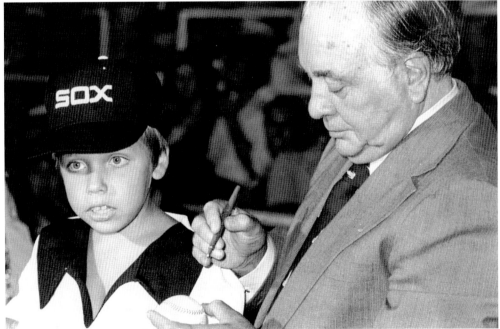

Mayor Richard Daley is seen in the last year of his life. Almost living in the shadows of Comiskey Park, Daley loved his White Sox. He was one Chicago mayor who could say that the White Sox played in a World Series during his lifetime. He set off the city fire sirens the night the Sox clinched in 1959, and people feared many things, including an attack from the Soviet Union. Unfortunately, the White Sox still hadn't been to a World Series by the time the Cold War was over and the Soviet Union had dissolved in 1989. (Leo Bauby collection.)

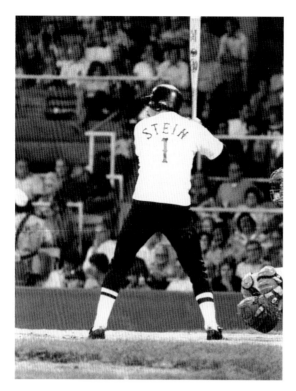

Third baseman Bill Stein looks foreboding at the plate in 1976. According to former *Chicago Sun-Times* reporter Joe Goddard, Stein was a lineup messenger for manager for manager Paul Richards. On one occasion, Stein examined the lineup card and saw that Richards had penciled in four outfielders. (Leo Bauby collection.)

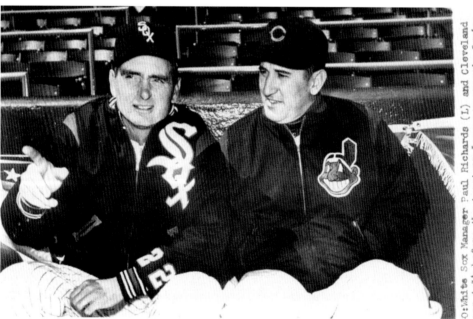

Paul Richards is shown here in happier with Indians manager Al Lopez in 1952. That year the Sox finished 81-73, 14 games out of first. Winning 81 games would have been a accomplishment for the 1976 team—even with the 162-game schedule. (Leo Bauby collection.)

A real rare occurrence in 1976 was a runner barreling for home plate. The runner in this case was Jorge Orta. From a certain angle, it appears that Orta will be tripping over a discarded bat. That would be just the type of the luck the Sox were running into during the mid-1970s. Although, it must be said that bad luck alone was the reason the Sox dropped 97 games in 1976. (Leo Bauby collection.)

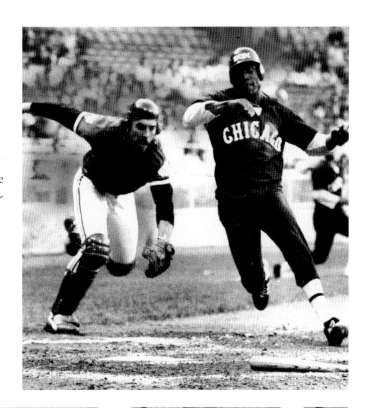

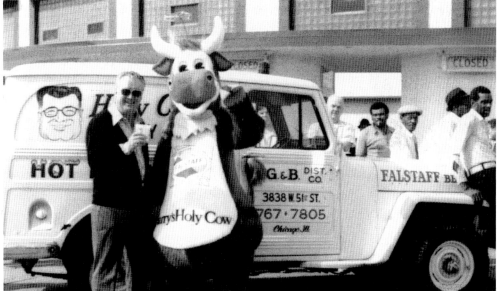

Before he was a Bud man, Harry Caray was a Falstaff man. Here Caray poses with the Falstaff mascot right outside Comiskey Park. Fans drank plenty of Falstaff during the early to mid-1970s. They had to. They needed something to kill the pain after seeing the White Sox playoff hopes dashed year after year. (Leo Bauby collection.)

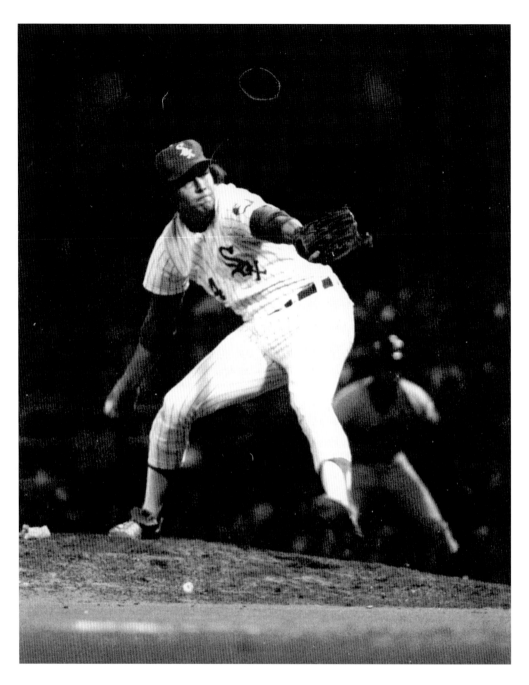

Rich Gossage is seen here in 1975 when he won American League Fireman of the Year Honors. He was a big man with a big windup. Gossage, unlike many of today's relievers, didn't wait until the last inning to enter game. Many times Gossage was there in the eighth or even the seventh. Can you imagine what a modern day pitcher would think if he knew he didn't have to get past the seventh before turning the ball over to Rich Gossage? (Leo Bauby collection.)

1976: BARELY HANGING ON

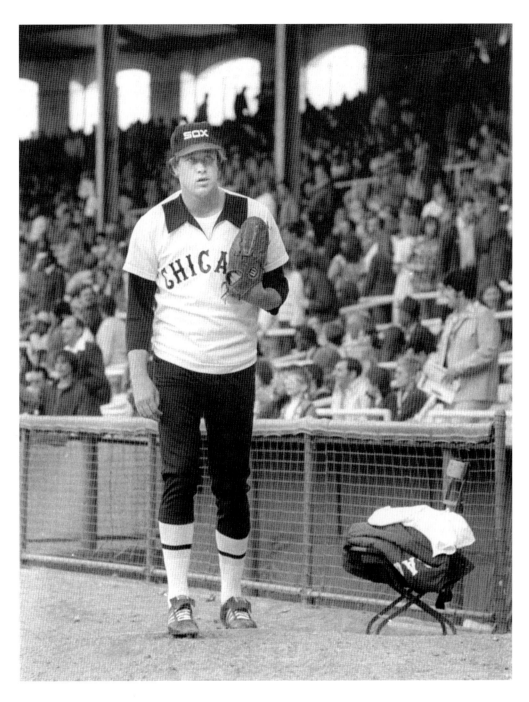

Rich Gossage tries to warm up in 1976. According to the Goose, warming up before game time in 1976 was next to impossible with the pre-game distractions caused by Bill Veeck promotions. When Gossage lashed out after being traded in December 1976, Veeck responded by saying Gossage was a very nice, young man. The nice young man had some great years for some other teams. (Leo Bauby collection.)

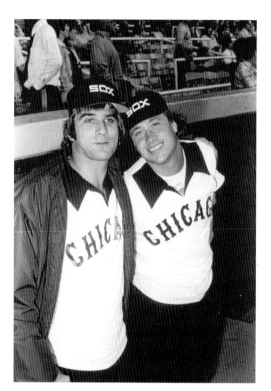

Two young pitchers that got away—Pete Vuckovich (left), who had some great years with Milwaukee, including a Cy Young year in 1982, and "Goose" Gossage. (Leo Bauby collection.)

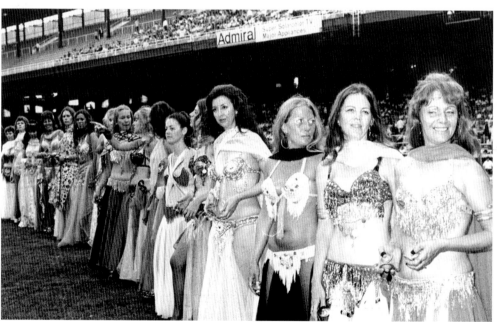

Are these the dancing girls Rich Gossage was talking about? What would have happened if one of them stepped in the box to face the Goose? Would she get a ball in the ear? (Leo Bauby collection.)

3

APRIL TO MAY

PROVING THEM WRONG

Very few White Sox fans had high expectations when the 1977 season began. It had been 10 years since the 1967 team had blown an excellent chance at the World Series by dropping the last five games of the season in the middle of a crazy four-team pennant race. In the next decade, the South Siders only contended in a serious manner once, in 1972. Even then they had a nearly impossible task of overcoming one of the best teams of the 1970s, the Oakland A's. Free agency had begun and big name players were going every direction but Chicago. White Sox fans—more accustomed to agony of defeat than the thrill of victory—expected 90 losses rather than 90 wins.

Very few in the media had any expectations for this team, either. Of the seven *Chicago Tribune* sportswriters making baseball predictions, no one picked the Sox higher than fourth. Rick Talley and Robert Markus even placed the Sox last, below the expansion Seattle Mariners. That wasn't much of a stretch considering that the 1969 White Sox actually ended one rung below the first year Kansas City Royals.

"Unhappy ballplayers, unsigned ballplayers, not enough ballplayers," Bob Verdi wrote, joining to chorus of Talley and Markus. "This will be a depressing summer for the White Sox."

Verdi picked the Sox to land in sixth, writing that the best thing the club had going for them was the first year Mariners. Even Verdi had some doubts Chicago could finish ahead of a team that had yet to play one major league game.

Across the street, longtime *Chicago Sun-Times* sportswriter, Sox fan, and Veeck admirer Bill Gleason wrote a desperate column about what he considered a desperate team. Gleason quoted a depressed Sox fan who had a fistful of opening day tickets, but didn't want to go. The discouraged fan was tempted to eat the money and stay home, atypical for a baseball fan in the hope-filled spring. Gleason almost pleaded with Bill Veeck to do something. It didn't matter what that something was, just do it.

When asked in 2005 about this column, Gleason naturally didn't remember specifics. But the feeling of desperation was nothing new for the veteran sportswriter, and Gleason replied, "Why should I have felt any different in 1977 than in any other year?" Gleason's pre-season prediction had the Sox in fifth.

Peter Gammons, in his preview of the American League West in Sports Illustrated, wrote that Veeck was a great innovator and salesman. But Gammons also thought Veeck would need more than a new paint job of Comiskey Park and gimmicky promotions to have any success in 1977.

Basically, the honeymoon was over for Bill Veeck. He had succeeded in keeping the team in Chicago, but was now faced with a group of championship-starved and cynical fans. And from the fans' mood and the media's Armageddon type predictions, the expectations for a championship were surpassed by the dread of another forgettable, losing season.

Fans didn't need the media or a sense of history to despair about the prospects of the 1977 White Sox. At third base, they had a guy with a bad knee that hadn't played in a year. At shortstop—well, after trading Bucky Dent for Oscar Gamble, they had no one. The Sox had little idea who was going to fill that giant hole, and then decided on Alan Bannister, a guy with an injured arm. And to complete the left side of the field was Ralph Garr. Known as the "Roadrunner," the speedy Garr often kicked up infield dirt behind him as he tore around the bases. Garr had won the National League batting title with a .353 mark in 1974 but saw his 1975 average drop over 70 points. He got back to exactly .300 during his first season with the Sox in 1976, but still hadn't met a cutoff man he liked.

The starting pitching staff was okay in spots with still-developing Steve Stone and a young Francisco Barrios. Yet was anyone predicting a Cy Young Award coming to the South Side of Chicago? They weren't, unless they wore a straight jacket.

Then there was the unhappy Oscar Gamble. Having come up in the Cubs system, Gamble understandably looked forward to playing with the Yankees in 1977. New York had gone to the World Series in 1976 and looked like they would be making a return trip in 1977. But Gamble now found himself traded to the White Sox right before the season started, a team that hadn't been to a World Series in 18 years. The outfielder began making salary demands before he played one inning for his new ball club, threatening retirement if his pay didn't increase from $75,000 to $100,000. In 2005, Gamble explained that he wasn't as angry as he was caught off guard. He said he fully expected to be with the Yankees in 1977, and Chicago was now un-familiar territory to him. He took solace in the fact that good friend Ralph Garr was with the White Sox.

There was a host of other players in contract limbo or battling with the White Sox for more money. Speculation about a championship didn't seem to fit in the mix; it centered around the type of string and baling wire Veeck would use to keep the team together.

The White Sox were chosen to provide the first competition for the expansion Toronto Blue Jays. Fans who thought playing a first year team, from a hockey town no less, was an easy way to start the year with a victory, but were sadly mistaken.

In a game where snow blurred the TV screen (Joe Goddard recalled Sox players squaring off for a touch football game and second baseman Jack Brohamer turning a pair of shin guards into make shift skis) the Sox left two runners on in the first, two in the second, three in the third, two in the fourth, two in the fifth, three in the sixth, two in the seventh, two in the eighth, and one in the ninth. The 19 stranded demonstrated a lack of clutch and opportunistic hitting and set a record for RBI futility for a single game. Chicago lost 9-5 despite—or maybe because—they had put 24 men on base. Of course it would have helped if they hadn't given up nine runs and 16 hits themselves.

The teams split the next two games, giving the Blue Jays their first ever series win.

With this dubious start and generous play to Toronto, the White Sox returned to Chicago for their home opener on April 12.

Bob Lemon took charge as manager in 1977 after working as pitching coach for the Yankees in 1976. Winner of 207 games as a pitcher for the Cleveland Indians, Lemon actually hit 37 career homers and had a career pinch-hitting average of .284 in an era long before the designated hitter. He won 20 games or more seven times and pitched a no-hitter against the Tigers on

June 30, 1948. His career ERA stood at 3.23, a mark many pitchers have a hard time achieving in a single season today. Lemon was elected to the Hall of Fame in 1976.

He looked more like the guy down the street than a big league skipper. With a portly body and an over sized nose, the middle aged Lemon could have easily passed for Sox fan on a barstool.

Bob Lemon's philosophy was simple: "The two most important things in life are good friends and a strong bullpen." With the departure of Gossage and Forster, it was doubtful that the Sox had a strong bullpen. Whether he made friends of Sox fans depended on the team record. Another 90-plus loss season would have the Sox fans calling for Barrabas.

"Bob had been a great player who didn't take himself seriously," according to Bill Gleason. "He enjoyed a drink, and enjoyed the give and take with the media. He was a free spirit which was one reason he appealed to Veeck."

His sense of humor was another good trait which Gleason felt Lemon would need "considering the team Veeck had given him."

"We were on a roll most of the year," third baseman Eric Soderholm later recalled. "Bob didn't have to do much. He just filled out the lineup card and let us play. And that's not a bad thing. Sometimes that's what you need."

Though optimism wasn't in full bloom with some fans threatening to eat their tickets, attendance exceeded 34,000 for the April 12 home opener against the Boston Red Sox. The White Sox prevailed 5-2 on the strength of a single, double, triple, and two RBIs from Jorge Orta. Chicago had scored one in the first and four in the second while pitchers Ken Brett and Dave Hamilton held off a potent Boston offense.

Although the White Sox home opening win had not quite dispelled the cloud that hung over the club, the team had one thing going for them: Richie Zisk.

Zisk, a Brooklyn native, came up through the Pirates organization. He had been developing into a power hitter from 1971 through 1976. His free agency status after the 1977 season had to be one factor in trading him to Chicago.

Zisk homered in his first at bat for the Sox with a 430 foot blast to straight away center and added three more hits in the otherwise forgettable game against Toronto. Two weeks later he clubbed two off Oakland A's left hander Vida Blue and drove in four in an 8-2 Sox win. Amazingly, the Sox were in first place at this point. Zisk became only the second hitter to hit two homers in a game off the flame throwing Blue.

Zisk hit a solo shot in Detroit four days later in a game in which the Sox overcame a 6-1 deficit and eventually won 10-7 in 14 innings. The right fielder finished the month of April with seven homers, and the Sox record was a decent 10-8.

"Chicago, like many of the great American cities," recalls Sox fan Gerry Bilek, "has its roots with great immigrations of the 1890s through the 1920s. Eventually, Chicago contained the second largest Polish population, second only to Warsaw. Being of Polish heritage, I certainly felt a connection to the slugging outfielder whose hard-nosed approach to the game appealed to the working class ethnic population of Chicago."

Ethnic pride and respect for hard work may have endeared Zisk to Sox fans. Unlike Oscar Gamble who didn't appear happy to leave New York, Zisk was content to be in Chicago and was willing to sign a new contract. But the Sox were cold to the idea, apparently almost resigned to the fact that Zisk would be leaving once he became a free agent at the end of the season.

Chicago Tribune reporter Bill Jauss was with the team on its initial visit to play the first year Seattle Mariners. The Kingdome, a matchbox of a domed stadium, was the new home to the expansion American League franchise. Jauss remembers Zisk being mesmerized by the hitters' ballpark.

"Wow," Jauss remembers Zisk saying as he gazed about the indoor park, "this is Wrigley Field with a dome on it."

Joe Goddard remembers Zisk striking out to end a game and just standing at the plate for a long time while everyone else left the field. The *Chicago Sun-Times* reporter later asked Zisk over drinks why he had stayed so long in the batter's box.

"He, [umpire Jerry Neudecker] didn't say 'strike three,'" Zisk told Goddard. "He didn't say 'you're out.' He told me to take a f—— hike."

So upset by what he considered unprofessional behavior by Neudecker, Zisk wanted to register a complaint about the umpire to the American League office. Goddard helped him craft his complaint, and Zisk was ready to mail the document to the American League main office. But before doing so, Zisk showed the letter to Bob Lemon and the White Sox manager emphatically told Zisk not to make any waves.

"Don't mail that," Lemon reportedly said. "Jesus Christ, if you do that every umpire is going to tell you to take a f—— hike." (Maybe it was a good thing there was no e-mail in those days.)

Goddard also recalls Zisk as a very thoughtful and intelligent man who may have been a little paranoid. In the late 1970s, a Soviet space satellite fell out of orbit and was on its way down to earth for a crash landing. Goddard said that Zisk feared the satellite would fall on his head.

"It landed somewhere in Australia," Goddard says. "When I called him to kid him about it, he said, 'that's not funny, that's not funny.'"

As Zisk became accustomed to American League stadiums or ceased fighting with umpires and recovered from his fear of falling objects from outer space, the right fielder began to enjoy playing in the American League. The White Sox traveled to Cleveland for a three game series on the weekend of May 6, 7, and 8. After winning the first game of the series 7-5, the Sox were set to face Wayne Garland, the Indians ace in the Saturday afternoon game.

Garland had a great year in 1976, going 15-3 for Baltimore with a 2.67 ERA. But the right-hander, having signed a then-astounding $2.3 million 10-year contract—felt the sting of a bitter fan backlash after getting off to an 0-3 start. During his last appearance, he was treated to an ovation of boos. A good start against the White Sox would help Garland regain his old confidence and at least get Indian fans off his back.

Garland actually was pitching fairly well as the game was tied at 2 in the eighth. Alan Bannister had led off with a single. The Sox were pretty much a station-to-station team in 1977, but this was a tough game against a tough pitcher. Zisk was up next and manager Bob Lemon called for a hit and run, a Sox rarity in 1977. Just trying to make contact, Zisk took a cut at a high fast ball that he normally would have taken for a ball. His drive went to straight away center. Indian outfielder Rick Manning drifted back but stopped just short of the wall and watched as Zisk's long fly cleared the center field fence by plenty, giving the Sox a 4-2 lead and an eventual 5-2 victory. The bargain basement Sox had beaten the millionaire pitcher Garland who saw his record fall to 0-4.

"It wasn't even a strike," Zisk said about the home run pitch. "You're not supposed to hit a pitch like that. I just muscled it. What can I say?"

Sox fans warmed up to Zisk, and the love affair between fans and player had begun. By the end of May, Zisk had 14 home runs, equaling the output of 1976 team home run leaders Orta and Spencer. The right fielder was overwhelmed by the enthusiasm of the White Sox faithful. Although he had some good years in Pittsburgh, he felt that he had really just come into his own in 1977, especially with the long ball.

Expectations rose during the next two months in ways that few could ever have imagined. June and July 1977 have to go down as the most exciting time of the decade for the franchise. Those two giddy months also defined the legacy of the South Side Hit Men, and produced some of the most intense emotions ever experienced in team history.

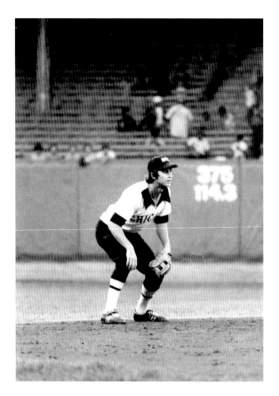

Alan Bannister is in at shortstop. Bannister was thrust into this role when the Sox traded Bucky Dent. He is often maligned for the defensive year he had in 1977. Who knows what he would have done if he had a decent arm? No doubt he would have committed less than 40 errors. (Leo Bauby collection.)

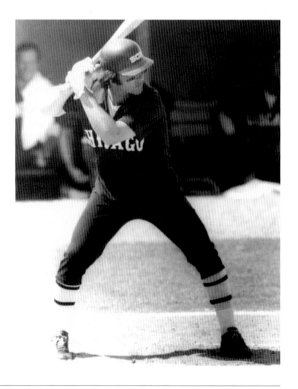

Bucky Dent stands at the plate during Spring Training in 1977. Rumors had surrounded Dent all during the pre-season. Trading him to the Yankees helped put the final touches on the formation the South Side Hitmen. The hole at shortstop would never really be filled until the arrival of Ozzie Guillen in 1985. (Leo Bauby collection.)

APRIL TO MAY: PROVING THEM WRONG

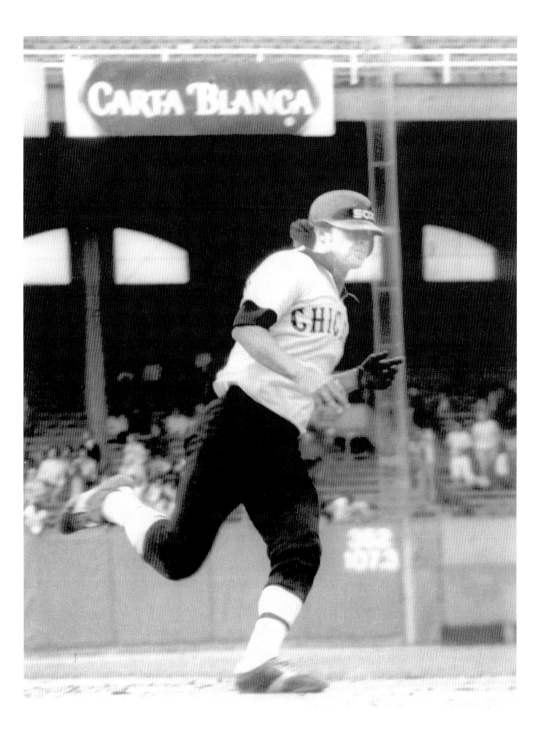

Alan Bannister rounds third. Defense was not Bannister's forte, but offense was. He scored 87 runs in 1977, providing a solid presence at the top of the lineup. He also hit a key homer against the Twins in a big July series. (Leo Bauby collection.)

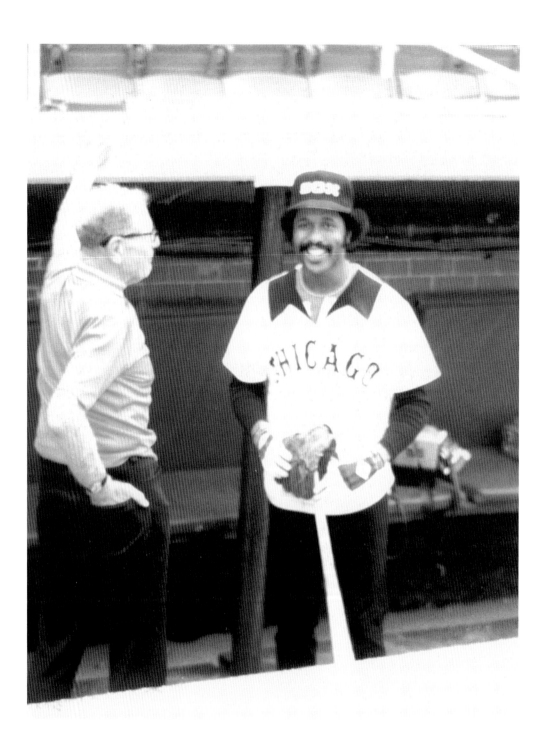

Bill Veeck (left) and Oscar Gamble—everything is all rosy. Veeck took a gamble on Gamble, at least for one season, and it was a short-term success. It is hard to imagine the South Side Hitmen without Gamble, who thought he was going the play the 1977 season with the New York Yankees. (Leo Bauby collection.)

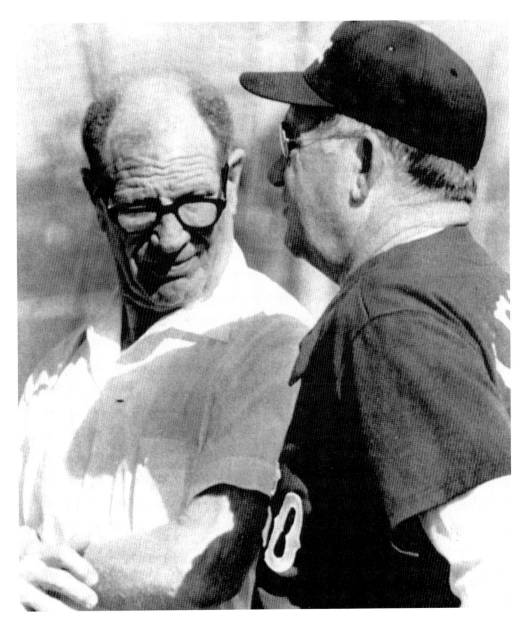

Pictured here is the brain trust of Bill Veeck and Bob Lemon. They were two free spirits who naturally attracted to each other. Lemon was probably just the right choice for the job. So many things worked in 1977. (Leo Bauby collection.)

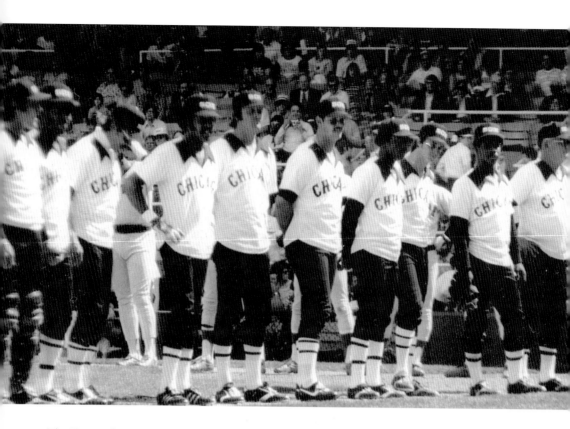

The Hitmen line up for opening day ceremonies at Comiskey Park. Did you ever see a more motley crew? The outcasts gave their fans a great and memorable season. What would have happened to the White Sox if they didn't have the lovable 1977 all-hit, no-field team? (Leo Bauby collection.)

APRIL TO MAY: PROVING THEM WRONG

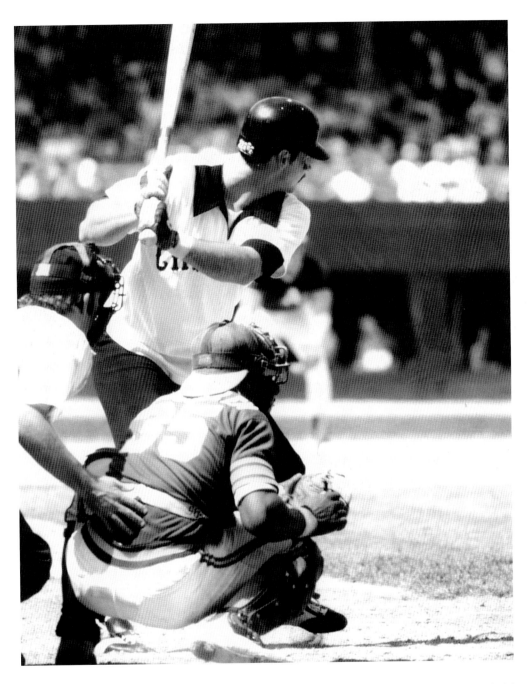

The early season hero was Richie Zisk. By the end of May he already had 14 homers and was bonding with Sox fans. He then picked up a roof shot after knocking a homer into the center field bleachers. Eventually fans held banners that read "Pitch at Risk to Rich Zisk." (Leo Bauby collection.)

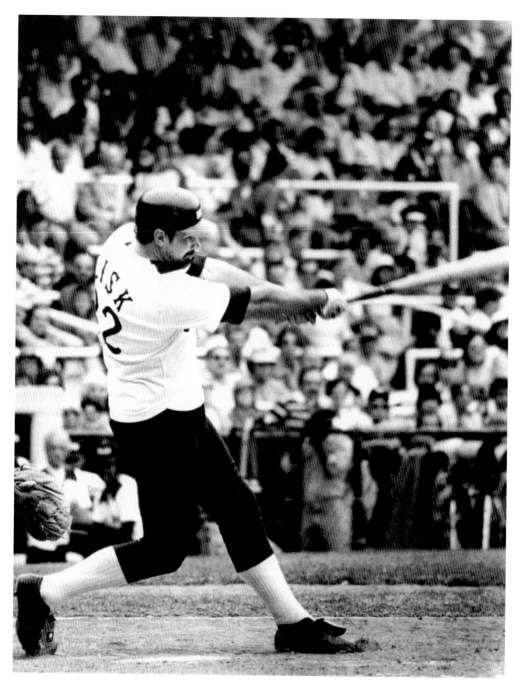

Richie Zisk follows through. His swing looks picture perfect, doesn't it? (Leo Bauby collection.)

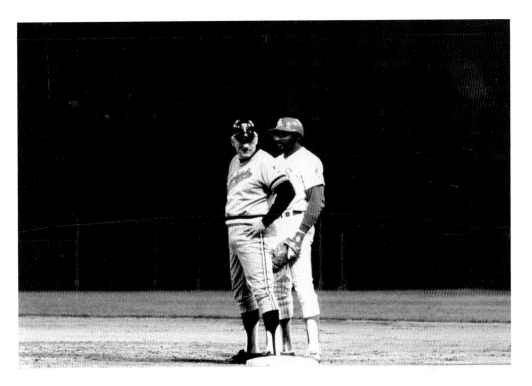

Dick Allen (right) poses with another feared, slugging first baseman, Harmon Killebrew. Killebrew was near the end of a career where he amassed 573 homers. Killebrew's compact swing had been something to watch. (Leo Bauby collection.)

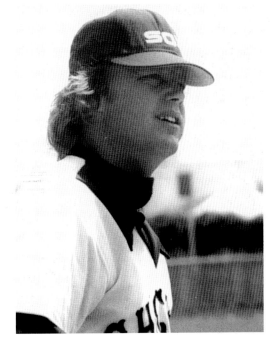

Dave Duncan is pictured during spring training 1977. Duncan would not make the club, but he would return as pitching coach during the early 1980s, which included the Winning Ugly year of 1983. (Leo Bauby collection.)

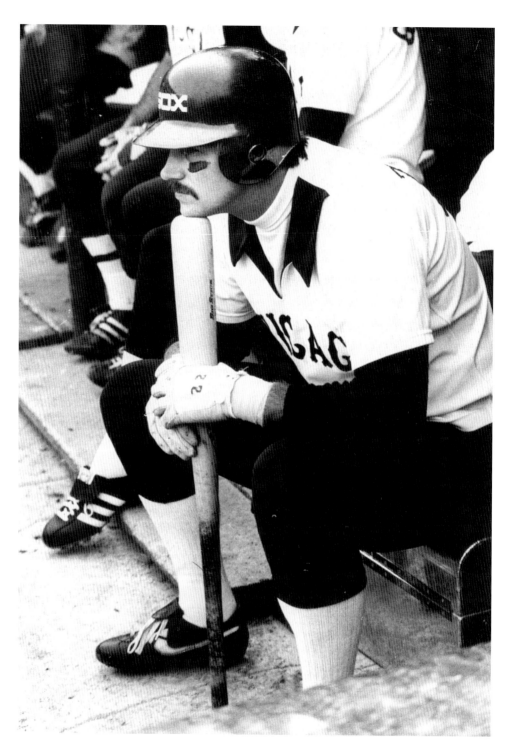

Richie Zisk is pictured in a pensive mood.   (Leo Bauby collection.)
Maybe he was thinking of another roof shot.

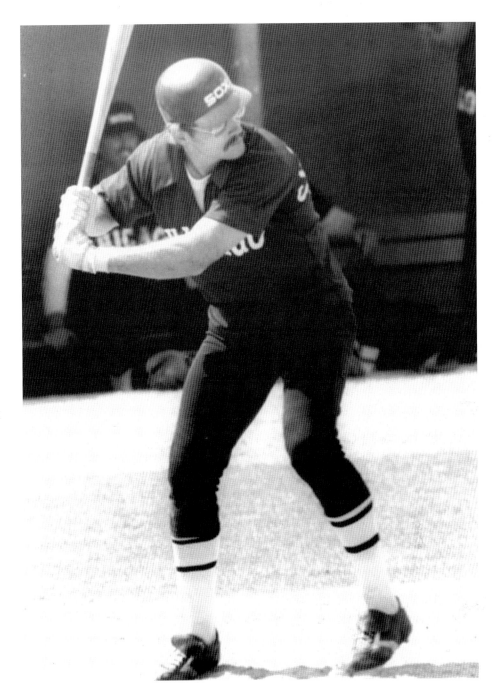

Eric Soderholm gets in shape during spring training. Soderholm was coming off a yearlong rehab stint for an injured knee. He felt he had a real chance to come back when he grounded deep in the hole at short and was thrown out at short. Making an out wasn't a great sign; running at full speed to first and slamming his foot down at the bag without getting hurt was the good sign. (Leo Bauby collection.)

SOUTH SIDE HITMEN

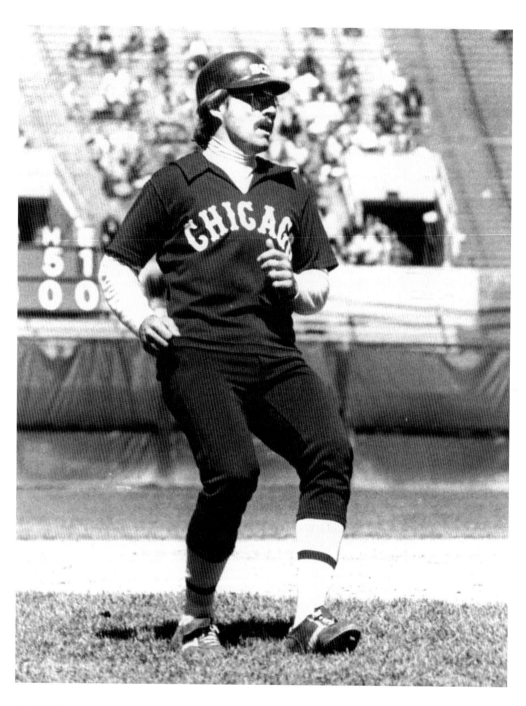

Soderholm is pictured during an early May series with the Cleveland Indians. The White Sox won two of three from the Tribe and slowly began to make believers out of their fans. (Leo Bauby collection.)

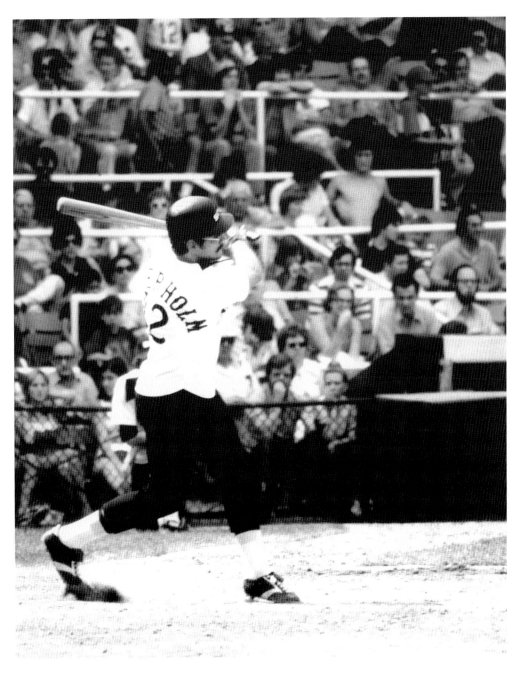

Soderholm takes a powerful swing for the fence. He hit 25 round trippers in 1977. (Leo Bauby collection.)

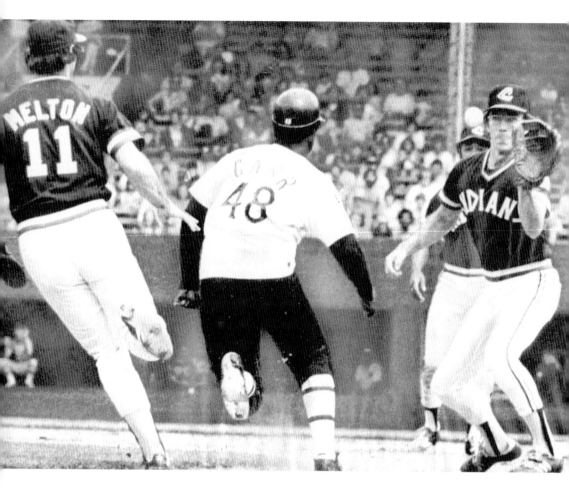

Ralph Garr is caught in a crowd of Indians. This was another Veeck brainstorm. Play a game in the morning and hopefully get done in time for brunch. The guy who was done in time for brunch was Jim Spencer who knocked in eight runs and had the day off after three at bats. The game was played on May 18, and had an 11:00 a.m. starting time. The White Sox won in a walk, 18-2. (Leo Bauby collection.)

4

THE JUNE NON-SWOON

The June Swoon. This Chicago baseball tradition breaks the hearts of both White Sox and Cub fans by derailing any chance of their favorite team playing into the later stages of October. Even though White Sox fans were pleasantly surprised by their team's decent start in April and May, attendance figures revealed they weren't believers quite yet. The fans had recent and painful memories reminding them not to fall in love with a .500 team masquerading as a contender. Both the 1973 and 1974 seasons had started off strong only to end in frustration.

The White Sox faced a good swoon test at home at the start of June 1977. They faced the Baltimore Orioles who had been to two World Series and had won two other division titles up to that point in the 1970s in a two game series. That was followed by a three game set against the Yankees, the defending American League champions.

The White Sox began by beating the usually unbeatable Jim Palmer. Taking advantage of the few scoring opportunities they had, the Sox scored two in the second and two in the seventh. They won 4-2 behind the complete game pitching of lefty Ken Brett. It was the last White Sox win for the lefty, as Brett was traded to California two weeks later.

Game two was more like the MO of the South Side Hitmen. The Sox scored one in the first, two in the second, and four in the third to run out to a 7-0 lead. Baltimore scored three in the seventh and one in the eighth to make it interesting, but the O's went down meekly in the ninth and the Sox had another win.

Although some fans began to believe in the Sox at this point, there were still plenty of doubters. For the two games against a good draw like Baltimore, only 18,125 showed.

After their defeat in the 1964 World Series to St. Louis, the Yankees lost their luster. But with their appearance in the 1976 series, they had returned to their old championship tradition. The era of Mantle, Maris, and Berra had transitioned to the late 1970s tradition of Jackson, Munson, and Randolph. Though each team was in second place in their division at the start of this three game series, the White Sox surprisingly had a slightly better record at 27-19 compared to the Yankees' 27-22.

The White Sox took game one 9-5. The difference was the seven runs they piled on in the fourth inning when they sent 12 men to the plate. New Yorker skipper Billy Martin was so flustered by the Sox onslaught that he was tossed out of the game as he came in to make a much-needed pitching change in the fourth inning.

After losing the next two games, the White Sox didn't appear to have made any statements in the series by losing two of three at home. However, in addition to drawing nearly 90,000 for the three games, they began to show that no team could relax against them even with a big lead.

The Yankees had a seven run inning of their own in the second inning and ran out to a 7-0 lead in game two. With tough lefty Don Gullet on the mound, Yankee fans probably thought the game was a walk through the park.

As it turned out, it was a like a walk through crazy Central Park. The Sox clubbed three homers including Zisk's shot that went bouncing around on the Comiskey Park roof. By the ninth, the 7-0 Yankee advantage had dwindled to 8-6. Sparky Lyle, who later won that year's American League Cy Young Award, was on the mound to mop things up, and, for a moment, it looked routine. Jim Essian struck out and Brian Downing flied out. One more out and the Yankees had their win.

But it wasn't routine. Alan Bannister and Jorge Orta singled and suddenly the winning run was at the plate in the form of Richie Zisk. It was the same Richie Zisk who had a roof shot in the second inning. Zisk flied out to left and Yankees had to be relieved that the Hitmen hadn't clobbered them to death.

In the series finale, New York again scored early by getting one in the first, two in the second, and three in the third. Again, the Sox wouldn't let the Yankees run away with anything. When the Sox plated a run in the seventh, the Yankee advantage was down to 7-6. A Bucky Dent homer in the ninth gave New York some insurance. Lyle again had to come in the ninth in nail down another 8-6 victory. Yankee fans breathed a little easier with this ending even though Chet Lemon represented the tying run when he tapped back to the mound for the final out.

Yes, they lost two of three, but the Sox scored 21 and pounded out 36 hits in the series against a team that once again was a contender. The series was lost, but it was just the beginning of a hit-barraged summer.

Dreams of first place; June is way too early to begin fantasizing about the playoffs, especially if you are a Chicago baseball fan. But almost right smack dab in the middle of June, the White Sox had their fans fantasizing of the near impossible after recent seasons of disappointments and finishes nowhere near first place.

In a mid-month weekend series against the once powerful and now 90-pound weakling Oakland A's, the White Sox more resembled the mild mannered offense of 1967 than the South Side Hitmen. They actually handled the A's with solid starting pitching allowing them to win three low scoring games in the four game set.

The White Sox began their winning by scratching out runs in the second and sixth during a Saturday afternoon game on June 18. In the second, two of the team's best home run hitters helped manufacture a run. Richie Zisk walked and went to third on an opposite field single by Eric Soderholm. Zisk then came in on a sacrifice fly by shortstop Kevin Bell.

In the sixth, Ralph Garr led off with a single. The Roadrunner would have been picked off by A's lefty Vida Blue, but Blue threw the ball away. Garr advanced to second, and, one out later, scored on a Jorge Orta single to center. The Sox led 2-0.

The Sox still led 2-0 going into the eighth inning. Lefty Ken Kravec had shut down Oakland on two hits and started the inning by getting Jim Tyrone to strike out looking. Then the A's threatened as they picked up singles from Rodney Scott and Manny Sanguillen, with Scott going to third. Kravec needed a strike out to keep Scott at third and got one when he set Mitchell Page down.

Dick Allen represented the go-ahead run with two out, and Bob Lemon summoned closer Lerrin LaGrow. Sox fans no doubt feared that Allen could clout one of his trademark Comiskey Park homers, but the former Sox slugger grounded out to short. For all their bluster, the A's came up with nothing.

THE JUNE NON-SWOON

LaGrow set the A's down quietly in the ninth, striking out the last two. The White Sox had one of their rare 1977 shutouts (they had three that year) and the young Kravec had earned his second win of the season.

The old man of the staff, Wilbur Wood, was slated to start game one of the next day's doubleheader. From 1971 to 1975, Wood was more than just the ace of the Sox staff. Often pitching with two days rest, the left handed knuckleballer logged in 1,681 innings during those five seasons, had 99 complete games, and won 106. But his May 9 injury ruined his 1976 season, and he was still rehabbing when the 1977 season started. The Sox rotation included the inexperience of Kravec, Chris Knapp, and Francisco Barrios. The more seasoned Steve Stone was coming off an injury himself although he felt he was completely healed when the season began. If the White Sox were actually going to contend, they needed iron man Wilbur Wood who had held up the staff during early and mid-1970s.

Wood looked like his old dominating self against the A's. In an eight-inning plus stint, he gave up one run on seven hits. He got a break in the fifth when Oakland's Earl Williams apparently had scored on a sacrifice fly by Rob Piccolo. But the Sox appealed, with Soderholm saying that Williams had left too soon. The third base umpire agreed, and instead of going ahead, Oakland saw its rally stifled when the embarrassed Williams was called out.

Very much unlike themselves, the Sox did next to nothing offensively. Except for Lamar Johnson, no one in the Sox lineup picked up a hit. Johnson, a multi-talented guy who sang the national anthem before the doubleheader, slammed two homers and a double. When closer LaGrow again set the A's down in the ninth after Wood walked the leadoff hitter, Chicago won another 1967 type nail-biter, 2-1.

"If Johnson sings the national anthem Monday night [the next date for the two teams], we're going to pitch around him," A's manager Bobby Winkles said.

Fan Mark Liptak had attended a Comiskey Park game a month earlier. Sitting in the first row of the box seats down the third baseline, Liptak picked up something coming from the dugout.

"I heard someone singing," Liptak recalls, "nothing fancy, just a few bars. It was Lamar Johnson. I think the Sox lost 3-2 or 4-3, something like that. Johnson, if memory serves, belted a home run that day, I want to say in the eighth inning."

Liptak's almost 30 year-old memory is pretty good. The White Sox lost 4-3, and Johnson hit a solo homer in the eighth.

Johnson had been hitting .300 in the White Sox farm system for several years but had a hard time breaking into the major league club because of Dick Allen and then Jim Spencer. In fact, Spencer would have been the more natural choice for this game against the righty Mike Norris, but he was injured. Johnson got more chances in 1977 and ended up having his best year home run-wise.

Yet the real story was Wood. It had to be frustrating for Wood to sit on the sidelines after starting 40 plus games for five straight years. On this day, he assisted his team when a tough pitcher kept them from knocking the ball around the park. In doing so, he picked up his first win in over 13 months.

"The big thing for us today was Wilbur's performance," Bob Lemon said. "I told Wilbur he pitched nine innings as far as I was concerned—with all those boots behind him." (The Sox committed three errors in a game they could have easily lost.)

In game two, a young pitcher stepped up for the Sox. Francisco Barrios had psyched himself up by talking to the ball during his no-hitter with John "Blue Moon" Odom to during his 1976 rookie year. His win that day wasn't as dramatic but just as effective. Going the distance and having a little more offensive support, Barrios threw a seven-hitter and won 5-1.

The doubleheader sweep was sweet, but it wasn't your ordinary sweep. Comiskey Park wasn't over-flowing, but the crowd of 24,161 more than appreciated the Sox that day. The old stadium began to rock as the White Sox vaulted into first place. Minnesota had been in first place since April 27.

First place. No, division titles are not won in June. Yet, very few expected the White Sox to be anywhere near first place any time after spring. Just who were these guys?

The suddenly front running White Sox traveled to Minnesota the next weekend. In the three game set, the Hitmen came alive again as they scored 26 runs on 41 hits, knocking out nine home runs. But they managed only one win, and that came on the heels of the only good pitching they had in the series. Chris Knapp threw a complete game in an 8-1 victory. In the two Chicago losses, Sox pitchers got lit up for 26 runs on 28 hits. Even the Hitmen couldn't overcome that.

The ugliest game of all was the last game of the series on June 26. The Twins scored 15 runs in the first four innings and never worried about losing. Steve Stone couldn't last past the second inning giving up eight runs on six hits. Minnesota scored six in the second, sending 10 men to the plate. They added four in the third and three in the fourth.

The White Sox had a six run rally in the third when they hit two of their four homers for the day. However, the Twins scored in every inning except the fifth and sixth, and won the game rather easily, 19-12.

The Minnesota series exposed the Sox somewhat as a one-dimensional team. And, even with the excitement of the doubleheader sweep of Oakland a week earlier, the fans still didn't totally believe in the Sox even though the team was more entertaining than many preceding clubs. Other than the New York series and the Oakland Sunday doubleheader, the Sox didn't break the 20,000 mark in a June home game. Their 15-13 record for the month wasn't a June swoon but was far from awe-inspiring. Giving up 19 runs in a game wasn't inspirational, either.

But as the month came to an end, the White Sox were 40-32. This was a good but not great record. On the plus side, they were in second place, but one game behind again front-running Minnesota. Summer had officially arrived, and Minnesota was coming to Chicago for the first four games of July. When had Chicago last truly played a meaningful game this close to the All-Star break? It had been too long, and usually the Sox saw their division hopes torpedoed by some calamity. The Minnesota series would be a far, far different story, starting an incredible month that would be a highlight show of the entire 1977 season.

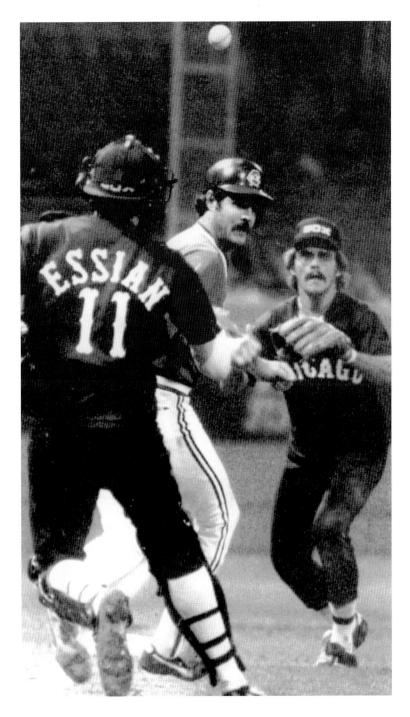

Caught in a rundown between Jim Essian and Eric Soderholm, former White Sox Bill Melton looks like he has nowhere to go. Ironically, Melton, who was booed loudly during the 1975 season, picked up his 1,000th career hit against the White Sox during the Hitmen season. (Leo Bauby collection.)

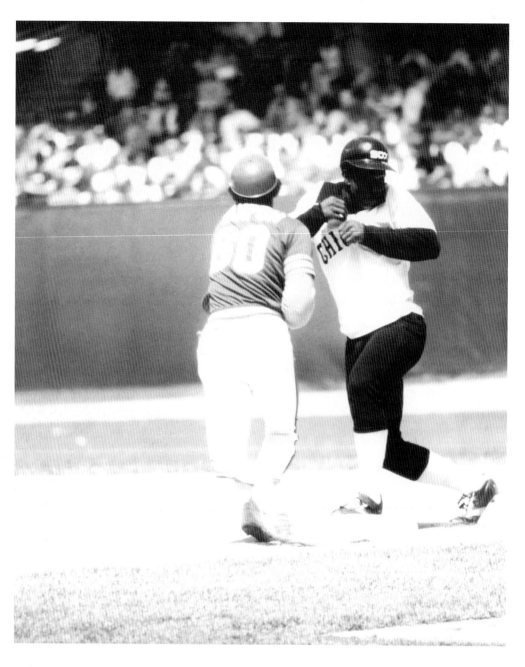

Pick off attempt goes awry as A's Dick Allen reaches around Ralph Garr. Garr scampered to second and eventually scored. It was one of the last games of Dick Allen's career, and was one of the first weekends that Sox fans began believing in the South Side Hitmen. (Leo Bauby collection.)

THE JUNE NON-SWOON

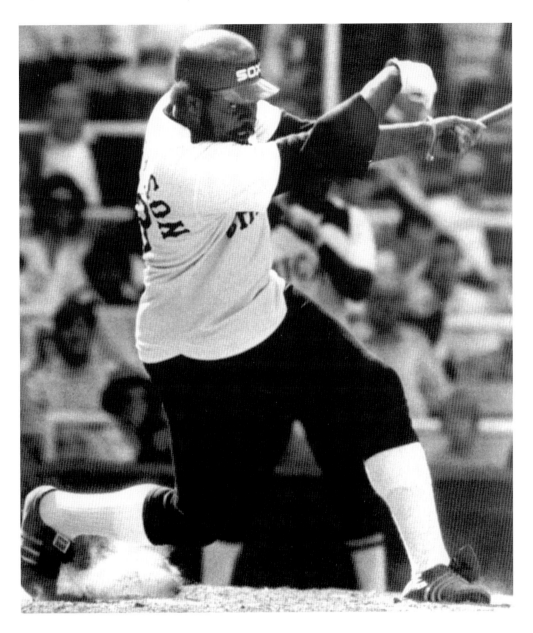

Lamar Johnson hits one of his two home runs against the A's in the first game of a doubleheader on June 19. His homers provided the winning margin in a 2-1 victory. The White Sox went in first place that day as they swept the A's. (Leo Bauby collection.)

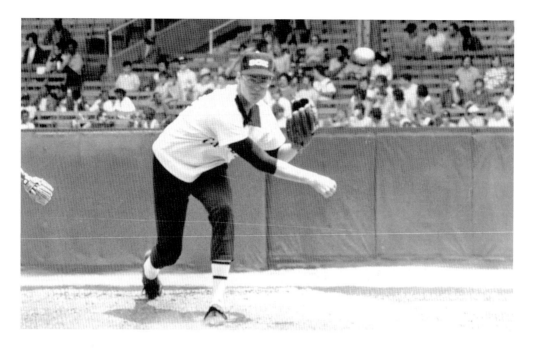

Chris Knapp, one of the young pitchers on the Sox staff in 1977, won 12 games during the Hitmen season. (Leo Bauby collection.)

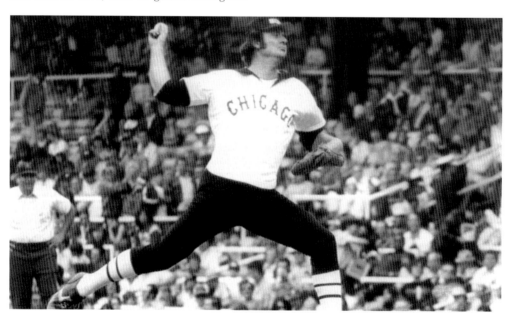

Lerrin LaGrow was another unlikely Sox hero in 1977. Acquired just before the season started, LaGrow had his best season as a reliever, saving 25 games. Very few would have thought of him as a closer but the righty did it time and again for the Sox as he posted a 2.45 ERA. (Leo Bauby collection.)

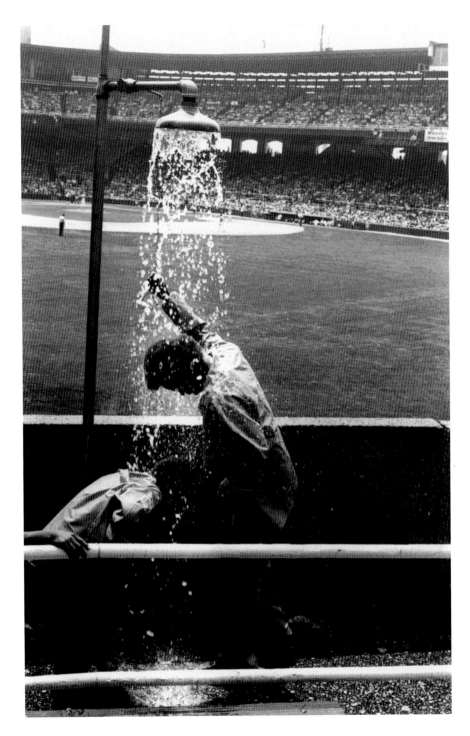

A fan cools off during the hot summer of 1977. The shower was one of the big symbols of the Hitmen year. It was situated in front of the center field bleachers, the spot where Richie Zisk hit one of his long home runs. (Leo Bauby collection.)

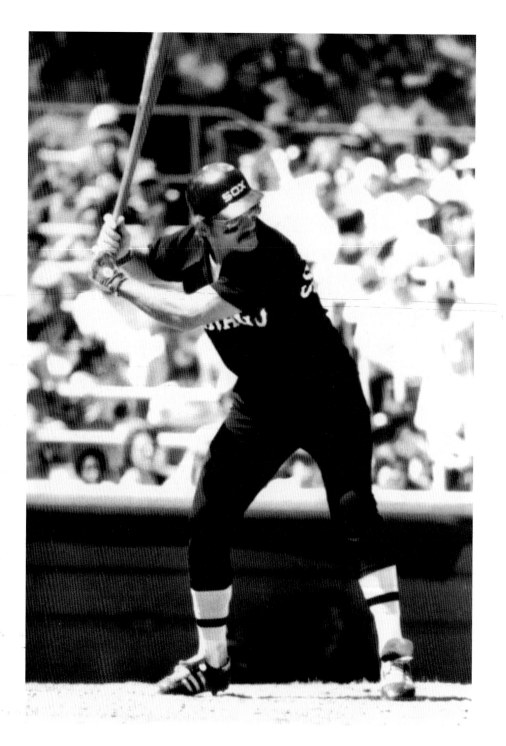

Eric Soderholm faces the Yankees in June of 1977. The White Sox lost the season series to the New Yorkers, but fought them tough in almost every game. The Yankees learned that most leads were not entirely safe from the South Side Hitmen. (Leo Bauby collection.)

THE JUNE NON-SWOON

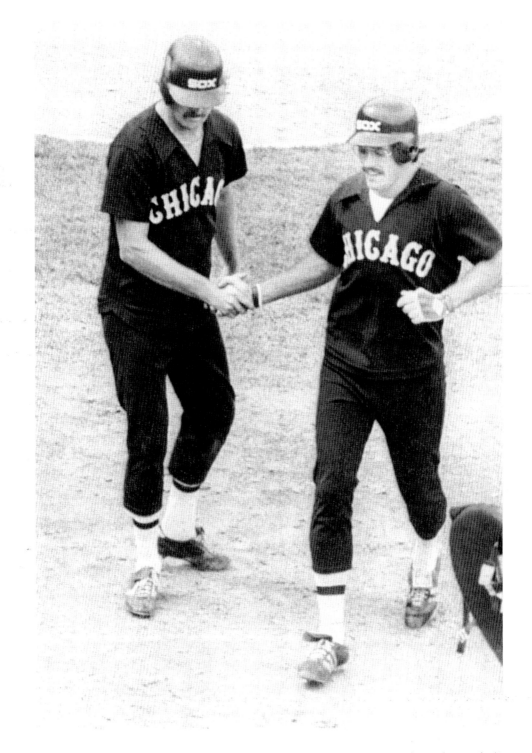

A very familiar scene at home plate in 1977, Jim Spencer (left) congratulates Eric Soderholm. This run is being scored on the road. (Leo Bauby collection.)

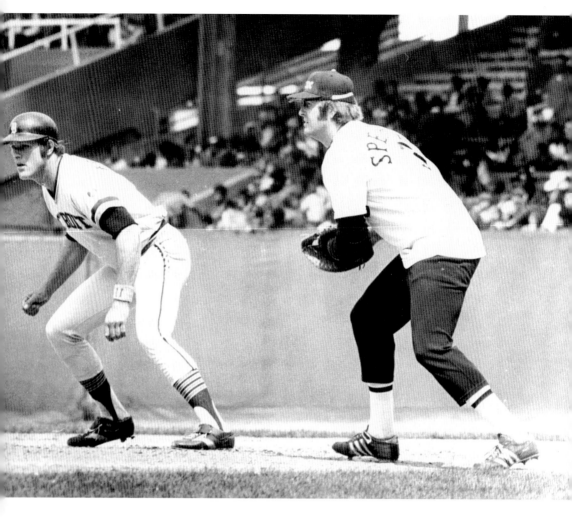

Jim Spencer holds a runner at first. Spencer was one of the few players who could play defense for the White Sox in 1977. His abilities were needed since throws from the infield that year had the potential to go just about anywhere. (Leo Bauby collection.)

THE JUNE NON-SWOON

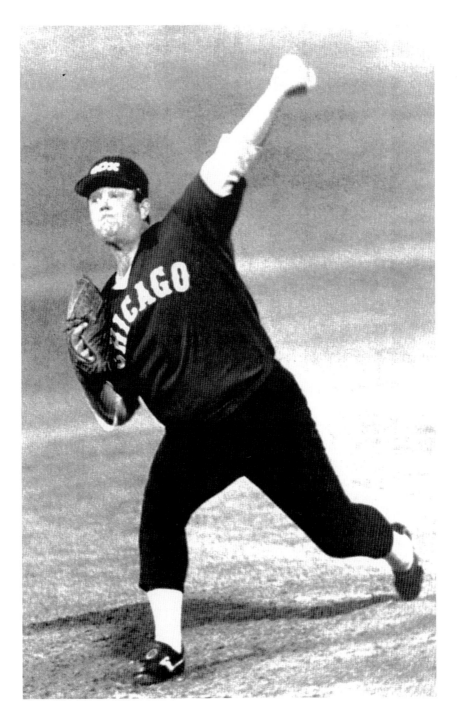

Wilbur Wood shows off his form on the road. In June, he won his first game in over a year, briefly giving fans hope that a pennant was possible. Unfortunately his ERA ballooned to nearly 5.00, and he won just seven games in 1977. He pitched his final game in 1978. (Leo Bauby collection.)

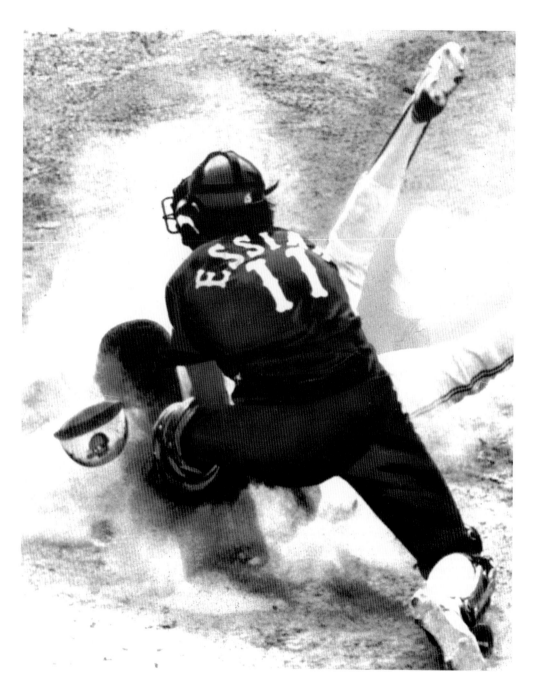

Sox catcher Jim Essian tags out would-be home plate stealer Pat Kelly. Kelly had supplied speed to the Sox during the early part of the decade when he played for the South Siders. The Sox ended up winning this June 12 game 6-4 in 11 innings. (Leo Bauby collection.)

THE JUNE NON-SWOON

5

JULY

A FAST, FURIOUS RIDE TO THE TOP

A playoff atmosphere. July 1 is still a little early to get hyped for the playoffs. Then again, White Sox fans had had nothing to cheer for since the Allen 1972 MVP season. Injuries ruined the 1973 club. The 1975 and 1976 teams contended for nothing. And July 4 is one date when fans begin judging their team. Are they for real or not? Ten years earlier the White Sox were in first place on July 4 and ended up only three games out at the end of a crazy pennant race. Even a split against the first place Minnesota Twins would leave the Sox within a game of first after the holiday weekend. Sox fans could feel free to have some hope after nearly a decade of almost total futility and frustration.

Minnesota had a formidable ball club, at least offensively. Although they would hit almost 70 fewer homers than the Hitmen, the Twins would score 23 more runs. They had the likes of Hall of Famer Rod Carew (who came into the series with a .411 average), slugger Larry Hisle, and up and coming star Lyman Bostock. The Twins led the Sox in hitting by a microscopic margin of .2844 to .2835. Their team ERA was slightly better by a .10 difference. No one could blame White Sox fans for having a bad case of nerves when the Twins came to Chicago for a four-game series. With these two evenly matched teams, a split would have been nice, demonstrating that the White Sox could play with the best of them.

Instead fans got more than what they bargained for in the series against the Twins, and during the month of July. In fact, July 1977 was one of the greatest months, winning percentage wise, in the history of the franchise. It was also a month that forever bonded fans with the South Side Hitmen.

In game one, the Friday night game, the Twins took a 1-0 lead on triples by Carew and Bostock. They never led again for the remainder of the game.

The White Sox responded in the first and the fans responded with a deafening noise from the very start. Alan Bannister picked up a bunt single and then Jorge Orta doubled Bannister to third. Then newly found hero Richie Zisk came to the plate.

Zisk brought the house down with a three run opposite field homer. He at first thought it would be a sacrifice fly caught against the wall in right center, but right fielder Bostock just watched as it landed in the seats. Zisk thought he had been a lucky, and that the wind had helped a little. The fans didn't care if luck was involved or not. They just roared right along with the exploding scoreboard.

"These folks," Zisk said referring to Sox fans, "are caught up in a pennant race. I've been through this with the Pirates, but later, in September."

Zisk got the fans revved up again in the third when he hit his second home run of the night. According to Bill Jauss of the *Chicago Tribune*, it was "no more than 20 feet off the ground, probably set a record for the least time zooming from home plate into the eighth row of the left center field stands."

The White Sox won 5-2 on the Zisk's 5 RBIs. Fans showed their appreciation later in the game, giving him standing ovations when he struck out twice.

"Every time I think I have Chicago fans figured out, they amaze me," Zisk said.

Chris Knapp, the righty who went the distance that night against Minnesota, was greatly affected by a crowd that only cared about the Sox climbing into first place, even if it was only by two percentage points as they did two weeks earlier.

"When I heard all those people in the ninth inning going, 'We're number one,' that made me want to go stronger," Knapp said.

The White Sox widened their lead against the once first place Twins the next day, thanks to the slugging of first baseman Jim Spencer.

"Jim was a real gentle type," Eric Soderholm recalled in 2005. "He was easy going, fun loving. When you [an infielder] released the ball and you knew it was too low or too high, you also knew Jim would get it. He was that good with the glove. He made infielders look good."

In 1977, he fit right in with the Hitmen because he was good with the bat as well. Fans began bringing banners that read, "C'mon Spence, Over the Fence." But who knew that Spencer would have an eight RBI day? On Saturday, July 2, the shell-shocked Twins found out.

Spencer hit his second grand slam of the year in the fourth. In the sixth, he singled to drive in Chet Lemon who had tripled. Finally in the eighth, Spencer hit a high homer in the right center field seats to drive in three more and put the game out of reach. The White Sox had actually been trailing 7-6 going into their half of the eighth, but in typical South Side Hitmen fashion, the offense exploded and made it look easy, winning 13-8.

Actually, it hadn't been all that easy. That seven run eighth inning might not have happened if Twins right fielder Dan Ford hadn't lost Alan Bannister's fly in the sun. As a result, all seven runs were unearned.

"This isn't the kind of team you give four outs or five outs," Bannister said. "These guys really hit with two outs."

In the first game of a Sunday doubleheader to close out the Twins series, Wilbur Wood dominated the hard hitting Minnesota club. The left hander gave up singles in the first, fourth, and ninth— and that was it. Again showing how they pile up runs, Chicago scored five in the second and won handily 6-0. Wood used only 93 pitches in a game that only took a little more than two hours.

"It was head high," catcher Brian Downing said in describing the movement of Wood's last pitch of the game to strike out Lyman Bostock, "but I caught it off the ground."

In the nightcap that mercifully ended the series for the Twins, the Sox used the big inning again to pummel the once first place Minnesota team. Jim Spencer did it again, this time with a first inning upper deck homer. His third homer of the series came after a Lamar Johnson triple, a Zisk double and Orta single.

The center field scoreboard, maybe because it was being used so much that summer, blew a fuse and didn't go off after the Spencer homer. It was repaired in time for later White Sox blasts that game. Yet, the fans made up for the silent scoreboard. *Chicago Sun-Times* reporter Joe Goddard called the ovation for the Spencer homer as one of the loudest of the season.

It also has to be said that one of the most memorable images of 1977 was Spencer standing right outside the Sox dugout acknowledging that ovation from the crowd. Many baseball people cringed at these "curtain calls" thinking the Sox were showing up their opponents with theatrics. However, others felt that the ovations were so loud and so long, that the players had to do something to acknowledge the fans. The fans and team reveled in it that Fourth of July weekend, even though the hard feelings caused by the curtain calls would cost them later.

In the midst of taking two that day and sweeping the Twins, few thought of any potential backlash. The Sox piled on more runs and Minnesota's pennant hopes took a real beating. Against Minnesota, Chicago scored 34 runs, hit seven homers, and now were in first place with a three game lead. The Twins had to leave Chicago talking to themselves.

All during the 1970s, the Sox struggled with attendance. They had some huge crowds like the record setting 55,555 on Bat Day on May 20, 1973. But inconsistency and dashed expectations had made things extremely difficult to keep a cynical fan base interested. For the series against Minnesota, they drew a paid attendance of 96,204 plus a little more than 9,000 who made their way in with a promotional giveaway. In addition to the numbers, the team had crowds that were emotionally charged. It would have been hard to believe, but the incredible month of July 1977 was just getting started and it would only get better.

"The series awakened the people," Bill Jauss said in 2005, remembering how he covered the four games for the *Chicago Tribune*. "They were beginning to think this team was for real."

Once Minnesota left town, Chicago kept winning, eventually extending their win streak to nine. One of their victims was Mark "the Bird" Fidyrich. Fidyrich had won 19 in his American League rookie year of 1976, and liked talking to the ball when he was on the mound. After this game Fidyrich wondered out loud to the media about what had happened to his stuff.

Detroit ended the White Sox win streak with a 6-5 win in 10 innings at Tiger Stadium. Chicago then split a two-game at home series against the Royals, but even in an 8-3 defeat began to believe in themselves. With that explosive offense, the South Side Hitmen felt they still had a chance even as they went into the bottom of the ninth trailing 8-1. But after scoring two runs, and loading the bases with one out, the Sox brought their fans back into to the game. Before Alan Bannister grounded into a double play to end the game, Oscar Gamble sat in the on-deck circle and dreamed about stepping up to represent the tying run.

"We've been bringing it all back," Gamble said after the loss. "Not all teams think this way. Last year's Yankees did." (The 1976 Yankees went to the World Series.)

A few days later, Boston came into town and, as was typical that year, the White Sox greeted their guests with a big inning, this one a six-run fourth. The Red Sox made a much needed pitching change in the middle of the fourth. Fan Mark Liptak was in attendance and recalls the "great atmosphere" and the feeling that along with it by seeing the White Sox in first place in the middle of July. (Over 41,000 were at Comiskey that night.)

"The entire lower deck was chanting, 'Red Sox suck, Red Sox suck,'" Liptak told the author in 2005. "During a pitching change, [Carl] Yastremski was talking to [Fred] Lynn. They looked at each other laughing because the fans were having such a good time."

The White Sox took that game 9-7 and won the series two games to one with a Sunday afternoon 3-2 win two days later. Steve Stone pitched one of his best games of the year, going eight innings, giving up two runs on a measly three hits. Stone walked two and struck out nine. The difference in this game was again provided by Jim Spencer when he homered in the right field upper deck directly over the auxiliary scoreboard. The game ended in dramatic fashion as catcher Brian Downing threw pinch runner Steve Dillard out trying to steal second. Lerrin LaGrow notched his 16th save.

One week later Chicago traveled to Boston and swept an oddly scheduled two-game series, scoring 17 runs on 23 hits which included six homers. Even the Red Sox were impressed.

Going into the last weekend of the month, the White Sox posted a 19-5 record for July. They faced the Kansas City Royals in a three-date, four game series. Kansas City, in second place, was the closest Sox pursuer. three and a half games out. They also had to be considered one of the teams to beat since they were the defending division champions. Could the Sox end the month in the same dramatic fashion as they began it?

July 29–31, 1977. There was nothing like it, not in that decade and very rarely duplicated before or since. Although White Sox fans can come up with other examples of great times at both ball parks, it is very doubtful that anything surpasses the last weekend of July 1977 (with the exception of the 2005 post season). It was a weekend that created high emotions and sent a strong message to the baseball world that something special was happening on the South Side of Chicago.

First, there was the attendance. Getting a ticket at Comiskey Park during the 1970s was not all that hard. Fans could arrive late and not worry about sitting behind a pole. During this weekend, Chicago drew 131,285, and for the month they drew a little more than 482,000. In contrast, the gate for the entire 1970 season was a little more than 495,000. Of course, it wasn't only the numbers; it was the noise and the intense fan emotion that created an incredible atmosphere typical only of 1977.

Secondly, the Sox won three out of four in the series, each time coming from behind. No, they didn't overcome huge leads, but they were playing a tough team in close games and it was never easy beating the likes of the 1977 Royals when they scored first. And naturally, Chicago used the long ball in dramatic style.

Finally, the four games capped an incredible month. The Sox finished July 1977 with a 22-6 mark, good for a .785 percentage. July 1977 ranks as a landmark 31 days. It was their best monthly showing since 1951, and the franchise third best winning record in team history. There is no question that the Chicago White Sox not only peaked that month for the year, but also for the decade, and almost for the century.

Game one on Friday night was so typical of South Side Hitmen contests. After giving up three Kansas City runs in the first, the Sox put together a six spot in the third, capped by a homer by Chet Lemon.

Not being wimps themselves, the Royals countered with a three run, George Brett homer in the fifth, and took the lead in the seventh with two more. But with the help of a hit batsman and an error, Chicago responded with four in their half of the seventh, and added another in the eighth. The Sox won 11-8, pounding out 17 hits and knocking around four Kansas City pitchers.

The White Sox trailed again the next day 3-2 in the seventh. Eric Soderholm turned the game around with a three run homer. When interviewed in 2000, Soderholm remembered that day as one of his best that season. He recalled touching second base and hearing and feeling the "roar" of the crowd. Although Old Comiskey Park had its many critics, there was one thing it had over many of the large modern stadiums: the then 67-year-old park was large but was enclosed and noise tended to stay in its confines. In 1977, there was plenty of noise at Comiskey and that day Soderholm not only heard it, he felt it.

Chicago won game two 6-4 with three more RBIs from Jorge Orta including a homer in the eighth. The nearly 35,000 in attendance went home very happy.

Sunday provided a usually unmemorable split for the Sox. However, game one provided an excitement that even went beyond 1977 standards.

Marty Pattin, generally considered a good but not great pitcher, started for the Royals. But Pattin had everything working for him that day, especially in the first five innings. He set down first 15 Sox in order, something completely unheard of in 1977. Fortunately for the Sox, Steve Stone continued his good pitching that month and Chicago trailed only 1-0 going into the bottom of the sixth.

Chet Lemon picked up the first hit of the game for the Sox leading off the sixth. The center fielder hit his 13th homer of the season to tie things up. Lemon would be heard from again later.

On two occasions it appeared that the Royals would win the game and take the crowd of a little over 50,000 out of it. Amos Otis homered in the seventh to give Kansas City a 2-1 lead going into the ninth.

But Jorge Orta singled in Alan Bannister who had reached on an error to send the game into extra innings. The normally powerful Sox had only three hits off the luckless Marty Pattin, but were still in the game.

Once more the Royals looked like they were going to win when they picked up two runs after two were out and no one was on in the tenth. In 1977, however, no lead was ever safe from the South Side Hitmen.

Jim Spencer singled and that man Chet Lemon came through again. Lemon lined a two-run homer into the lower deck in left to tie the game one more time. One out later, Ralph Garr singled in Eric Soderholm with the winning run. It had to be one of the most exciting wins during a month with nothing but exciting wins.

Now no matter what happened in game two, the Sox had won another four-game series against a contender that month, and with the sweep of the Twins in the beginning of July, provided victorious bookends for that historic 31 days. It was quite a transformation from the previous year when the only anticipation the end of July brought was a game in August where players wore short pants.

Kansas City averted the sweep, winning game two 8-4 by slugging three homers. The Royals left Chicago in an angry mood, and losing three out of four was only part of it. They had little respect for the White Sox as a team and even less for the curtain calls. The Good-bye song only soured their mood further. In short, the Royals thought the Sox fans and players were making fools out of themselves with the ovations and the singing. Kansas City vowed they would catch and pass the White Sox.

This type of bitterness didn't take anything away from the euphoria that accompanied July 1977. The South Side Hitmen were in first place, by a comfortable but not an overwhelming margin. They seemed to be alleviating the disappointment and letdown in the entire Chicago sports city. The crybaby Royals, a team Sox fans liked to call annual pennant chokers, couldn't dampen the spirit of 1977.

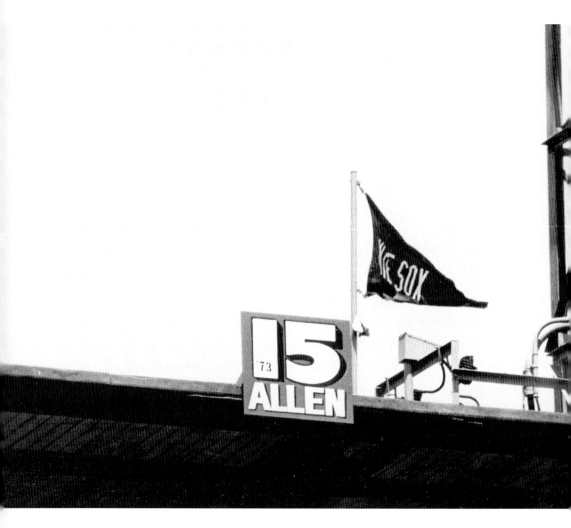

Plaques were placed where roof shots were made. Zisk added to the rooftop history in 1977. It was amazing only one blast made it up there during the 1977 season. Leo Bauby collection.)

Spencer holds Twin Dan Ford on first. Ford made a huge error in the second game of the exciting July four-game series at Comiskey. Spencer made him regret it with a three-run homer that broke open a tight game. Sox won the contest 13-8. (Leo Bauby collection.)

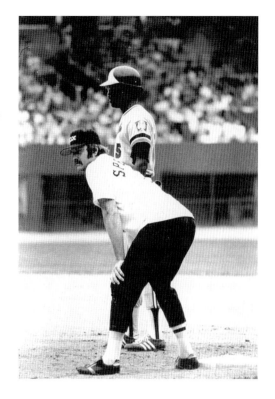

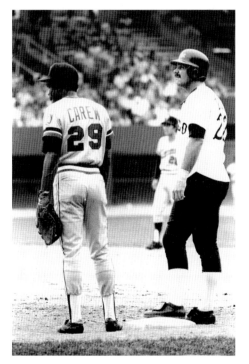

The Twins' Rod Carew does the honors of holding the not-do-fast Richie Zisk at first base. Carew was elected to the Hall of Fame in 1991. Richie Zisk, at this writing, is the manager of the Daytona Cubs in the Florida League. (Leo Bauby collection.)

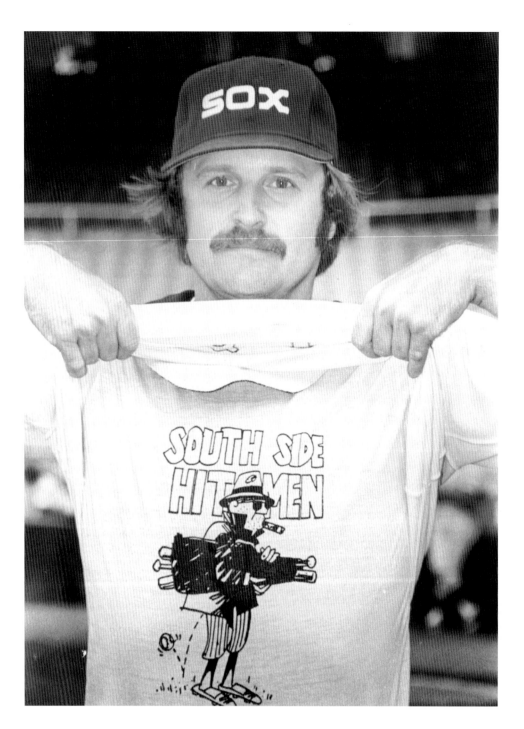

Jim Spencer holds a 1977 souvenir T-shirt bearing the "South Side Hitmen" nickname. The shirt was very popular, as was the team. The name has its own meaning with Sox fans and its mere mention brings back memories of the White Sox offensive onslaught of 1977. (Leo Bauby collection.)

JULY: A FAST, FURIOUS RIDE TO THE TOP

Jorge Orta does some mean looking hitting at Fenway Park. Boston was one of the few teams that didn't scoff at the Hitmen in 1977, and actually got a kick out of Comiskey Park fans. The Red Sox were also impressed with the hitting prowess of the White Sox. (Leo Bauby collection.)

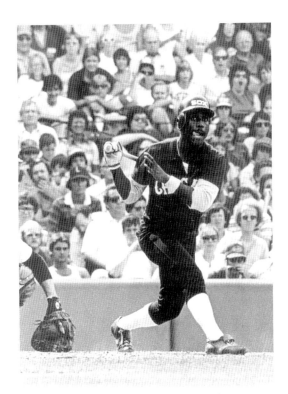

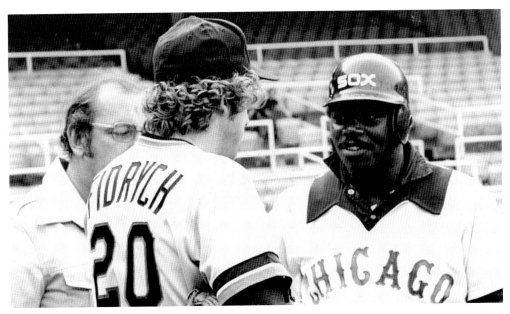

Pictured here, from left to right, are White Sox radio announcer Lorn Brown, Tiger pitcher Mark "the Bird" Fidrych, and Sox first baseman/singer Lamar Johnson. The Sox tamed Fidrych in a July 8 game 10-7, leaving the poor guy wondering what happened to his stuff. (Leo Bauby collection.)

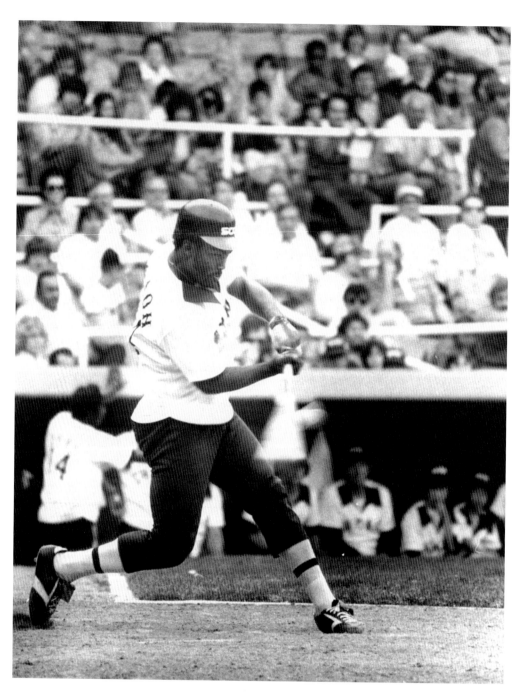

Chet Lemon unloads a powerful swing during July. The young center fielder began to come into his own during the summer of 1977. His two home runs in the first game of a July 31 doubleheader against Kansas City capped off an incredible month. Fans didn't know it, but his second homer that game, which tied the game in the tenth, would turn out to be the last great moment of the decade. (Leo Bauby collection.)

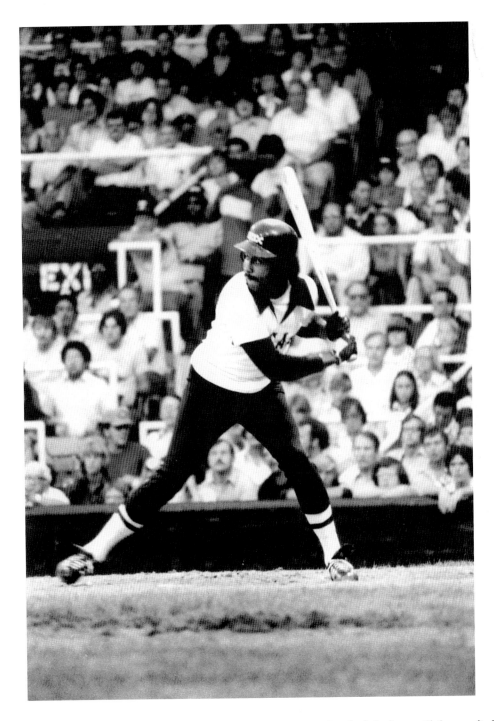

Oscar Gamble stands at the plate. Gamble became the first White Sox left handed hitter to knock out 30 homers in a season. Though he would only play two seasons with the White Sox, South Side fans will forever link his name with the team and the summer of 1977, as if Gamble had spent his entire career in Chicago. (Leo Bauby collection.)

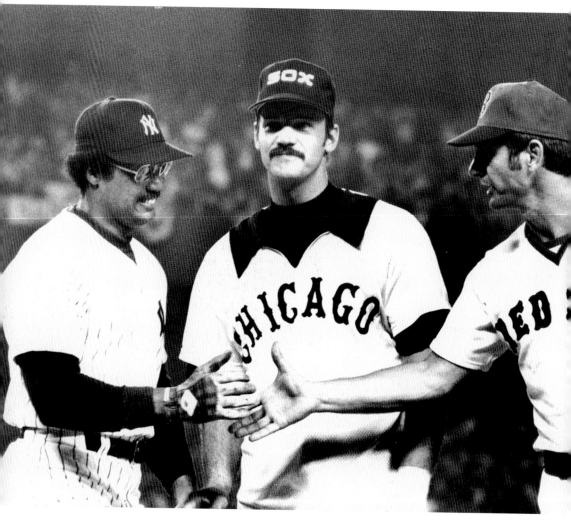

Richie Zisk was the only representative for the White Sox on the 1977 All-Star game. Here he is standing next to Reggie Jackson (left) and a Red Sox player. The American League lost the game 7-5. The game was played in Yankee Stadium. (Leo Bauby collection.)

JULY: A FAST, FURIOUS RIDE TO THE TOP

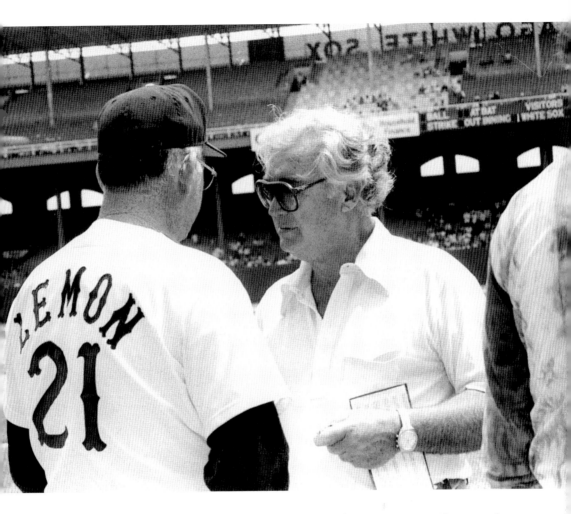

Manager Bob Lemon and play-by-play man Caray enjoy Comiskey on a nice summer day in 1977. It was a great summer for baseball on the South Side of Chicago. With his statue in front of Wrigley, it is sometimes forgotten that Caray began his Chicago broadcasting career with the Sox. (Leo Bauby collection.)

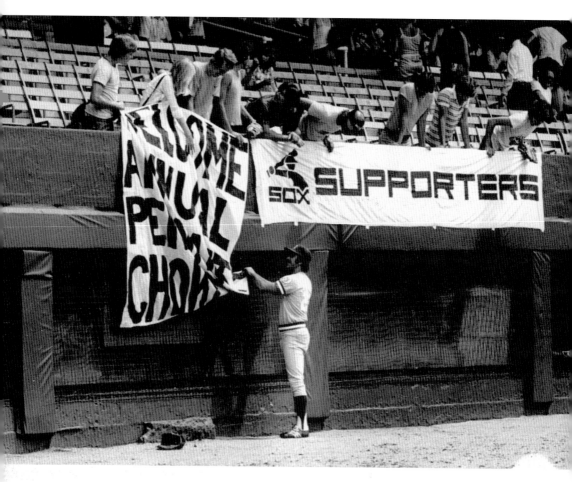

Banners were popular in the left field seats during the 1977 season. This one was not exactly a love note to the Kansas City Royals. It read, "Welcome Annual Pennant Chokers," for Kansas City's inability to win a playoff series. According to Sox fan Paul Duffy, the Royals confiscated the banner and destroyed it. The Royals were not impressed and even resented the success of the South Side Hitmen. Duffy is one fan who to this day cheers for a Kansas City last place finish. (Leo Bauby collection.)

JULY: A FAST, FURIOUS RIDE TO THE TOP

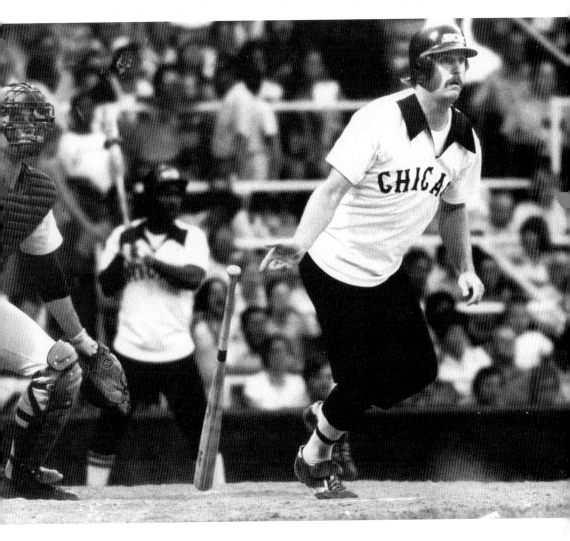

Jim Spencer follows through on a swing. Spencer had a big month in July, starting with the exciting series with the Twins. He also hit a game winning home run against the Red Sox in the July 17, 3-2 contest. Sadly, he died way before his time in 2002. (Leo Bauby collection.)

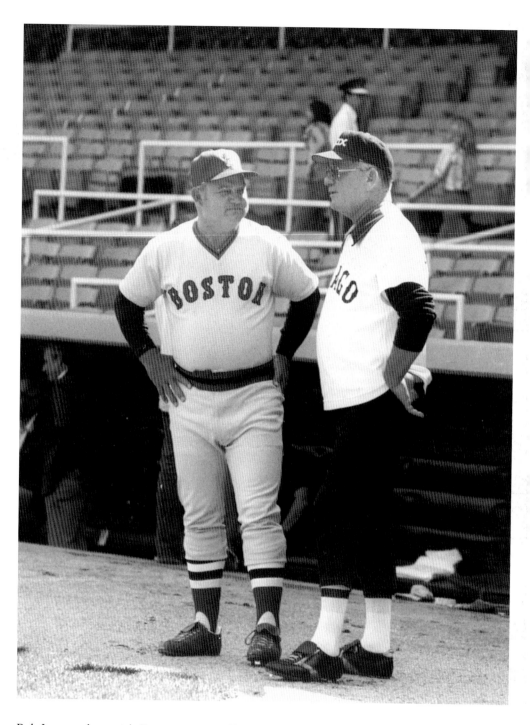

Bob Lemon chats with Boston manager Don Zimmer. Zimmer, unlike the angry Kansas City Royals, actually respected the 1977 Sox. The Hitmen had traveled to Boston that month and knocked the ball all around Fenway. They did the same when the Red Sox had visited Comiskey. (Leo Bauby collection.)

JULY: A FAST, FURIOUS RIDE TO THE TOP

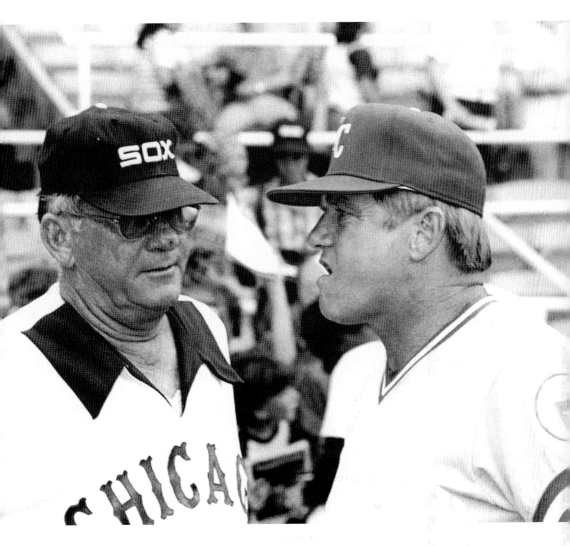

All looks great here between Bob Lemon (left) and Royals manager Whitey Herzog. The same can't be said for the feelings between their players. (Leo Bauby collection.)

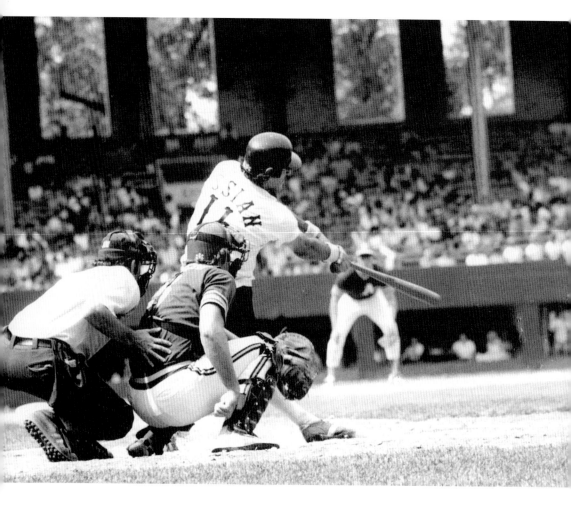

Jim Essian takes a healthy cut. He was part of back-to-back homer combination in the emotional Fourth of July weekend series against the Twins with Alan Bannister. He was one of nine South Side Hitmen to break into double figures for home runs. (Leo Bauby collection.)

6

AUGUST TO SEPTEMBER

WINDING DOWN

Bonafide contending teams contend in the last part of the season. Though technically later season games don't count any more than games in April or May, their importance is magnified as top teams play head to head and there is less time to bounce back from slumps and losing streaks. Teams in mid-season form must turn it on during late-season hysteria or they return to the middle of the pack from whence they came.

After the exciting three of four series over the Royals to end July, the Chicago White Sox seemed ready to go where no Sox team since 1959 had been. They were in first place, 5 ½ games in front of the second place and defending division champion Royals. Everybody on the club seemed to be veterans having career years or young players coming into their own. The story looked like it was going to be a great one; one where a once financially strapped and talent-impaired team had a great chance to get into the post-season.

Before facing an angry Kansas City team again, the Sox were scheduled to finish a 10-game home stand with a four-game set against the fourth-place Texas Rangers.

Winning Ugly would become the battle cry of the 1983 Sox. The first week of August 1977 was plenty ugly with winning only a small part of it. Chicago dropped three out of four to the Rangers, lucky not to be swept in their own ballpark as they salvaged the last game 5-4. With Texas amassing 36 runs in the four games, the Sox were lucky they didn't let the last game get away from them as they almost blew a 5-1 lead in the late innings. Their lead in the American League West was beginning to shrink.

Playing on the road is tough. The visiting team has to face a variety of disadvantages including not being able to sleep in their own beds, playing in a park that is not tailored for them, and the always hostile atmosphere of someone else's hometown crowd. The hostile atmosphere was the biggest obstacle they faced heading into Kansas City for a three-game weekend series.

The Royals were still seething. Not only were they angered by good-bye songs and curtain calls, Kansas City had little respect for the unexpected and first-place holding Sox. Before leaving Chicago, Royals outfielder Amos said he wasn't impressed with the overall Chicago lineup except for a few hitters. "We'll catch them," he predicted.

The first game on August 5 set the tone for the series. Young pitcher Chris Knapp came in with a 9-5 record, but the right hander was knocked out in the second inning. The Royals did some South Side hitting of their own with Otis and catcher Darrell Porter hitting back-to-back homers in a five-run second inning. John Mayberry homered to lead off the third and tipped his cap to the crowd as he returned to the dugout. Before the Sox knew it, they were down 8-1. The final was 12-2 in one of the most humbling losses of the season for the South Siders. Three Sox pitchers had been pounded for 17 hits.

Kansas City won games two (6-3) and three (3-2) to finish the sweep. The worm had begun to turn. Manager Lemon was left in the dugout after game three to ponder the powerful shift in momentum. Over 118,000 Royal fans had come to see their hometown heroes take the air right out of the surprising White Sox. Chicago was still in first place, but their lead stood at a half game ahead of the second place Twins, and one and a half in front the vengeful Royals. Fourth place Texas was not too far back, three games behind. The four-team race brought back memories of 1967.

By August 13 things began to look bleaker. For the first time since July 1, when they beat the Minnesota Twins in that memorable series, the White Sox were no longer in first place. Blowing a two run lead in the eighth, the Sox lost to the Rangers 10-7. And while the Sox had endeared themselves to their fans with an unexpected pennant run, opposition in their division continued to show lack of respect for them and their fans.

"I haven't seen too many teams bludgeon their way to a pennant," Ranger manager Billy Hunter said.

"It's catching up with them—finally," said Texas reliever Darrold Knowles. "It's a little surprising to me they were up there this long. Even if you hit the ball like they do, and score seven or eight runs a game, you gotta get hurt in the long run if you can't catch it that good or throw that good."

The White Sox climbed back into first place with a 6-5 win in the second game of this three game series, but lost the finale as they were again beaten by their own tactics losing 12-9. And again the South Siders felt the backlash as a result of their fan celebrations. Ranger fans had a sing along to serenade the Sox. The good-bye song was played over the loud speaker and the Ranger faithful gladly joined in.

"Whatever happened to that Chicago World Series?" wondered Ranger reliever Dock Ellis. "The Cubs have gone down the tube. You don't suppose the White Sox will be next, do you?"

The Cubs, uncharacteristically, had been playing well but went into their usual slide and would end up dead even for the season. Unfortunately for the White Sox, they were next, as the entire Chicago baseball scene went down the tube as Dock Ellis so eloquently put it.

In an August 16 game against the Yankees, it looked like the Sox would pull out a win in 1977 South Side Hitman style. Chicago went into the top of the ninth down 9-4. They then rattled a barrage of hits. Chet Lemon started off things with a single and was homered in by Spencer. Brian Downing singled to left and one out later Bannister doubled Downing to third. Orta singled in Downing and a Zisk sacrifice fly brought in Bannister. Lamar Johnson singled and Soderholm walked to load the bases. Gamble batted for Lemon and singled in two. When it was all said and done, the Sox had piled on six and took a 10-9 lead.

But as Texas manager Billy Hunter said, not too many teams bludgeon their way to a pennant. The Yankees won the game on a two run homer by Chris Chambliss in their half of the ninth. The inspiring ninth inning rally was rendered meaningless by a heartbreaking loss when the relief pitching couldn't hold the lead. Randy Wiles was the losing pitcher for the White Sox. Wiles never pitched in another major league game.

August 20 was another benchmark in the 1977 season. The Kansas City Royals, as many of their players had predicted, moved into first place. They would never relinquish that position.

By the end of August, the White Sox were still in the hunt, two and a half games behind the Royals. But August had been a terrible month, their only losing month of the season. (Other than the three games in October.) Just what had happened in those dog days?

In an article for http://www.ESPN.com in 2003, writer Keith Scherer analyzed what had gone wrong for the White Sox. His statistics and analysis pretty well mirrored what so many others had been saying about the South Side team.

The ugliness began with the pitching. White Sox hurlers allowed almost six and half runs per game that month. Obviously any team, even a team with great hitting would have a hard time winning over any long stretch if it needed to average seven runs a game to do it.

Even uglier, the Sox staff gave up at least 10 runs eight times. That fete had occurred only three times in the three previous months. Giving up runs in double figures will do it to you most of the time.

The maligned defense lived up to its criticism in August 1977. The Sox gave up 30 unearned runs during the 11-18 month. That is one unearned run a game, and that is pretty hard to overcome. Scherer put it this way: "Balls were slipping through and dropping in, double plays weren't being turned –the pitchers were under constant pressure, and under duress they allowed 33 home runs, again the worst for any month."

Scherer also believes that Orta and Bannister made for a terrible double play combination. The White Sox were last in the number of double plays turned that year.

And on the days the team wasn't knocking the hell out of the ball, they were having a hard time manufacturing runs. Scherer pointed out that the Sox were last in number of steals and stolen base percentage in 1977. They stole a meager 42 while being caught 43 times. Bunting was also a big problem for White Sox. They had but 33 sacrifice hits, again the least in the major leagues.

In essence, their lack of balance caught up with the team in August 1977. Their fans' enthusiasm was thrown back in their faces, and used as a psychological ploy against them. The most lovable thing about them—that they could hit and do nothing else—had exposed the Sox as a team that could not go wire to wire. A foreboding September awaited them.

Much has been said about winning games in September. Being in contention in the last full month of the season is an excellent indicator of how that season has gone and just how good a team is. The 1977 White Sox entered September 73-56, their best record for starting that month since 1965. For a pleasant change, White Sox fans looked forward to that stretch month of September and had some hope of a championship. The White Sox did have one huge disadvantage. Since they no longer had any games with front running Kansas City, they would have to depend on weaker teams in the Western Division to beat the Royals to help the Sox gain ground.

Contending teams make late season acquisitions to push themselves over the top. The Sox went out and picked up ex-Cub Don Kessinger to shore up their not-so-good infield defense. They then re-acquired reliever Clay Carroll from St. Louis. Carroll had valuable post-season experience, winning the decisive game of the classic 1975 World Series for Cincinnati by throwing two hitless innings including a three-up three-down ninth inning in Boston.

Bill Veeck felt he did all he could with his limited resources to shore up his ball club and give Chicago fans a chance to experience their first World Series since 1959.

September 8 was a day that helped seal the fate of the South Side Hitmen. The White Sox started the month with an okay 4-3 mark, but they continued to lose ground to the Royals. The euphoria and hope of July 31 now seemed like it had happened in another season.

First there was symbolism. In the first game of a doubleheader against the California Angels, and in the 137th game of the season, the South Side Hitmen were shut out for the first time. Nolan Ryan, author of many shutouts and no-hitters, earned his 19th win of the season by throwing six and one third innings of three-hit ball. Chicago actually had a great opportunity to score in the first inning when Ralph Garr led off the game with a double and advanced to third on a fly out to right by Alan Bannister. Jorge Orta came up needing only a decent fly to the outfield to score Garr. But before Orta could even attempt to deliver, Garr got himself picked off third by Ryan. Orta did fly out to right but it only ended the inning.

The Sox actually chased Ryan in the seventh when Zisk and Orta singled with one out. Lefty Dave LaRouche relieved Ryan, and got Gamble to fly out to center. Lamar Johnson, pinch hitting for Spencer, fouled out. The last threat of the game for the Sox produced a goose egg.

Game two went beyond symbolism. The Sox blew a 2-0 ninth inning lead and lost 3-2. A wild pitch by Lerrin LaGrow brought in the winning run. Lefty Ken Kravec had given up three hits in eight plus innings, but a succession of three relievers couldn't protect the lead. The hard-hitting Sox had been held to two runs and 12 hits in the doubleheader which was enough to evoke memories of Black Wednesday, 1967.

To compound the misery of this double loss, Kansas City won by knocking out five homers and easily beat Seattle 7-2. The Royals now had a seven game lead over the Sox with 24 remaining. In recalling how the Royals netted a 12 ½ game gain in the standings against the Sox in a little less than six weeks, Steve Stone used the old cliché in 2005 saying they "passed us as if we were standing still."

The Sox were not actually standing still. They had it in reverse, now playing eight games under .500 since the historic July 31 doubleheader. In the reversal, the defending division champs had a foot on the throat of the White Sox.

Chicago rebounded a little with a win the next day. However, Wilbur Wood tied a major league record by hitting three batters in one inning on September 10. None of them were really hurt by the slow moving knuckle ball, but the White Sox felt the pain of a 6-1 loss. A three-run homer by Bobby Bonds provided the Angels with more than enough runs against the suddenly offensively impaired White Sox.

Four days later, the Hitmen were shut out for the second and last time. They again had an opportunity to score when they loaded the bases with one out in the fifth. But Garr forced Bannister at the plate with a grounder to first and Lemon forced Garr at second with a grounder to short. Twins pitcher Dave Goltz went all the way for the win, the only pitcher to throw a complete game shut out against the Sox that year. More importantly the Sox fell to nine games behind the now runaway Royals with only 15 left to play. Only a person with a Cubs fan view of the world would think the Sox would have any chance at a division championship.

All that was left was a little team history. On September 17, Oscar Gamble became the first left-handed White Sox batter to hit 30 homers in a season and only the third South Sider to perform that feat. (Bill Melton and Dick Allen had been the others.) Chicago was down 3-0 in the seventh when Gamble tied the game with a three run shot after Lemon and Orta had walked. No one seemed to care that Gamble took a curtain call for the 15,378 in attendance. Unfortunately the White Sox lost the game when the Angels pushed a run across in the ninth and then made it hold up. Regardless, it was somewhat fitting that Gamble came through in the clutch to get the Sox back into the game. Gamble's final homer of the season came on the next day, giving him the team lead for the season.

On September 27, just days before the season ended, Zisk joined Gamble in the 30-homer club when the Sox exacted a little revenge on Dave Goltz. Zisk's eighth inning solo shot proved to be the difference in a 4-3 win. It was also the first time in the 77-year history of the franchise that the White Sox had two 30-homer players in one season.

But personal achievements were all that was left for the South Side Hitmen. Two days earlier Kansas City clinched their second consecutive Western Division title. While the Sox had cooled down considerably during the last two months of the season, the Royals had an even more incredible month in September than the Sox did in July. Kansas City went an amazing 25-5 in September. They, without a doubt, proved they were the best team in the division, and one of the best teams in baseball. Because of Kansas City's surge, the division race was not even competitive. Even second place Texas finished eight games behind the Royals.

Chokeitis. Many Chicago sports fans thought their teams were forever inflicted with it. But on the last day of the 1977 season, White Sox fans didn't think their team had let them down or choked away a great chance to go to the playoffs. The White Sox, which had been at the top or near the top of the standings since July 1, had actually fallen to third. Texas, with a near Kansas City type September, had taken over second place. No matter what the Sox did that day, they were going to end up in third.

Eric Soderholm recalls how he wanted to achieve two little milestones. He wanted to end the season with a .280 average and have 25 homers. He was able to do both, picking up his 25th homer in the fifth inning. He also remembers the ovation the crowd gave him after his last round tripper. It was as if the White Sox were still in the division race.

The White Sox clowned around and enjoyed the crowd of a little over 20,000. As they took the field for the last inning and when they came in for their last at-bat, they received ovations. As in the season opener, the White Sox finished against an expansion team, this time the Seattle Mariners. Seattle won the game 3-2 as the South Side Hitmen hit very little that dark and rainy afternoon.

No matter. The fans didn't want to leave Comiskey once the game was over. They cheered and Bill Veeck cheered right along with them. It was such a rare day since the decade of disappointment that began in late September 1967. The South Side Hitmen were just different. They knocked the hell out of the ball like no other Sox team before them and allowed their fans to actually think a Chicago World Series was possible. The fact that they didn't get to the Promised Land didn't matter. After the game, White Sox fans chanted, "We want the Sox, we want the Sox."

"Bill Veeck and I were in the depths of despair at this time a year ago," Soderholm said after that final game. "The Sox were in financial trouble and I didn't know if I would ever play again. We both had great comebacks." (Soderholm would win the American League Comeback Player of the Year Award.)

"Win, lose or draw, we put on a show," Alan Bannister chimed in. "Then again the fans put on a show, too."

At mid-season, Richie Zisk had made it clear that he wanted to stay with the White Sox.

"I would love to make my home here and raise my family here," Zisk said. "I'm hopeful something can be worked out. I honestly mean that. But at the same time I realize that with each day that goes along puts me closer to free agency—not that I am looking forward to that."

Unfortunately that last game of the season was the last for Zisk as a White Sox player. It would be the last for others, too. And also unfortunately, the reign of the South Side Hitmen would last for just one year.

"People don't realize what offensive balance we had," Oscar Gamble recalled in 2005, referring the power from the right and left as he ticked off the names of Zisk, Spencer, Lemon, and Soderholm. "If we could have stayed together when the pitching came later, we would have been in the Series."

Looking back in 2005, Soderholm summed up the team in a different way. He referred to himself as a "step and dive" at third, alluding to his reduced range. Alan Bannister had "to sling it at short" because of his bad shoulder. He also remembered that Jorge Orta was not too hot at turning double plays. Soderholm described Lamar Johnson as "a big target at first," and recalled Zisk's non-range in right. He felt Ralph Garr was at the end of his career and had a hard time chasing down fly balls. But the combination of this rag tag bunch was just the right mix—at least for one year.

"We felt we had something to prove," Soderholm says now. "People told me and Bannister that we would never play again. Zisk felt as if he wasn't wanted in Pittsburgh."

At the center of the improbability of the South Side Hitmen was owner Bill Veeck. The baseball powers that be had speculated that Veeck and his group didn't have the resources to run a major league franchise. As free agency began in the late 1970s, that was probably true. Veeck didn't have the ability to sign a marquis star like Reggie Jackson to a long-term contract. Instead, Veeck tried to buy time by trading a player or players that he wouldn't be able to sign for other players he wouldn't be able to sign. This rent-a-player strategy didn't work in the long run. But in 1977, some players may never have been available to Veeck if it wasn't for the dynamics of free agency. It certainly was the case regarding Soderholm and Stone and probably in the cases of Zisk and Gamble. Today Stone and Soderholm are grateful for the faith Veeck had in them when others had been skeptical.

Yet the newly found freedom of players exploring the market place worried fans as they enjoyed the summer of 1977. From all indications, the South Side Hitmen were not going to stay together. Most of the speculation centered around Zisk and Gamble, the team's leading home run hitters. In the middle of all the excitement, it was becoming apparent that a winning team was going to be intentionally split apart once the season ended. Fans appealed to the players to stay, but it wasn't a matter of loyalty. Gamble said in 2005 that the Sox did make him an offer as he tested the free agent market after the 1977 season. In comparison to other offers he received, Gamble said the Sox offer "wasn't even close."

There was a parallel to the early 1960s when bitter Veeck critics savaged him for trading away talent and potential costing the Sox future pennants. During the late 1970s, the Sox had a net loss when they traded one player they couldn't sign for another whom they also would not able to resign. As a result, the success of the 1977 Hitmen was short lived.

Still, the South Side Hitmen have to be credited with helping the Sox remain in Chicago. Couldn't anyone imagine what kind of interest Chicago would have had in a team that in any way resembled the 1976 squad? In 1978, the White Sox drew a little over 1.4 million and in 1979, they had a little more than 1.2 million. By 2005 standards, that isn't overly impressive. In comparison to the Sox attendance in the early part of the decade, it was quite an achievement. The afterglow of 1977 had to be partly responsible.

Even the most cynical and hard boiled fan will get defensive if anyone accuses the South Side Hitmen of "choking." Most will say that the 1977 White Sox didn't have the depth to win a division championship or World Series. Fans know that the defense wasn't there, and the pitching was only so good. They knew that, in the end, good pitching stops good hitting in the long run. So many fans felt they got what they paid for. The 1977 South Side Hitmen gave them the most exciting moments of the decade, and that was enough to endear the team to its faithful for decades afterward. Only the passage of time and a World Series team like the 2005 edition will push the memories of 1977 to the back burner.

"They didn't want the whole field, they wanted the whole grandstand," says Bill Jauss who many times covered the Sox for the *Chicago Tribune.*

Jauss referred to the resentment and anger the Kansas City Royals felt toward the Hitmen after that season-defining series at the end of July. Jauss said that he understood the resentment the Royals felt since they looked at themselves as a team that paid its dues and weren't ready to take a back seat to the upstart White Sox. Kansas City followed the philosophy of batting instructor Charlie Lau (whose last batting coach job was with the White Sox before he died in 1984) and used the whole field to pick up hits. It irked the Royals to see this one-dimensional team swing from the heels and then bow to their fans like an actor who was just too full of himself.

The Royals may have used that resentment to rally themselves, but they were wrong if they thought the Sox were grandstanding. The Hitmen had awakened a slumbering fan base that had not been impressed with .500 records or .241 hitters. The decade between 1967 and 1977 had been a long one with only a few highlights. The year 1977 was different in that it was unexpected and thus exceeded the hopes of fans who had grown tired and frustrated with a team that sometimes played like a contender but finished as an also-ran. More importantly, there was an excitement at Comiskey Park that lasted the whole summer when other White Sox teams could only occasionally stir such emotion. A case can be made that the 1977 White Sox are more loved and revered than the division winners of 1983, 1993, and 2000, and that only the 2005 World Series squad will produce a team that can generate similarly charged emotions.

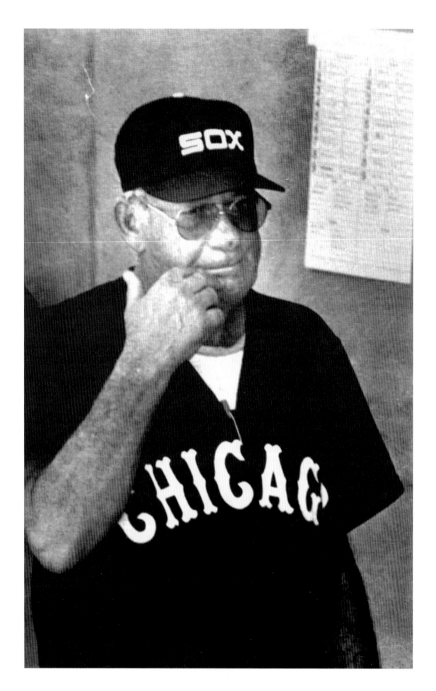

Almost in a state of shock, Bob Lemon muses in the dugout after the Royals had swept the Sox in a three-game series during the first weekend of August in Kansas City. The White Sox were crushed in game one, and couldn't win close games two and three. The Royals had their revenge for the previous weekend in Comiskey when White Sox fan hysteria was at its 1977 peak. Worse yet, Kansas City was on its way to division championship. (Leo Bauby collection.)

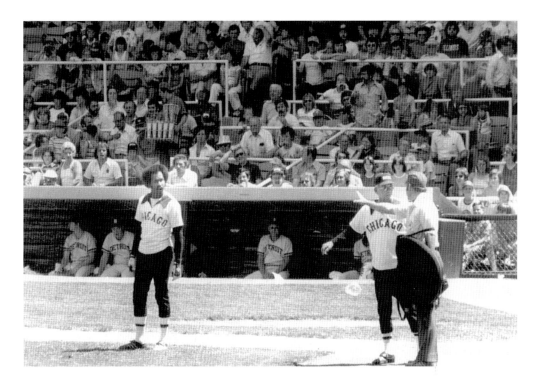

Oscar Gamble (left) and Bob Lemon have a disagreement with the umpire. Nothing much went right during the month of August. (Leo Bauby collection.)

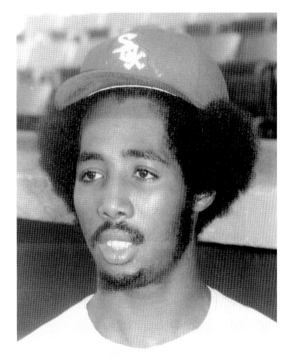

There is one other thing that went right in 1977. The White Sox signed Harold Baines after making him the overall first pick in the amateur free agency draft. A key member of the 1983 Winning Ugly team, Baines could always be counted on for a late inning hit that drove in a big run. Fans loved Baines because the quiet guy let his bat do his talking for him, finishing his career with 2,866 hits. He received a long-standing ovation during his last career at bat on September 27, 2001, at Comiskey Park, now called U.S. Cellular Field. (Leo Bauby collection.)

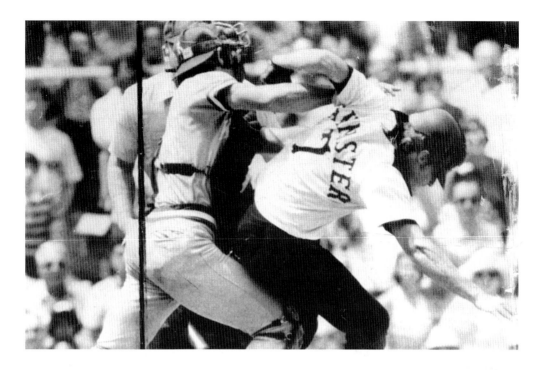

Darrell Porter puts a rough tag on Alan Bannister. Tension between the White Sox and Royals was high during the summer of 1977. Porter ended up getting into an altercation with Sox pitcher Bart Johnson during the momentum changing series in Kansas City. (Leo Bauby collection.)

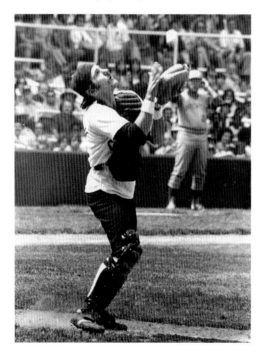

Catcher Jim Essian gets under a pop-up. The White Sox could have used a few more plays like this in August. Instead their pitchers got hit around for over six runs a game and their defense didn't help matters much. They paid for it with their 11-19 record that month. (Leo Bauby collection.)

Harry Caray poses with broadcast partner Mary Shane. Veeck, who liked to be different, broke ground by bringing a woman into the booth. Her Sox broadcasting career was short. (Leo Bauby collection.)

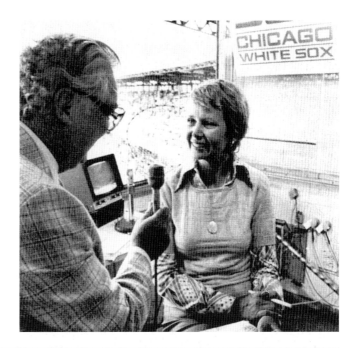

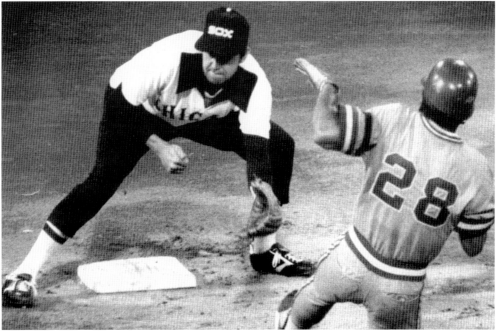

To shore up the weak White Sox defense, Veeck went out and got Don Kessinger in August 1977. Kessinger, a key component of the 1969 Cubs, was known for his great range at short and his incredible off balance throws from deep in the hole. He would later manage the White Sox until the beginning of August during the not-so-memorable 1979 season. (Leo Bauby collection.)

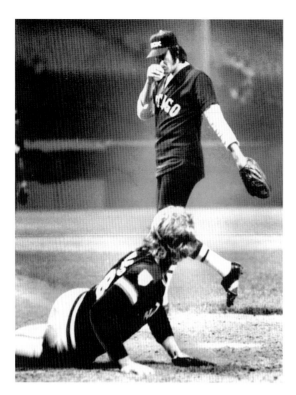

The mercurial, but talented Francisco Barrios won 14 in 1977. Here he is gesturing to an opposing player in a kind of un-sportsmanlike way. Barrios never came close to fulfilling his potential after the 1977 season. He died of a heart attack in 1982 two months short of his 29th birthday. (Leo Bauby collection.)

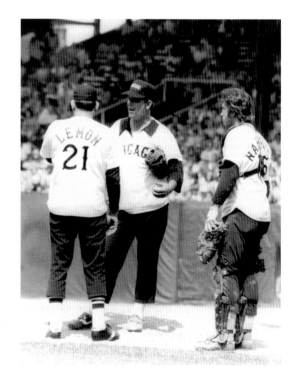

Unfortunately, in a too familiar scene in August of 1977, Bob Lemon comes out to the mound to make a pitching change. (Leo Bauby collection.)

7

THE 1977
HITMEN REMEMBERED

Fan Memories of the South Side Hitmen

<u>David Sheputis:</u> This is my favorite all time Sox team and the best games I ever attended were that season. I was 13, we were living in southern Illinois at the time, and I listened to almost every game on the radio. My most memorable game was July 31. The Sox played a doubleheader against the Royals wrapping up a four-game first place showdown of which they had already won the first two. It was banner day and my brother, stepfather, and I stayed up all night making a banner for the doubleheader. We had to leave around 4:00 a.m. and basically slept all the way to Chicago. We got there before the gates opened and there were already big crowds outside the ballpark. We ended up sitting in the right field upper deck, halfway up, against the rail looking down into the center field bleachers. It was extremely hot that day, and the whole atmosphere in the park was electric. I can remember when the Sox took the field for the first game; they were given what seemed like a ten minute standing ovation delaying the state of the game. The crowd was just at a fever pitch that whole first game, without a scoreboard telling them to cheer. It was the loudest I can ever remember it being in the old ballpark. Marty Pattin started for the Royals, and I seemed to remember he had a perfect game for six innings. Then in the seventh someone for the Sox (I think Chet Lemon or Alan Bannister) hit a homer to break up the perfect game. Then in the tenth Chet Lemon hit a homer and I swear the upper deck was shaking it was so loud. It gave me goose bumps. We went down to the field between games to line up for the banner parade, and it was like an English soccer game with spontaneous chants/cheers just breaking out. By the time the second game started, the heat and probably a lot of booze has just taken it out of the crowd. I remember the Royals won it easily. Hal McRae and Al Cowens incited the crowd by tipping their caps to the crowd mocking the Sox curtain calls during the first game. I watched a lot of fights in the center field bleachers in the second game and security continually getting pelted with garbage when they would try to break it up.

<u>Richard Brook:</u> I typically attended at least 20-25 games annually. Back in 1977, with a surging, exciting team on the field, I attended over 40 home games. One of the most vivid memories I have of that season, while usually seated in the left field stands, was how Sox fans started singing, "Na, Na, Hey, Hey, Good-bye." It was the last week of July and the Sox were heading into a weeklong home-stand against the Twins and a four game weekend series against the Royals. The left field grandstand fans started taunting the Twins by singing, "Na, Na, Na, Na, Na, Na, Na, Minnesota, good-bye." That carried over when the Royals were here, and as they

were being knocked from first place, the left field fans again sang, only this time saying "Royals." By Saturday, Nancy Faust picked up the song and played it all weekend long. The rest is history, and the song remains a fixture today whenever an opposing pitcher is removed. As usual, the fun didn't last past August, and we continue to wait for a championship season. [Fan quoted before the 2005 playoffs.]

Paul Duffy: I was in high school and my dad took my brother and sisters and me to a Friday night game on May 13. It was "Anti-Superstition Night" because it was Friday the 13th. It was one of Bill Veeck's ridiculous over-the-top pre-game carnivals. They had 13 people who called themselves "witches" on the field before the game to put a "spell" on the other 13 AL teams. People broke mirrors on the field with baseball bats. They set up a ladder and announced beforehand that they'd make the visiting Cleveland walk under before the game, but I think the Tribe players refused. The Sox beat the Tribe easily. [Actually it was a 5-3 Sox win.]

Bill Veeck was like a rock star in 1977. I saw him arrive in a cab at the park a couple times that summer and people always yelled nice things to him and wanted to shake his hand or get him to sign something. He always looked happy to be talking to people and was very nice. He'd walk around the ballpark during the games and there was a buzz when he was nearby. He co-hosted the "Mary Frances Veeck & Friend" show with his wife Sunday mornings and we'd never miss it; often we were on our way to the ballpark when it was on the radio. Mary Frances Veeck was a very gracious and intelligent person and they were great together.

Howard Cosell was doing Monday Night Baseball for ABC and Harry Caray did an interview with him (I think on radio) before a game. Cosell was effusive in his praise during the Caray interview and both basically complimented each other. Then Cosell went on the national telecast and just savaged Caray, calling him unprofessional for being a cheerleader, etc. Caray ripped Cosell afterwards about being a back-stabber. It became fashionable for national announcers, players, and others to rip on the behavior of the Sox fans, Veeck, and Caray/Piersall. I took offense to it; the Sox had never won anything in my life and what was wrong with having fun with it?

Leo Bauby: The early season Sunday doubleheader vs. the A's. I watched all five hours on my grandparents' TV as the Sox won the first game 2-1. Lamar Johnson cracked two homers in game one and the Sox had a well-pitched game. The Sox won game two and I specifically remember Dick Allen pinch hitting [for the A's] in a key situation and striking out. After the game Harry did his post game recap from the Channel 44 booth and the Sox fans were loud. He repeatedly waved his microphone in an attempt to let the fans voice themselves on the air. [So he could resume his recap.] The noise actually got louder and Harry was having a ball. Soon the "We're Number One" chant began and Harry commented how the best fans in the world have waited a long time for this. The TV crew caught Harry's interaction with the fans a good five minutes after he was through recapping the game. I believe this was a defining moment in 1977, as the fans' excitement for the Sox became infectious from this point on.

I caught Greek Night Vs the Red Sox on the radio as there were terrible thunderstorms where we lived. The White Sox bashed the Red Sox and cruised to a big lead. Wilbur Wood again held a very potent Red Sox lineup to a couple runs until he tired. Our radio crackled with every bolt of lightening. I remember Harry Caray asking the audience to stop by Comiskey Park that night if they wanted to earn money. There were not enough beer vendors to service the 45,000 person crowd.

A fan next to us offered my friend and me sips from his whiskey bottle. We declined as we were only eight years old. [Bauby and his friend were at the July 31 doubleheader. He vividly remembers Chet Lemon's first of two homers in game one going into the left field upper deck.]

Nancy Faust—The Person Entertaining the Fans

In two interviews that she has given the author, Nancy Faust never claimed to be a lonely woman. To the contrary, with all the attention fans have given her during the past 35 years, it would be hard to believe that Faust would ever feel unpopular.

Yet when she was hired as the third organist for the White Sox in 1970, she may have considered joining a lonely hearts club, at least after spending so much time at the vast and sometimes lonely looking Comiskey Park. Stationed out in center field close to 500 feet from home plate, Faust played to an empty house most of that summer. Bill Melton once described that 106-loss experience as "hard to be humiliated in front of 5,000 people."

Sometimes the White Sox didn't draw that much, and there wasn't much applause for a team going down to one defeat after another. It couldn't have done much for a musician's ego to constantly entertain a small audience.

Then there was the White Sox organization's idea of getting fans involved in the game. Front office man Stu Holcomb gave Faust a list of players and their native state songs. They could be played when a player was at bat or entering the game. No doubt Chicago fans would feel the chills when they heard the state song of Oklahoma. (Oklahoma was the birthplace of Virle Rounsaville. Remember him?)

Additionally, Faust wasn't welcomed with open arms by some, expressing their belief that the ballpark was no place for a woman organist. A petition was passed around calling for her ouster.

"That has been the only negative thing about my job," Faust recalls.

But Faust became more known as attendance improved during the early 1970s. Not taking Holcomb's advice, Faust was a little more imaginative about entertaining White Sox fans. And in 1977 she cemented her place in team history by starting a tradition that has endured for almost 30 years with no signs of dying.

"It wasn't the first time I played it," Faust says, referring to a song that was a hit for a group named Steam. It made it to number one for two weeks in Billboard's Top 100 chart in December 1969.

The Kansas City Royals visited Comiskey Park almost eight years after Steam had its 15 minutes of fame. No doubt group members had no idea that their song, a ballad about a guy who is the third part of a love triangle and desperately wants to see the object of his affections kiss another guy good-bye for good, would ever become a theme song for a major league baseball franchise.

"The mood at the park was at a fever pitch," Faust recalls. "The Sox were vying for first and it was a free for all at the park. The fans were into the game and they started singing. You can't dictate something like that.

"Later on people asked me, 'What was that song?'"

The actual title of the song is "Na, Na, Hey, Hey, Kiss Him Goodbye." It was played to serenade opposing pitchers as they left the game after being once again pummeled by the South Side Hitmen. Faust also played it at the end of White Sox victories when the opposition had no choice but say good-bye to any chance of getting a victory that day.

Mercury Records re-released the "45" and it became a hit once more. The record company presented Faust with a gold record as a token of its appreciation.

"Harry Caray told them to 'forget the record and just give her the gold,'" Faust said.

"He [Caray] promoted every side of the game," Faust added. "And that included me. When he sang during the seventh inning stretch, he always said, 'Let me hear you, Nancy.'"

Faust, who has missed only five White Sox games since 1970 due to the birth of her son, doesn't believe she ever alone caused any adverse fan reaction by playing a song, especially during the 1970s.

"In the old days, you didn't need any stimuli," Faust says. "It was a natural excitement. What I do is to enhance the emotion and prompt people to respond. There were times I got cues from the fans."

"There are still organists in five or six parks, and two or three are full time," Faust says, referring to the dying breed of organ players. "It is not a popular instrument. I have the edge. Not a lot of people are doing what I am doing."

Faust has added technology and other instruments to modernize her act, but she says, "I long for days and years that have gone by. You can never replace the good old days."

No, one cannot relive the past. However, Sox fans still feel an attachment to Faust and she remains a symbol of the team. How many organists are still remembered by a team's fans? Betcha you can't name one of them.

Steve Stone Remembers the South Side Hitmen

Every team has a defining game in a memorable season. Steve Stone, who led the Sox staff with 15 wins in 1977, thinks the second game of the July 31 doubleheader was the pivotal game that helped put an end to the White Sox division hopes that year. While third baseman Eric Soderholm believes that Hal McRae's slow home run trot and angry post-game remarks to the media put the White Sox on the defensive about the curtain calls, Stone questions the lineup that manager Bob Lemon put on the field when the White Sox had a chance to sweep the defending Western Division champion Royals.

"When you have your foot on their throat," Stone said in the summer of 2005, "you better kill them."

Stone remembered Lemon using a great deal of the Sox bench in that game and thought it was not a good time to rest the team's players. (In fact, regulars Garr, Orta, Zisk, Gamble, Spencer, and Chet Lemon were in the contest. Regulars Soderholm, Essian, and Bannister didn't start though Bannister was late inning replacement and got one at-bat. These three regulars were replaced by part-time players Jack Brohamer, Brian Downing, and Tim Nordbrook. The three went a combined one for nine, although that hit was a two-run homer by Downing in the ninth that made the score a little more respectable.)

"I don't know why he did it," Stone said of Lemon, who died in 2000. "Managers didn't explain why they did things back then."

However, loss of momentum or no loss of momentum, Stone believes the best team won the Western Division Title in 1977. He described Kansas City as "a complete ball club," and the White Sox, even with nine players in double figures in home runs, didn't have the depth to be there at the end of a six-month season.

"We were short on skills." Stone recalls. "In a 162 game-season, whatever you have suspect will come out. You can't win the pennant with 10-9 wins. We were a bit shaky on defense. Jorge Orta is still waiting to complete his first double play of 1977."

Stone signed as a free agent with the White Sox after spending three seasons with the Cubs. He labeled himself as the cheapest of the first crop of free agents, making $60,000 a year. He quickly calculated that the White Sox paid $4,000 a victory, wondering out loud if the Cubs would like to pay Kerry Wood that much for each of his victories. Regardless, Stone was grateful to Bill Veeck for giving him a chance to perform for the White Sox, and credits the Sox owner for creating the excitement during the summer of 1977.

"Harry Caray talked about having fun at the ballpark," Stone said, "and that was Bill's idea. He lived that phrase. That is what he gave them that year. It was exciting."

Stone also recalled Veeck saying, "If you don't have money, you should err on the side of offense."

Stone also has fond memories of Caray who had spent 11 seasons on the airwaves describing failed White Sox attempts to go to the World Series.

"Harry would come up to me after a loss, and say 'what happened to you,'" Stone recalled. "I never made any excuse to him. He respected that."

As a result, Stone says, it was Carey who put Stone's name on a short list when the Chicago Tribune Company was looking for a color man in the WGN-TV broadcast booth for Cub games. And Stone felt that the relationship between players and announcers and the rest of the media was more healthy in 1977 than now when "thin skinned" players get offended about what is written or said about them.

"We viewed the media as our friends," Stone remembers. "There was no 24-hour sports cycle with people trying to uncover dirt."

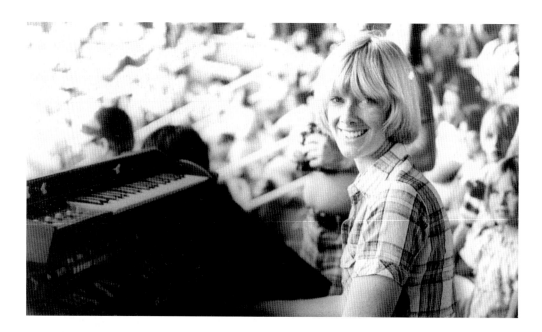

Nancy Faust is seen here one year before the Hitmen. Throughout the years, Faust has said, "I try to make myself accessible to the fans." It is one reason that she has been able to remain a fixture with the White Sox through two ownership changes, two stadiums, and over three decades. It is amazing how she is associated with the 1977 team almost in the same way the players are. (Leo Bauby collection.)

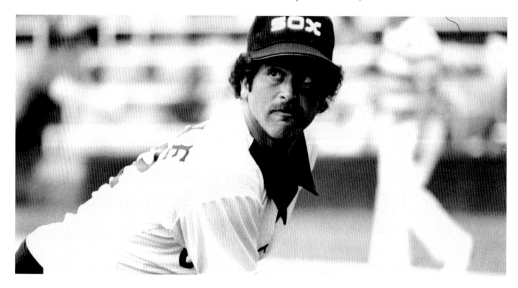

"But I didn't get any hits," Steve Stone said when contacted by the author in 2005. Like many others, Stone associated the 1977 White Sox with hits and homers and not pitching. He still led the White Sox with 15 wins that year. His best year was in 1980 when he won 24 for Baltimore and won the American League Cy Young Award. (Leo Bauby collection.)

Stone felt that Bob Lemon had not put in his "A" lineup against Kansas City in the second game of the infamous July 31 doubleheader. Brian Downing, shown here chasing a pop-up, started game two, which was one of 69 games he appeared in that season. He went on to have an "A" type career with the California Angels. (Leo Bauby collection.)

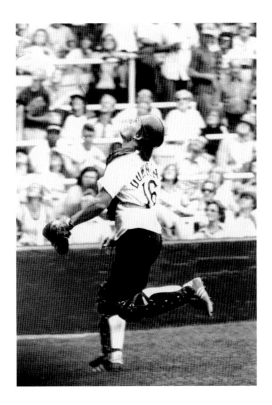

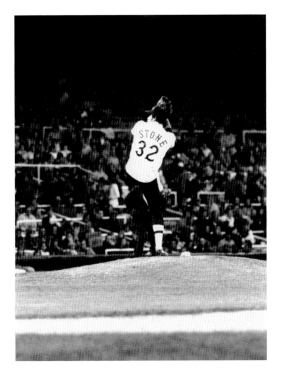

Steve Stone is in pitching form against the New York Yankees. Very few of the games between the Sox and Yankees were pitching duels in 1977. Stone and the Hitmen had their problems against the team that went on to win the World Series. Yet the Yankees always knew they had to come to the park to play when the White Sox furnished the competition. (Leo Bauby collection.)

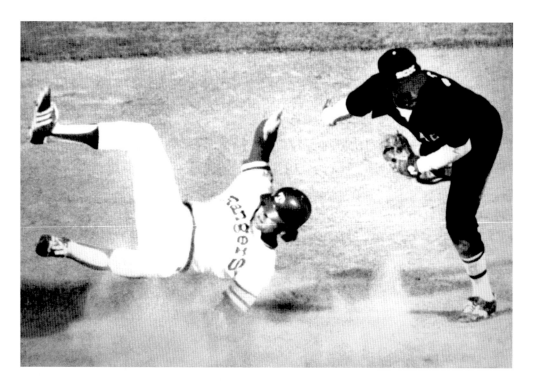

Stone jokes that Jorge Orta is still waiting to complete his first double play of 1977. Well, not quite. He is turning the trick here in May of that year. (Leo Bauby collection.)

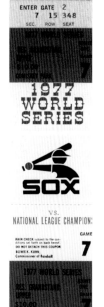

Another printed World Series ticket never used. It would have been a great series if the Hitmen had a chance to do their thing on the national stage, if only to get even with Hal McRae. (Leo Bauby collection.)

Chet Lemon was still swinging the bat well in September. However, it was all over pretty quickly during that month. The White Sox wouldn't play another meaningful September game until the Winning Ugly season of 1983. (Leo Bauby collection.)

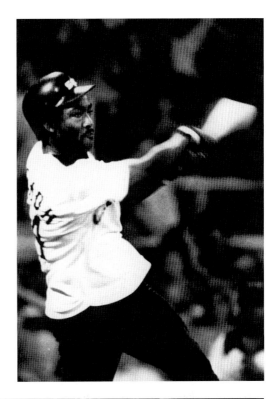

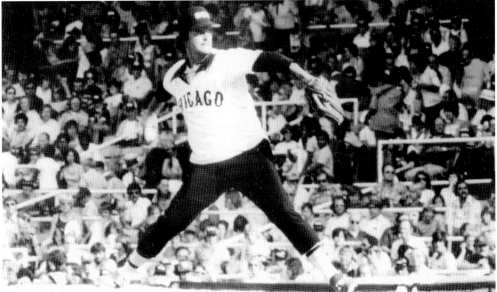

Clay Carroll looks to be in good form in September. He had been traded away right before the season started and re-acquired for the stretch run. His numbers were not that great for the month. It didn't really matter. Kansas City was so good that month that no one was going to catch them. (Leo Bauby collection.)

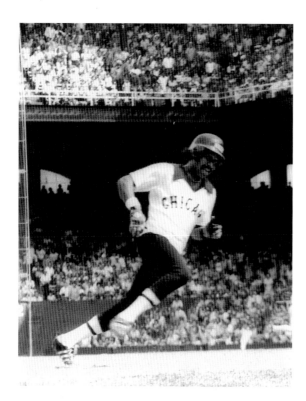

Oscar Gamble rounds third and heads for home. In the background is a pretty good looking crowd. The Hitmen brought many out to the park, because they were the most entertaining Sox team in a long time. Entertaining, yes. Championship winning, no. (Leo Bauby collection.)

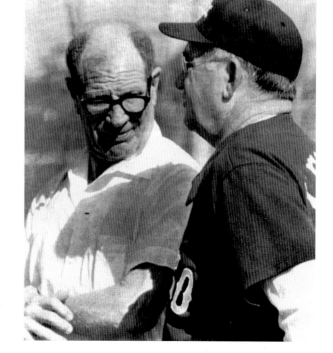

Bill Veeck (left) and Bob Lemon are conferring again and looking fairly relaxed. No conferring could keep the Royals from taking the division. (Leo Bauby collection.)

Richie Zisk was one of the most popular players during the Hitmen season. Here he is signing autographs for some fans. The last game of the season wasn't over for long when he cleaned out his locker and left, never playing for the White Sox again. (Leo Bauby collection.)

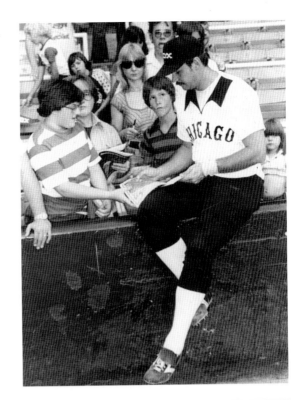

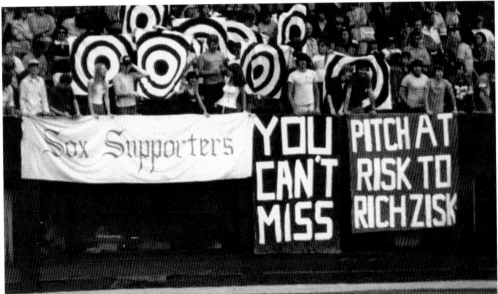

Banners were very popular during the 1977 season. Here we have the Sox Supporters, the bull's eyes, and the warning of pitchers of the risk of throwing to Richie Zisk. The emotion at the ballpark has been rarely matched since 1977, and in some ways, will never be matched. (Leo Bauby collection.)

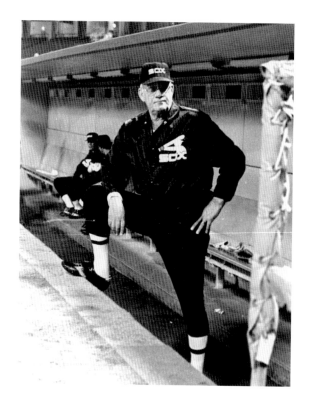

Bob Lemon sits on the dugout steps during an away game in September. The body language tells it all. (Leo Bauby collection.)

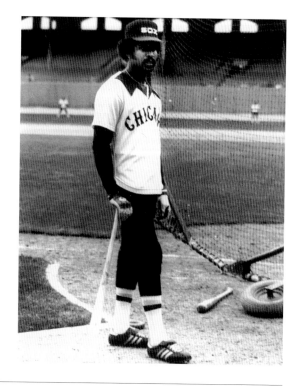

Oscar Gamble stands by the batting cage symbolizing the hit in South Side Hitmen. Gamble became the first left handed hitter for the Sox to hit 30 homers in a season and ended leading the team with 31 round trippers. (Gerry Bilek collection.)

8

THE SOUTH SIDE
HITMEN — AFTERMATH

There is no question that the 1977 Chicago White Sox left an everlasting mark on Chicago baseball history. No Chicago baseball team on either side of town that decade created the memories of the South Side Hitmen. Part of the charm of the 1977 team was that they had a different hero almost every game.

Other teams and their fans didn't understand the emotion that engulfed Comiskey Park that summer. They couldn't stand the curtain calls and the taunting good-bye song. Even six years later, after the bitter American League Championship series, the Baltimore Orioles taunted the Sox and their fans by singing the same song during their locker room pennant celebration.

There were several reasons why fans latched on to the team. The first has been stated many times in this book: the 1977 White Sox could hit. After decades of the go-go way of manufacturing runs, the 1977 team just hit the hell out of the ball. Reporter Bill Jauss recalled Veeck thinking he was a hitter or two short from winning it all in 1959 and vowed not to make that mistake again. Remember the 1990 White Sox? They won 94, but couldn't come close to the dominating Oakland Athletics. Many Sox fans look back at the 1990 team with great affection, but the atmosphere at Comiskey Park didn't have the emotion that was generated during the summer of 1977. The exception was the last game ever to be played at the old ball yard when fans bid Comiskey an emotional good-bye. The Sox won that day 3-2 when a bad hop single turned into a triple, plating the eventual winning run. That team of over-achievers hit a whopping total of 106 homers with old guy Carlton Fisk leading the way with 18. Nothing else needs to be said here.

Lack of expectations was another reason fans fell in love with the 1977 Sox. At season's start, no one picked the Sox to do anything but finish in the lower half of their division. Once the team looked like it was going to contend, a reverse psychology took place. The team became the blue collar Cinderella, taking on a different aura from recent Chicago baseball teams who were looked upon as choke artists and late season party-poopers.

Also there was the fan backlash to free agency. As was earlier stated in this book, free agent turned Indian pitcher Wayne Garland was booed mightily when he made an early season return trip to Baltimore. Though fans probably sympathized with players more then than now, purists abhorred the idea of buying a pennant. What happened to building a farm system and using one's guile to assemble a ball club? Why should someone like George Steinbrenner be able to take the Yankees to the World Series just because he had the money to do it? And the Yankees? Hadn't they been there before? The 1977 White Sox, seemingly a bunch of misfits discarded by the rest of baseball, were more lovable than a bunch of rich guy carpetbaggers.

Yes, it was old-fashioned baseball and a great change of pace at Comiskey. There was no hoping some little guy would steal a base and come home a sacrifice fly. Instead, the exploding scoreboard was used as never before.

Bill Veeck was praised for his "Rent-a-Player" scheme. Under this plan, Veeck would trade a player or players that he knew he was not going to be able to sign for another player he knew he would also not be able to sign. So instead of merely losing a player, he would gain the services of another player who just might have a career year before moving on. In the case of Richie Zisk and Oscar Gamble, it worked well enough to give the Sox one of the most exciting seasons ever.

"Nobody's asking about my finances now," gloated Bill Veeck in the middle of the July excitement.

No, no one was asking his financial picture that almost kept him from buying the team in late 1975. However, maybe someone should have because the fallout from the 1977 season was coming and another White Sox decline was on the way.

Rich Gossage, Terry Forster, Bucky Dent, Richie Zisk, and Oscar Gamble. These players were traded for each other, and so essentially when Zisk and Gamble were not resigned, the White Sox lost five players. Then, in December of 1977, Jim Spencer was traded to the Yankees in an essentially cash deal that netted the Sox two players (Stan Thomas and Ed Ricks) who never played one inning for the team. The South Side Hitmen had been dismantled before the fans' eyes.

To offset the loss of Zisk, the Sox acquired Bobby Bonds from California. To replace the left handed hitting hole created by the departure of Gamble, Ron Blomberg was signed as a free agent. Blomberg had been first player to play the role of designated hitter in 1973, but had only two at-bats in 1976 and none in 1977. Even in 1975, Blomberg had only 106 official plate appearances. He was signed to a four-year guaranteed deal.

Additionally, the White Sox felt that Lamar Johnson was ready to fill in as the every day first baseman. From appearances the Sox had the firepower to replace the combined 79 homers of three players (Zisk, Gamble, and Spencer) who had played such a vital role in the 1977 season.

The good feelings of the South Side Hitmen carried over to the beginning of the 1978 season. Veeck ran commercials of happy fans singing the good-bye song. The gloom and doom of an almost move to Seattle and an embarrassing 1976 season was gone.

A total of 50,754 fans came to welcome the new season on April 7 against the Red Sox. And for a day, the 1977 excitement was back, and there was the good feeling generated by an underdog player, all of which was so typical of the previous year as the Sox won 6-5.

Yet, the chemistry and excitement were not back. Bonds, heavily relied upon to replace the popular Zisk, got off to a slow start. After hitting only his second homer of the year in a May 16, 8-3 loss to the Yankees, Bonds learned he had been traded to Texas for Claudell Washington. Washington inspired fans to hang "Washington Slept Here" signs in right field while playing nearly three uninspired baseball seasons in Chicago.

The Blomberg gamble didn't pay off. The former Yankee hit .233 for the Sox in 1978 and was released just prior to the 1979 season. The team chose to pay him the remaining three years of his contract without benefiting from his services. And with Steve Stone leaving for free agency in November 1978, the 1978 team was dismantled as quickly as its 1977 counterpart.

One 1977 South Side alumnus did quite well for himself. Manager Bob Lemon was fired on June 30, 1978, and landed on his feet by taking over the New York Yankees. By late July, the Yankees were 14 games behind division leading Boston. New York caught the Red Sox, forcing a one-game playoff for the Eastern Division Championship. Ironically, it was ex-Sox Bucky Dent who hit one of the most memorable homers in playoff race history to help the Yankees into the playoffs and eventually the World Series. Bob Lemon's team vanquished the annual pennant-choking Kansas City Royals in the American League Championship Series and beat the Dodgers in a tough six-game World Series.

The most memorable thing about the White Sox 1979 fifth-place finish was, of course, Disco Demolition. Most White Sox fans of that time know the details about the promotion that drew a great crowd for a July 12 doubleheader against the Detroit Tigers. Films depicting the atmosphere in Comiskey show that an eruption was just waiting to happen. While the crowds of 1977 carried an excitement because of an entertaining club, the electricity before the blowing up of disco records between games was a different type altogether. In 1977, Sox fans held up banners like "Pitch at Risk to Rich Zisk." The disco haters flagged the upper deck railings with "DISCO SUCKS" signs. While the 1977 crowds cheered on the Sox to demolish the opposition, the July 12, 1979, crowd attempted to demolish Comiskey Park.

The Veeck era was coming to a close. His sale of the White Sox to a group headed by Eddie Einhorn and Jerry Reinsdorf was completed on January 30, 1981. (This was after a failed attempt to sell the franchise to Edward DeBartolo when the American League owners looked down on DeBartolo's gambling interests.) The popular shower was ripped out of center field. Einhorn made comments about the new ownership running a class organization, taken by some that Veeck had not. The new owners also claimed Comiskey was in deplorable condition, and thought the team's TV contract was a disgrace. Free TV would still be available to fans but not like before.

Stung by the criticism, Veeck stayed away from Comiskey Park for a good deal of the time during the last couple years of his life. He appeared on a local PBS TV show about baseball produced and aired on WTTW-Channel 11. Veeck sat with other guests, drinking beer and criticizing Major League Baseball. He died on January 2, 1986, having spent his last years as a true baseball outsider.

Whatever can be said about Bill Veeck, one accomplishment cannot be taken away from him. Veeck was the architect of the 1977 South Side Hitmen. The crowds were large and loud. Even if a fan wasn't at the game, he could still feel the adrenaline and excitement engulfing him as if he were sitting in the left field seats. Unlike past Sox teams, the Hitmen pasted one hit after another, with few bloopers or grounders sneaking through in the infield. Line shots were fired all over Comiskey which could rip a fielder's face off if he was stupid enough to get in front of it. The scoreboard went off time and time again, blowing fuses and firing duds from exhaustion. Sometimes the smoke from the fireworks hung over the field, no doubt stinging the opponents' eyes and rubbing salt in the wound. In 1977, Sox fans reveled in it, because after all, the scoreboard fireworks had been used so rarely in the past.

It all seemed to be in defiance of White Sox critics everywhere. You don't like the home run fireworks? You don't like the fact that the 1977 Sox contended longer than anyone thought they had a right to? You don't like names on the backs of uniforms? You don't like curtain calls and serenades? You don't respect a team that hit and not do much else? Then the hell with you, for the 1977 Chicago White Sox gave their fans an excitement and hope that had been missing for so long, and what other people thought didn't matter.

And in the Channel 44-WSNS-TV broadcast booth, Harry Caray pounded Budweisers or whatever was available. He sang "Take Me Out to the Ballgame" during the seventh inning stretch. He led the cheers with his main rallying cry, which, more often than not, was portentous of excitement to come. This cry was echoed by a banner held by fans in the left field seats that read, "Oh-H, For The Long One."

Yet, in 1977, the fans didn't need Harry Caray or anyone or anything else to get them excited. The noise and the intensity of the emotion fed on each other and provided memories that have lasted decades. No round the clock coverage from ESPN or rooftop seats were needed.

Bill Veeck was sometimes called the PT Barnum of Baseball. His promotions and gimmicks were often criticized, frowned upon or scoffed at as a con game to divert the fans from remembering how bad the team was. But, unlike some of Goose Gossage's laments, baseball on the South Side of Chicago in 1977 was no circus. The 1977 Chicago White Sox were not just the Chicago White Sox. They were the South Side Hitmen.

Banners were again popular at Comiskey Park during the beginning of the 1978 season. This one could have been right if Bonds hadn't been traded away to Texas. (Leo Bauby collection.)

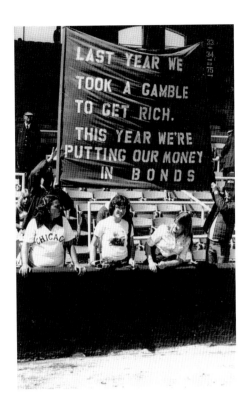

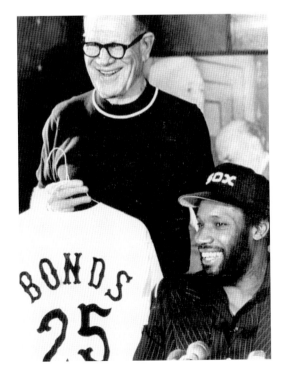

Bill Veeck (left) and Bobby Bonds look happy after the trade that brought Bonds to the White Sox. Bonds hit 31 home runs in 1978—too bad that 29 of them were with Texas. (Leo Bauby collection.)

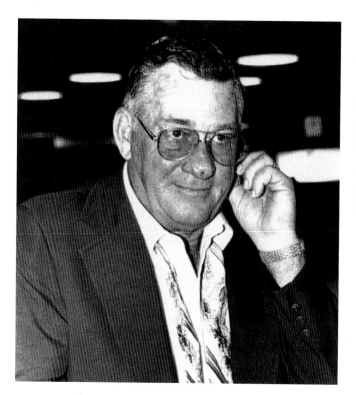

Bob Lemon was let go on June 30, 1978, after it was becoming obvious that the Sox season was going nowhere. He landed on is feet and is shown here after being hired by the Yankees. New York again won the World Series. The White Sox finally did the trick in 2005. (Leo Bauby collection.)

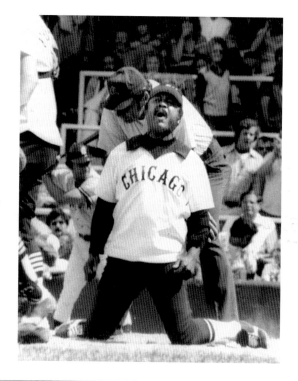

Larry Doby took over after the departure of Bob Lemon. He is taking issue with an umpire here, not that it did any good. Doby lost this argument, but more importantly, the Sox lost many more ball games. Their record was almost a complete reversal of 1977 as they lost 90. Doby wasn't around for the 1979 season. He should have been thankful for that. (Gerry Bilek collection.)

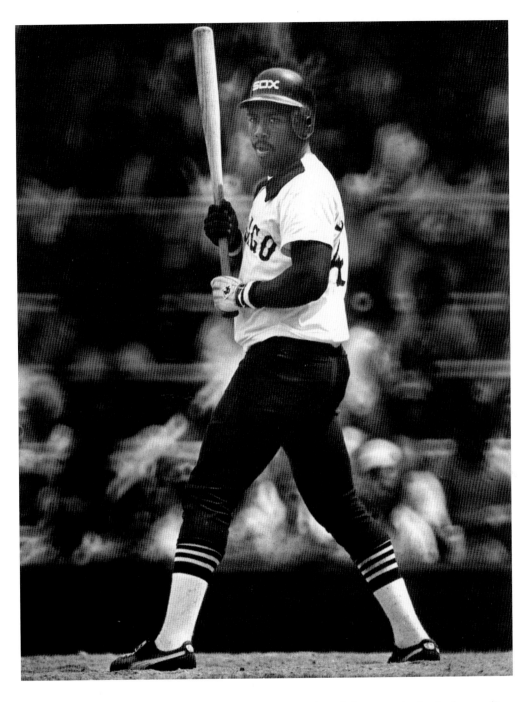

Chet Lemon had his best year with the Sox in 1979, hitting .318, walloping 17 homers and knocking in 86. Too bad most of the remainder of the team had a bad year. (Leo Bauby collection.)

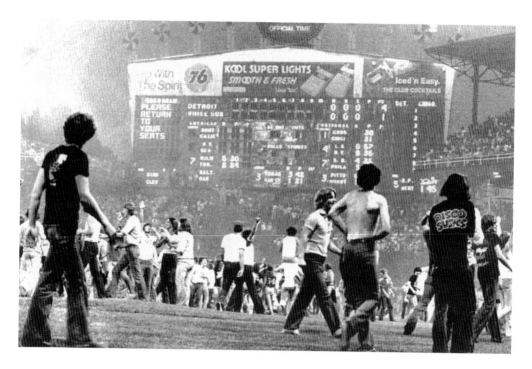

Would this be a White Sox book without a picture of Disco Demolition? The franchise has not been able to run away from the legacy even though it happened a little over a quarter of a century ago. Worse yet, just think if one of these fine gentlemen showed up at your door asking for your daughter's hand in marriage? (Leo Bauby collection.)

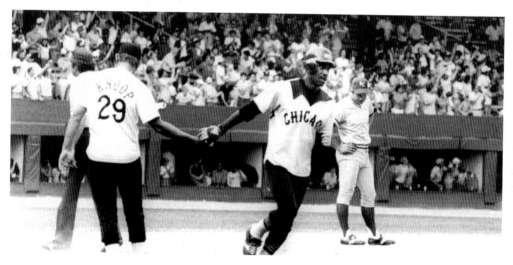

Claudell Washington makes his way for home. Washington was picked up in a trade for Bobby Bonds in May of 1978. He hit three homers in a game just a few days after Disco Demolition. Most fans agreed that Washington had talent, but also figured he went right back to sleep after slugging the three homers. (Leo Bauby collection.)

THE SOUTH SIDE HITMEN—AFTERMATH

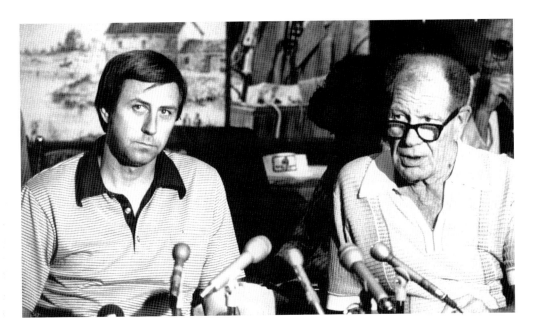

Don Kessinger (left) appears with Bill Veeck to announce his resignation as Sox manager in August of 1979. He is pretty somber looking, but the failure of the team that year couldn't be hung on his shoulders. Even Veeck admitted that Kessinger was not armed with enough talented players. Kessinger was one of the classiest players to put on a Chicago baseball uniform, and he deserved better. (Leo Bauby collection.)

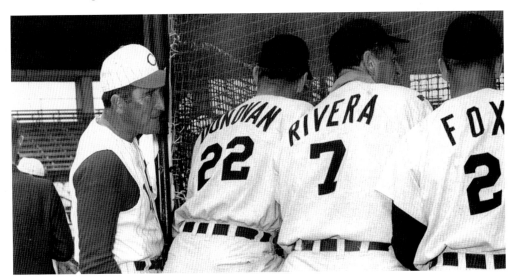

What was the big deal about names on the backs of uniforms? Bill Veeck took a great deal of heat when introducing the concept in 1960. With all the expansion during the last 40 plus years, it is probably a very good thing that names are on the backs of uniforms. (Leo Bauby collection.)

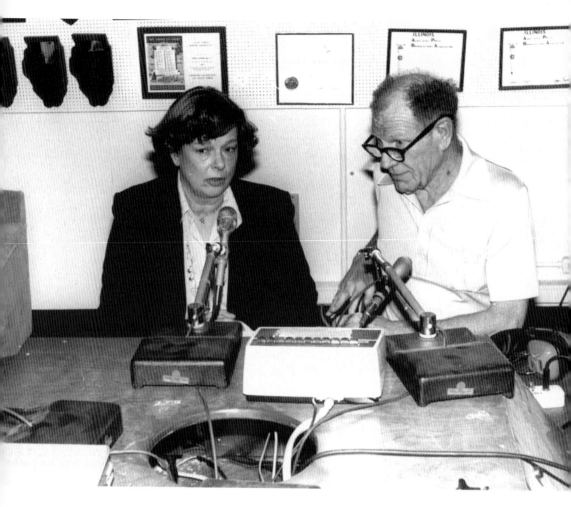

Sometimes people wondered why Bill Veeck was so popular even when his teams weren't so good. The simple answer was that Veeck was a charismatic man who was accessible to the fans. This included a Sunday morning radio show where he and his wife, Mary Frances, took calls. By 1980, some of those calls were getting hostile. (Leo Bauby collection.)

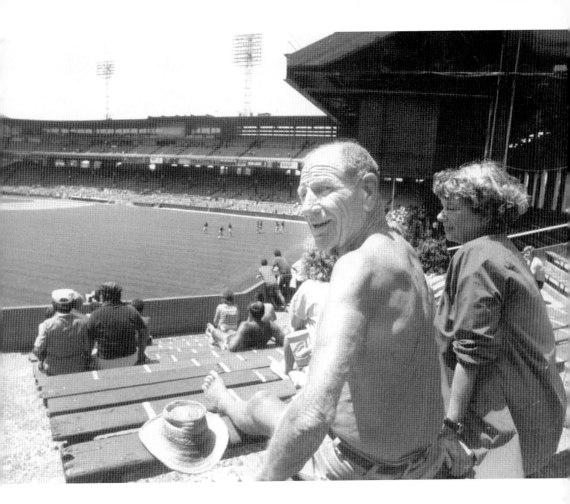

The shirtless Bill Veeck is seen sunning himself during his last game at Comiskey. He is sitting in the center field bleachers. Veeck had spent more time during the last years of his life at Wrigley than Comiskey. (Leo Bauby collection.)

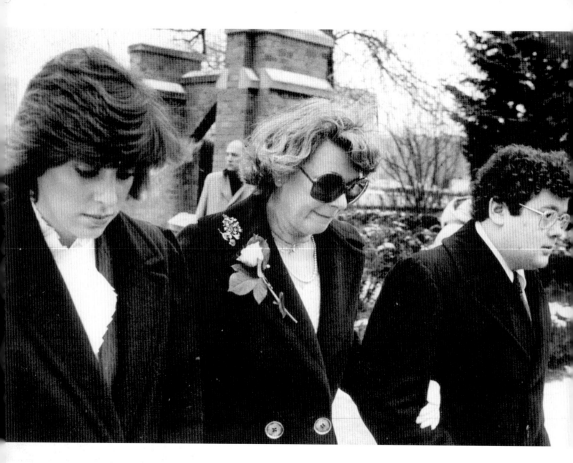

Bill Veeck died on January 2, 1986. His baseball legacy is still being debated. That legacy is considerable. Here, mourners remember a man who had lived a full life. (Leo Bauby collection.)

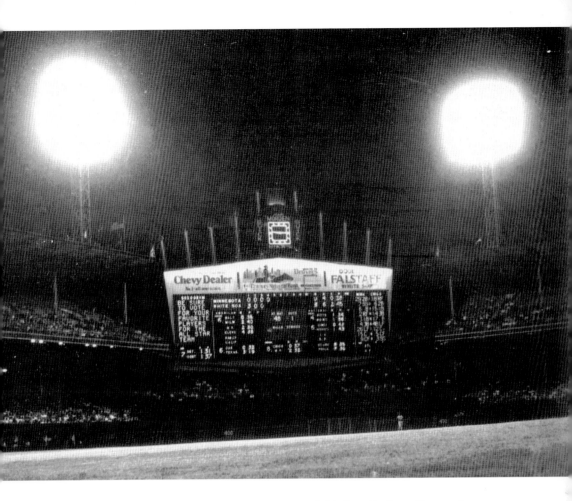

One of Bill Veek's most endearing gifts to the Chicago White Sox fans was the Monster in center field. (Leo Bauby collection.)

How the 1977 South Side Hitmen Were Dismantled

- Ralph Garr was sold to California Angels on September 20, 1979.
- Chet Lemon was traded to the Detroit Tigers for outfielder Steve Kemp on November 27, 1981.
- Richie Zisk was signed as a free agent by the Texas Rangers on November 9, 1977.
- Oscar Gamble was signed as a free agent by the San Diego Padres on November 29, 1977.
- Jim Spencer was traded to the New York Yankees with pitcher Bob Polinsky and outfielder Tommy Cruz for pitchers Stan Thomas and Ed Ricks on December 12, 1977.
- Eric Soderholm was traded to the Texas Rangers for pitcher Ed Farmer and infielder Gary Holle on June 15, 1979.
- Alan Bannister was traded to the Cleveland Indians for outfielder Ron Pruit on June 14, 1980.
- Jorge Orta was signed by the Cleveland Indians as a free agent on December 19, 1979.
- Jim Essian was traded to the Oakland A's with pitcher Steve Renko for pitcher Pablo Rorrealba on March 30, 1978.
- Brian Downing was traded to the California Angels along with pitchers Chris Knapp and Dave Frost for outfielders Bobby Bonds and Thad Bosley and pitcher Richard Dotson on December 5, 1977.
- Ken Kravec was traded to the Chicago Cubs for pitcher Dennis Lamp on March 28, 1981.
- Lerrin LaGrow was sold to the Los Angeles Dodgers on May 11, 1979.
- Lamar Johnson was signed by the Texas Rangers as a free agent on January 15, 1982.
- Wilbur Wood was granted free agency on November 2, 1978.
- Francisco Barrios was released by the White Sox on September 1, 1981.
- Steve Stone was signed as a free agent by the Baltimore Orioles on November 29, 1978.

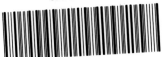

DEATH IS THAT MAN TAKING NAMES

DEATH IS THAT MAN TAKING NAMES

INTERSECTIONS OF AMERICAN MEDICINE, LAW, AND CULTURE

ROBERT A. BURT

UNIVERSITY OF CALIFORNIA PRESS · Berkeley · Los Angeles · London

THE MILBANK MEMORIAL FUND · New York

University of California Press
Berkeley and Los Angeles, California

University of California Press, Ltd.
London, England

© 2002 by the Regents of the University of California

Library of Congress Cataloging-in-Publication Data
Burt, Robert A.
  Death is that man taking names : intersections of American medicine, law, and culture / Robert A. Burt.
     p.   cm. — (California/Milbank books on health and the public ; 7)
  Includes index.
  ISBN 0-520-23282-8 (cloth : alk. paper)
    1. Death. 2. Terminal care—United States. 3. Death—Social aspects—United States.
  [DNLM: 1. Attitude to Death—United States. 2. Death—United States. 3. Jurisprudence—United States. 4. Right to die—United States. BF 789.D4 B973d 2002]. I. Title. II. Series.
  R726.8 .B875 2002
  306.9—dc21

                                   2001007071

Manufactured in the United States of America

10 09 08 07 06 05 04 03 02 01
10 9 8 7 6 5 4 3 2 1

The paper used in this publication is both acid-free and totally chlorine-free (TCF). It meets the minimum requirements of ANSI/NISO Z39.48-1992 (R 1997) (*Permanence of Paper*).♾

There's a man going round taking names.
There's a man going round taking names.
He has taken my father's name,
And he's left my heart in pain.
There's a man going round taking names.

Death is that man taking names.
Death is that man taking names.
He has taken my mother's name,
And he's left my heart in pain.
Death is that man taking names.

There's a man going round taking names.
There's a man going round taking names.
He has taken my brother's name,
And he's left my heart in pain.
There's a man going round taking names.

Traditional Spiritual

CONTENTS

FOREWORD

The Milbank Memorial Fund is an endowed national foundation that engages in nonpartisan analysis, study, research, and communication on significant issues in health policy. The Fund makes available the results of its work in meetings with decision-makers, reports, articles, and books.

This is the seventh of the series of California/Milbank Books on Health and the Public. The publishing partnership between the Fund and the Press seeks to encourage the synthesis and communication of findings from research that could contribute to more effective health policy.

Robert Burt contributes to more effective policy for the care of persons who are near death by arraying evidence that in American society "ambivalence about death can be denied" but "it cannot reliably be suppressed." The results of developing and implementing policy to "bring public visibility and rationality to death-dispensing decisions" have included "new guises for public concealment and implicit acceptance of irrational impulses."

Burt challenges policymakers to acknowledge persistent ambivalence about the acceptability of death. He argues that law and clinical policy should insist that persons making decisions that bear on death—including dying persons themselves—should recognize and "amplify" this unavoidable ambivalence. To do otherwise, he argues with elegance and eloquence, is to risk "renewed (and perhaps even more virulent) abuses of dying people."

Daniel M. Fox, President
Samuel L. Milbank, Chairman

ACKNOWLEDGMENTS

Good friends have read the manuscript of this book at various stages; I have accepted many of their recommendations, resisted some, and benefited throughout from their attention and support. My thanks to Bruce Ackerman, Steve Arons, Lee Bollinger, Bob Butler, Anne Burt, Linda Burt, Randy Curtis, Owen Fiss, Kathy Foley, Dan Fox, Jay Katz, Rogan Kersh, Michael Lauder, Howard Markel, Ted Marmor, Eric Muller, Tom Murray, Shep Nuland, Marty Pernick, Jim Ponet, Mark Rose, Paul Schwartz, Wayne Ury, Kenji Yoshino, participants in a Milbank Memorial Fund day-long meeting in May 2001 (Dan Callahan, Carolyn Clark, Michael DeLucia, Nancy Dubler, Marvin Frankel, David Schuman, Jack Schwartz, William Williams, Lynne Withey), my seminar students at the University of Michigan in fall 2000 (Mary-Grace Brandt, Richard Horenstein, Nikhil Parekh, Marina Reed, Elizabeth Repko), and, for her superb editing, Ellen F. Smith. I am also grateful for research support in 1997–98 from a John Simon Guggenheim Fellowship and continuously from Yale Law School and Dean Tony Kronman.

CHAPTER ONE

GOOD DEATH

I Fear No Evil

As a man going round taking names, death appears threatening, uncontrollable, robbing the living of their identity and leaving pain in his wake. There is no comfort in this vision, and American culture has not embraced it. We have sought comfort by imagining death in another format: a different man taking names, one might say—a man administering a checklist of rationalized criteria for admitting death. "Has Mr. G—— voluntarily agreed to disconnect his respirator?" "Did the unconscious patient in 216, when he was mentally competent, fill out an advance directive about terminating life-prolonging treatment?"

This new format is intended to rebut the disturbing premise that death dissolves personal identity. It reflects an ambition that individuals should rationally confront and control the approach of death—that death should not be something that happens to you but something that you do. This ambition is admirable; but it is also potentially dangerous and destructive, because death cannot ultimately be controlled— because the competing image of the man inflicting pain by taking names cannot be entirely suppressed.

The new format first took shape as a supposed antidote to physicians' relentless warfare against death and their consequent infliction of terrible suffering on people who were inevitably and uncontrollably dying. Some critics, content simply to blame physicians for these inflictions, have imagined that new rules favoring patient choice and self-control would be an adequate protective response. Others have placed the blame in broader cultural attitudes shared by most physicians and patients—a relentless fear of death and a common com-

I

mitment to the scientific ambition of postponing death indefinitely. Compelling moral principles lie beneath both of these critical perspectives: advocates for patient choice invoke powerful ideals of individual autonomy; the cultural critique rests on the proposition that death should not be understood as an inherent evil but seen instead as a natural event in the cycle of life and an experience that can be satisfying in its own terms. Both of these moral ideals are attractive. I suspect, however, that the intensity of our wishes to attain these ideals obscures the practical possibilities for their achievement—and even worse, that the recommended pathways toward these ideals in fact lead back in circles toward the old abuses, the old inflictions of pointless, terrible suffering on dying people.

The conviction that a "good death" is a "chosen death," that this ideal can best be achieved through rational self-determination, rests on a cultural critique: that American society has been "death denying" and that this denial explains our medical and general social mistreatment of dying people during the past century.[1] From this diagnosis, the prescription appears to follow that we should bring death out from its closet, that we should openly acknowledge the inescapable reality of death and unmask the prior hidden practices by which abuses flourished. This diagnosis and its curative prescription have not been limited to the treatment of dying people, but have also been applied in two other contexts involving purposefully chosen death: abortion and capital punishment.

In the treatment of dying people, physicians were accused of unilaterally exercising all decisional authority by refusing to inform patients of their treatment options or, even more fundamentally, of the fact that they had a terminal illness. Through this refusal to inform patients—so the charge goes—physicians implemented a professional role as the active agents of the death-denying cultural imperative; physicians, that is, removed the burden of decision making from patients in order to protect them from unwanted knowledge about the reality of death.[2] The reform prescription of informing patients about their terminal condition in order to implement the new ethos of patient self-determination accordingly rested on a rejection of the cultural denial of death.

For abortion practices during the past century, it appears that physicians played an even more direct role as cultural agents in denying death. Immediately following the Civil War, as will be discussed in chapter 3, every American state enacted legislation to forbid abortion except to protect the mother's life; but these laws left individual physicians free to interpret this exception as broadly as each might wish, and, accordingly,

an invisible practice flourished of physician discretion to "kill fetuses" (for that was the cultural definition provided by each state statute). In the 1960s, public attention began to focus on this hidden physician discretion; and abortion practice exploded into full public visibility with the Supreme Court's 1973 ruling in *Roe v. Wade.*[3] In this context, as in treatment of dying people, the old pattern of hidden, though implicitly acknowledged, physician decision-making authority suddenly seemed inappropriate. (Some pro-choice advocates dispute whether abortion does indeed involve death, by insisting that the fetus is not a "person" capable of dying as such; but, as I will develop in later chapters, this dispute in itself illuminates central features of American society's changed attitudes toward death.)

In administration of the death penalty following the Civil War, physicians were not the critical actors; but the same cultural impulse to conceal the enterprise of dispensing death from public view was expressed in a different form. During the course of the nineteenth century, the previous practice of well-attended and festive public executions was abolished, as state legislatures moved executions behind prison walls and permitted only small numbers of official observers. The decision-making apparatus for imposing the death penalty also was altered toward public invisibility, as legislatures repealed criminal statutes providing automatic death sentences for large numbers of specified criminal convictions; in place of this more visible regime, new laws provided that juries should have complete discretion, in a limited number of serious crimes, to choose for or against the death penalty with virtually no external supervision. By the 1960s, this hidden discretion by anonymous jurors was widely seen as promoting arbitrary and abusive results—an accusation that reached climactic expression in the 1972 Supreme Court decision in *Furman v. Georgia,*[4] overturning every state death penalty law for failure to provide publicly visible standards and regulatory supervision to ensure rational, responsible decision making.

The same theme has thus dominated contemporary reform efforts in these three death-dispensing contexts—end the prior practice of concealment (and overturn the underlying cultural imperative of "denying death") by bringing decisions about death into public visibility. This new public visibility was, moreover, understood as a way toward promoting rational decision making. Rationality was the explicit goal embraced by the Supreme Court for reformed administration of the death penalty; and capacity for rational decision making was the explicit precondition envisioned by courts and legislatures in the new regimes for patient self-

determination regarding terminal illness and for the woman's choice regarding abortion.

The intertwined reform banners of public visibility and rational decision making were held high, in an especially revealing turn of phrase, by the legal philosopher Ronald Dworkin in advocating self-determination for terminally ill patients and pregnant women. At the very end of his book *Life's Dominion,* Dworkin cites La Rochefoucauld's maxim "that death, like the sun, should not be stared at," and continues, "We have not taken his advice: we have been staring at death throughout this book."[5] Dworkin rejects La Rochefoucauld's advice without any argument—as if it were self-refuting or perhaps sufficiently contradicted by the fact that Dworkin himself had stared at death and emerged unscathed. But in this rejection, Dworkin—like most participants in the contemporary debates—confuses two separate questions: whether death-related matters can be rationally discussed and whether these matters are amenable to purposeful rational control.

I believe, however, La Rochefoucauld's maxim conveys a deeper truth that has been ignored by exponents of this shared assumption regarding the possibility and desirability of public visibility and rational control in the current controversies about death-dispensing decisions. The proposition "that death, like the sun, should not be stared at" does not mean that death cannot be observed, that human psychology is somehow grounded on denying the existence of death. The maxim suggests that death can be directly faced just as the sun can be stared at—but that in both cases the prolonged effort will induce a kind of dazzled blindness.

In the course of this book, I will examine, in separate chapters, the unfolding of reform efforts since the 1960s to bring public visibility and rationality to death-dispensing decisions in the three different contexts I have identified: treatment of dying people, abortion, and the death penalty. I will show how, in each of these contexts, the avowed goals of the reform efforts were only momentarily embraced and were ultimately superseded by new guises for public concealment and implicit acceptance of irrational impulses. I will also offer an explanatory hypothesis about the persistence of the impetus both for concealment and for infliction of abuse in death-dispensing decision making. My speculation arises from the following premise: notwithstanding the rational plausibility of believing that death is a morally neutral biological fact or even a morally preferable outcome in some circumstances, we cannot readily erase a persistent contrapuntal conviction that death as such is inherently

wrong—a logical and moral error. This contrapuntal conviction may not be an eternal verity, but it is so deeply rooted in our Western tradition, at least, that the current American reform efforts have little effective power to refute it. The reform efforts may succeed in suppressing this conviction from general social awareness; but this suppression, I will argue, can only temporarily contain the coiled impulses for renewed (and perhaps even more virulent) abuses of dying people.

In the final chapter I will argue that public efforts to overcome, to forcibly suppress, the persistent contrapuntal sense of death's wrongfulness can and should be abandoned—that we should purposefully embrace acknowledged ambivalence about the acceptability of death, and to this end we should design decision-making structures for the administration of death with the conscious goal of amplifying this ambivalence in the minds of all participants in such decisions.

The underlying premise of this conclusion is my belief that death in itself provokes ambivalence, no matter how fervently we wish it were not true. I believe that the struggle to deny ambivalence—by efforts to control one's own death or the death of others, to find moral justification and emotional satisfaction in embracing death for oneself or for others—can never be more than a temporary palliative. I believe that the effort to banish ambivalence by rigidly embracing the positive valuations in the ideals of autonomy, of a good death, or of physicians' benevolence leads ultimately to the intensified eruption of their inherent negative valuations into guilt-ridden, hurtful conduct.

Some anthropologists claim that negative attitudes toward death are an artifact of Western or even only of American cultural attitudes and that other cultural practices, especially in Asia, reflect calm acceptance of death. Some historians claim that contemporary American fears, often expressed as "denial of death," are only a recent development in our own culture, and that nineteenth-century American practices also reflected calm acceptance.[6] It is difficult to evaluate the descriptive accuracy of these anthropological and historical accounts. Calmer attitudes toward death might have predominated in other cultures and in other times, perhaps because early deaths were a more familiar experience than in our time or because religious beliefs in an afterlife were more firmly entrenched. It is also plausible, however, that these calm self-depictions were more in the service of wishful thinking, of a strenuous effort to deny ambivalence. The ostentatious serenity in these practices may itself be grounded in an unacknowledged strategy of denial; but we, standing in a different culture or a different time, see only the unambivalent public

face—which we single-mindedly embrace in our own eagerness to deny ambivalence.

Whatever the degree of equanimity toward death in these other times and places, these alternative attitudes simply are not available to us today. Our problem is to unravel the intense hostility toward death that has been characteristic of American culture for at least the past hundred years, since scientific medicine took exclusive custody of death and the dying process. Driven by this hostility, scientific practitioners in medicine and public health have had dramatic successes in averting death, effectively doubling the average life span in America during the course of the twentieth century. During much of that century, the suffering imposed on dying people was a hidden cost of that relentless warfare; during the 1970s, this cost suddenly emerged into public view. This was when the hospice movement was imported from Britain into the United States, with an avowed mission of holding back physicians from aggressive but pointless efforts to cure and instead providing comfort to those who were inevitably dying.

The hospice movement has had an important influence on American practices and attitudes generally; but it would be difficult to find, even among the most ardent advocates of the hospice philosophy, any campaigners for wholesale abandonment of our previous efforts to forestall death. Perhaps we can temper these ambitions in order to foster a more serene attitude toward death when it is truly unavoidable; but this adjustment can only occur for us in the context of persistent contrapuntal ambitions to expand the range of avoidable death. Some shift away from the intense negative valuation of death, some accentuation toward a positive perception of death, is the only cultural pathway available to us in America today. Ambivalence in some significant measure will persist for us, no matter how fervently anthropologists extol other cultural attitudes or historians praise alternative past practices.

The inevitable persistence of ambivalence does not mean that we must necessarily acknowledge it; but refusing this acknowledgment is likely to be costly, to breed some version of the past abuses inflicted on dying people. A central ambition of this book is to identify the reasons that refusal to acknowledge ambivalence toward death is likely to lead to this result and to suggest some possible remedial strategies.

The beginning of wisdom, I believe, is to concede—at this moment, at least, in our cultural history—that the very thought of death clouds rational judgment in many, and perhaps even most, peoples' minds. This proposition was demonstrated by an elegantly simple psychological ex-

periment published in the *New England Journal of Medicine* in 1982, in which patients who had experienced serious illness, physicians, and graduate students in business school who had taken courses in statistical analysis were asked to decide whether they would choose surgery for lung cancer. Within each of these categories, one half was told that the surgery had a 90 percent likelihood of survival for more than one year; the other half was told that the therapy carried a 10 percent likelihood of death within one year. Though the information was, of course, identical, the responses among the two groups of patients, physicians, and graduate students were strikingly different. Where the information was presented as a probability of survival, 75 percent of the subjects opted for the surgery; where the information was presented in terms of probability of death, only 58 percent chose surgery.

In formulating their initial hypothesis for the experiment, the researchers anticipated that lay patients would be much more influenced by the differential framing of the information than would the physicians or the graduate students; "much to our surprise," they reported, the differential effect was virtually the same for the physicians, notwithstanding "their considerable experience in evaluating medical data," and for the graduate students, all of whom "had received statistical training." As the researchers observed, "this effect of using different terminology to describe outcome represents a cognitive illusion" that clouded the rational decision-making capacity of physicians as much as laymen.[7] Both had a powerful, irrational aversion to the simple mention of the word "death."

The contemporary reform agenda to replace physician control with patient self-determination is peculiarly vulnerable to this obscuring cognitive illusion. Self-determination for many people, perhaps for most, is likely be derailed in confronting death not simply by a preexisting aversion but by the intensification of that aversion. The basic reason for this cognitive derailment was evoked by Leo Tolstoy in his account of the death of Ivan Ilych:

> In the depth of his heart [Ivan] knew he was dying, but not only was he not accustomed to the thought, he simply did not and could not grasp it. The syllogism he had learnt from Kiezewetter's Logic: "Caius is a man, men are mortal, therefore Caius is mortal," had always seemed to him correct as applied to Caius, but certainly not as applied to himself. That Caius—man in the abstract—was mortal, was perfectly correct, but he was not Caius, not an abstract man, but a creature quite, quite separate from all others. He had been little Vanya, with a mamma and a papa, with Mitya and Volodya, with

the toys, a coachman and a nurse. . . . "Caius really was mortal, and it was right for him to die; but for me, little Vanya, Ivan Ilych, with all my thoughts and emotions, it's altogether a different matter. It cannot be that I ought to die. That would be too terrible."[8]

A psychological explanation for Ivan's illusion of immortality was offered by Sigmund Freud, an explanation which does not depend on his elaborate and often unconvincing systematized theoretical scaffolding. In a 1915 essay on war and death, Freud observed that "it is impossible to imagine our own death [because] whenever we attempt to do so we can perceive that we are in fact still present as spectators." This was Freud's causal explanation for his assertion that "at bottom no one believes in his own death, or, to put the same thing in another way, that in the unconscious every one of us is convinced of his own immortality."[9] Both Tolstoy and Freud imagined, however, that this logical fallacy could be overcome. For Tolstoy the antidote was embodied in his literary creation of Ivan's manservant, the wholesome, open-hearted peasant Gerasim, who was able to accept the inevitability of death in a way that Ivan was not; Gerasim alone was able to comfort Ivan as he lay dying, to approach him with compassion rather than the aversion, fear, and denial of his physicians, his family, and his entire social circle. For Freud, rational mastery of unconscious processes seemed to offer a similar transcendent possibility; at the end of his 1915 essay, Freud opined that it would "be better to give death the place in reality and in our thoughts which is its due"[10]—as if the logical impossibility he had identified could somehow yield to "reality."

Faced with reality, however, both men seem to have wavered. Tolstoy's prolonged flight away from his home to the remote railway station where he finally died belies his own possibility at least of attaining this cherished goal of calm acceptance.[11] Whatever Freud's personal achievement in his death, to which I return later in this chapter, his general thinking about the issue after 1915 assumed a darker hue. For much of his career, Freud believed that rational inquiry could cut through the distortions of illogical thinking to a clear-sighted view of "reality." This was the fundamental goal, as he conceived it, of psychoanalytic excavation of the workings of unconscious mental processes—hence his frequently cited dicta, "where id is, there ego shall come into being again."[12] Over time, however, he modified his rationalistic optimism as he became more convinced of the stubbornness of unconscious mental processes, of the persistence of what he called "primary process think-

ing" in juxtaposition—and even as a defining counterpoint—to rational or "secondary process" thinking.

Freud became, moreover, especially impressed with the role of the idea of death itself in the deepest recesses of human thinking. The existence of a mysteriously termed "death instinct" and its continuous opposition to a "life instinct" became increasingly central to his conception of the human psyche.[13] There is, however, a more convincing way to understand Freud's hypothesis about the continuity of human psychological struggle between self-preservation and self-destruction without relying on some extrinsically endowed "instinct," some externalized "Heavenly Power," as Freud poetically imagined.[14]

We can begin with Freud's simple observation in his 1915 essay, that denial of death is built into the very processes of human cognition because, when we try to imagine our own death, we still remain "present as spectator." From this observation, we can see how there is an emptiness, a kind of conceptual "black hole," in the way that human beings conceive of themselves as a "self"—and this emptiness exerts a continuously (one might say, a "logically") unsettling pressure on the sense of coherence and solidity of that conceptualized "self." This unsettling pressure is, moreover, not simply a matter for detached philosophic contemplation. In times of individual or social stress, this conceptual pressure can impel destructive action—aimed outward and inward, in aggressions toward others and toward oneself. In the conceptual logic of the "self," both philosophically and psychologically, there are internal contradictions that correspond to Freud's hypothesis of a continuous opposition between a death and a life force—contradictions that become translated into action in times of stress and that testify to the inherent fragility of the ideal of self-determination in the administration of death.[15]

These philosophic contradictions have been most trenchantly analyzed by Charles Taylor in his book *The Sources of the Self*. For our purposes, we can summarize Taylor's perspective in two propositions. First, the core logical difficulty, the basis for the "continuing philosophic discomfort," with the modern conception of self is its unstable conceptual conflation of a first-person and a third-person perspective, a continuous and inherently confusing shift between "radical objectivity" and "radical subjectivity" within the conceptual structure of the Self.[16] Second, the modern conception of Self does not stand on its own but is instead a kind of proxy for the pre-Enlightenment worldview in which God's existence subsumed the conceptual confusion that has now clearly emerged

in the modern shift between first- and third-person perspectives. God, that is, embodied the third-person perspective through which first-person Selves could observe themselves (or understand themselves as being observed) without imagining (as Freud understood) that their own self-observational capacities were somehow immortal. The post-Enlightenment secular removal of God from this conceptual centrality meant, as Taylor vividly stated, that "the disengaged subject [that is, the modern Self] stands in a place already hollowed out for God; he takes a stance to the world which befits an image of the Deity." [17]

I would argue that the Enlightenment project of emptying this hollowed space, of secularizing the world, was liberating, exhilarating, even heroic in its implications; but it also was an experience of loss and even carried some implication of wrongdoing. Nietzsche's observation that God was dead in the post-Enlightenment world conveyed this conjunctive sense of liberation, loss, and suspected wrongdoing. Whatever its various virtues, moreover, this secularization creates special problems for making sense of human death.

The cosmic characteristics of the modern conception of the self-determining Self can also be seen in the developmental pathways by which each individual comes to shape his or her own mature and culturally prized sense of self. As individuals pass from infancy toward adulthood and reconceive themselves as self-determining adults, they must separate themselves from their parents' influence. This occurs not only in obvious rationalist terms of resisting their parents' commands and expectations but in deep psychic structural changes by which new distinctions are made that in infancy and childhood had no direct correspondence in individual thinking—most notably, for our purposes, distinctions between self and other. The self-other distinction is not a self-evident natural fact, and the radical conceptual separateness—the sense of "uniqueness" and "freedom" between individuals in the Western mode—is, in particular, not a necessary fact of nature. Whatever its various virtues, the path that each individual follows in forging this personal conception of self carries with it a sense of loss and even of wrongdoing at the same time that it conveys an exhilarating liberation—one might say, in a virtual parallel track with the cultural development of cosmic modern Self.

For individual psychological development, the sense of loss is in the individuating divergence from a nurturant feeling of unity with parents, and the sense of wrongdoing is in the implication of a combative wrenching, even a violent act of separation, from the parents in the process of in-

dividuation. In psychoanalytic understanding of individual development, this self-individuation is seen as inevitably involving parricidal implications and thereby carrying some unavoidable sense of guilt as well
as pleasurable self-mastery and freedom. Freud himself imagined, quite
unconvincingly, that there was some actual historic moment in human
tribal life when a band of brothers united to kill their father and that this
primal act is responsible for the burden of parricidal guilt that somehow
conveyed itself to every individual alive today.[18] Freud's more persuasive
successors, staying closer to observable data in the patients whose inner
lives they have painstakingly explored, have found recurrent parricidal
fantasies and haunting guilt as part of the normal process of individual
maturation.[19]

This conjunction of feelings—of self-mastering liberation, of lost
nurturance, and of violent wrongdoing—does not occur at one specific
moment in individual psychological development and then disappear
forever (as if, that is, the mature, culturally prized sense of Self emerges
like a gorgeous butterfly from its discarded chrysalis). These conjoined
feelings are instead a recurrent characteristic of self-evaluation among
mature adults—felt with differing intensity and relative emphases both
among different individuals and at different times for the same individual. For many people, perhaps for most, the imminent prospect of death
brings special prominence and intensity to all of these conjunctive elements in their sense of themselves as "independent, self-determining
selves." The prospect of death means that this prized Self will disappear,
will be lost, is threatened in some primal way. This unaccustomed jeop-
ardy inspires for many, perhaps for most, an intense restorative effort, a
self-renewal that throws the individual backward on the developmental
pathway previously traveled and requires that the individual encounter
once again the various landmarks, the feeling states, that marked his or
her original passage toward the mature sense of self.[20]

Thinking about death at a distance is a far more intellectualized exercise than is the confrontation when death looms imminent. Especially
when serious illness is the immediate precursor, the individual's loss of
an accustomed sense of bodily comfort and intactness itself disrupts his
or her ordinary self-conception.[21] In the impassioned confusion of this
imminent confrontation, an individual must recapture his ordinary sense
of self; and it is not, as in ordinary times, easily available for the asking.
This recapturing is possible—but it involves a recapitulation (however
rapidly or even smoothly accomplished) of the psychological voyage by
which the individual's sense of self was originally achieved. In this retrac-

ing, fragments reappear of mourning for the loss of early oneness with caretakers and of guilty feelings about the imagined violence involved in this separation. The experience of these vagrant emotions—however fleeting, however much they are buried in unconscious mental processes—projects an aura of wrongfulness surrounding death.

In one sense, this wrongfulness is understood as a logical error akin to a grammatical mistake: this is the impossibility, the illogic of imagining one's own death. In another sense, this wrongfulness is understood as a grievous event in personal psychological development—the mourned loss of a sense of oneness with a nurturing world, as we come to think of ourselves as separated individuals. Neither the logical nor the developmental sense of death's wrongfulness is understood as a moral judgment in the conventional vocabulary of morality. But these two senses of error, of wrongdoing, establish the conceptual basis or breeding ground for the persistent moral condemnation of death.[22] This is the connecting link between the modern, secular sense of the individuated self and the traditional Western conviction of the evil inherent in death.

In our Western cultural tradition, death is not viewed simply as a fearful event; there is an aura of wrongfulness, of intrinsic immorality, attached to the very idea of death. In the Western religious tradition specifically, death made its first appearance in God's created universe as a punishment for wrongdoing. If Eve and Adam had not eaten the fruit of the tree of knowledge, if they had obeyed God's specific commandment, they would have lived forever; but they disobeyed, were expelled from the Garden of Eden, and lost eternal life.[23] This traditional explanation for the universal human experience of death—as a punishment for wrongdoing—reaches a climactic expression in the final book of the Christian Bible, the book of Revelation's prediction that when "a new heaven and a new earth" will appear entirely cleansed of sinfulness, then "death shall be no more, neither shall there be mourning nor crying nor pain any more."[24]

Although this tradition speaks directly only to believers, the cultural conviction about the inherent wrongfulness of death did not disappear when formal adherence to religious belief retreated in response to the Enlightenment progression of secular rationality. Our secular culture may not provide the same unequivocal data as the Bible provides for equating death and wrongdoing. But strongly suggestive data can be found in several contemporary contexts to the same effect.

A clear connection can be seen, in particular, in the common attitude among modern physicians toward death—not simply that they are

passionately committed to forestalling it for their patients but that, when death does occur, someone has failed, has behaved in a blameworthy fashion. For some physicians, this aura of wrongdoing expresses itself in self-blame. Thus one physician, who sees himself as a representative figure within the profession, has observed:

> Seriously ill, hospitalized patients . . . require of doctors almost continuous decision-making. Although in most cases no single mistake is obvious, there always seem to be things that could have been done differently or better: administering more of this medication, starting that treatment a little sooner. . . . The fact is that when a patient dies, the physician is left wondering whether the care he provided was adequate. There is no way to be certain, for it is impossible to determine what would have happened if things had been done differently. . . . In the end, the physician has to suppress the guilt and move on to the next patient.[25]

This vague but persistent sense of physicians' culpable responsibility for patients' deaths can also be seen in the widespread difficulty among practitioners in accepting the propriety of withholding life-prolonging medical treatment. A 1993 national survey of physician attitudes found that 87 percent, an overwhelming proportion, agreed that "all competent patients . . . have the right to refuse life support, even if that refusal may lead to death" and that thus allowing patients to die "by forgoing or stopping treatment is ethically different from assisting in their suicide."[26] At the same time, however, two-thirds of the physicians saw an "ethical difference between forgoing (not starting) a life support measure and stopping it once it has been started" and three-quarters found it "helpful" to distinguish "between extraordinary (or heroic) measures and ordinary treatments . . . in making termination-of-treatment decisions."[27] These distinctions had been uniformly rejected by courts, government commissions, and working ethicists as essentially irrational—as distinctions without a difference.[28] The authors of this survey suggested that this variance with the views of "ethical opinion-leaders" may exist because medical practitioners are "unaware of . . . pertinent national recommendations." Based on their open-ended interview data with a sample of practitioners, however, they identified other reasons much less amenable to rational refutation: "psychological discomfort with actively stopping a life-sustaining intervention; discomfort with the public nature of the act, which might occasion a lawsuit from disapproving witnesses even if the decision were legally correct; and fear of sanction by peer review boards."

Even these stated reasons, however, conveyed the sense of a rationalizing structure erected over vague but powerful misgivings; as the authors noted regarding one of the seemingly erroneous distinctions, "for many practitioners, it does feel worse to withdraw than it does never to have initiated a course of treatment."[29] These physicians, as I see it, were struggling with the question of their responsibility as a function of their direct participation in their patients' deaths. They could understand, but they could not accept, the rational proposition that the underlying disease was responsible, or that the patient who refused medical treatment was responsible, for the ensuing death. The physicians could not shake loose from a vague sense not only of their own responsibility but of their culpability unless they rigorously distanced themselves from any suggestion of participation in the act of dying.

This sense of wrongdoing, this vague but persistent aura of guilty conduct, surrounding the confrontation with death can also be seen in another aspect of medicine's custodial role before the 1970s. The initial breach in this custodial role occurred in the 1976 decision of the New Jersey Supreme Court in Karen Ann Quinlan's case.[30] While attending a party in April 1975, Karen Ann had inexplicably fallen unconscious and stopped breathing; she was rushed to a hospital where her breathing was restored with the assistance of a mechanical respirator. Permanent brain damage had, however, apparently already occurred; it seemed that her capacity for cognitive functioning had been destroyed although some neurological reflexes remained intact. Thus she was not dead by ordinary medical criteria but was instead diagnosed as having fallen into a "permanent vegetative state." After some three months during which her condition remained unchanged, Karen Ann's physicians suggested and her parents agreed (with the support of the family's priest) that the mechanical respirator should be removed. The hospital administrators, however, balked at this suggestion; Karen Ann's parents then initiated a lawsuit, and the New Jersey Supreme Court ultimately authorized the removal of the respirator. It quickly became apparent, however, that Karen Ann did not need the respirator to survive; in fact, she lived almost ten years after the respirator had been removed, though she never recovered consciousness.

This confounding result was in fact foreseeable; but the aura of wrongdoing surrounding death in effect blocked its acknowledgment. The state court imagined that the central problem to be solved in Karen Ann's case was the unwillingness of hospital authorities to relent from the pointless, technologically driven prolongation of her life. There was

enormous press attention to this case, and this was also the overwhelming popular understanding of it—not simply in Karen Ann's particular situation but as a general matter, that physicians always aggressively deployed every conceivable instrument of medical technology to prolong life, notwithstanding the absence of any sensible hope for cure or even a tolerable circumstance for living, and even when this aggressive treatment imposed terrible (and pointless) suffering on helpless patients. This was not, however, an accurate portrayal of most physicians' conduct, at least in the circumstances of a patient like Karen Ann Quinlan.

At the original trial in 1975, Dr. Fred Plum of Cornell Medical College testified that he had examined Karen Ann and had concluded that she did not need the respirator to survive. Plum was one of the most knowledgeable physicians in the United States about her condition (he had coined the term "persistent vegetative state"), but the judges and other testifying physicians ignored this aspect of his testimony. Plum also testified that in his experience no patients like Karen Ann survived longer than six months after a diagnosis of this condition; but he was not asked why they died and he did not volunteer an answer to this question. I met Dr. Plum at a panel discussion on the *Quinlan* case in the late 1970s, and he told me then that if the lawyers or judge had asked him at the trial, he would have explained that most vegetative state patients develop recurrent respiratory infections and that the common practice among physicians at the time was to withhold antibiotics from them.

The problem of relentlessly aggressive medical treatment and the iatrongenic imposition of considerable, pointless suffering on inevitably dying people did exist in 1975—as it continues to exist today. The irony of the *Quinlan* case is that it was mistakenly understood by the judges and the lay public as epitomizing this problem, when, in fact, it represented a different, and in many ways more revelatory, characteristic of the social role of medicine in dealing with death: that is, a public commitment among physicians to preserve life at virtually any cost coupled with a private willingness to embrace death but without public acknowledgment—one might even say, a secret willingness to embrace death so long as the secret was never admitted. Dr. Plum's testimony was typical of physicians' attitudes and their accepted social role—physicians could inflict death so long as everyone obeyed the social ethos, "don't ask, and we won't tell."

This unacknowledged dispensation of death by physicians is a confirmatory marker for the persistent aura of wrongdoing that has surrounded death since it came under medical custody. The reality was ac-

cessible to anyone who chose to inquire; but the lay public did not ask and physicians did not volunteer the hard truth that sometimes they accepted, and even acted to hasten, their patients' deaths. Although this was clearly understood among physicians as acceptable professional conduct, the etiquette of public disavowal underscored the social function of a widespread conspiracy of secrecy, of refusal to acknowledge what almost everyone knows: a shared understanding that there is something wrong, something shameful in actions which, if publicly acknowledged, would inspire and deserve condemnation. Notwithstanding the scientifically based conviction that death is natural and inevitable, notwithstanding the rational plausibility of the proposition that prolonged life can be more burdensome than death, the secret character of physicians' embrace of death betrayed the contradictory condemnation of death, the ambivalence that persisted in the supposedly new era of scientific, secular rationalism.

This underlying connection is implicitly revealed by the essential similarity between the format for medical dispensations of death—the "open secrecy," the ethos of "don't ask and we won't tell," which conveys the shamefulness of the death-dispensing enterprise—and the new regime of self-determination in choosing whether to prolong life or to hasten death. On the face of the new regime, it might appear that death is no longer hidden from public view—that there is a new ethos of public acknowledgment and the old denial of death has been repudiated by the new norms of advance directives and open conversation among physicians, patients, and families. Yet the fact that advance directives have manifestly failed to affect the course of end-of-life medical treatment and the documented reluctance of most physicians, patients, and families to discuss death even when it is obviously imminent and unavoidable provide considerable grounds for skepticism.[31] These shortcomings might only demonstrate that we have not yet embraced the new norms of self-determination with sufficient rigor and that redoubled effort is necessary and appropriate to this end. But there is a more fundamental ground for skepticism. The new regime of patient self-determination contains an impulse toward secrecy within its own internal premises—an impulse toward secrecy which, I believe, betrays the same sense of shamefulness, of guilty concealment, that bedeviled the old regime of medical custody.

The secrecy at the heart of the self-determination ideal is expressed in the substantive emptiness of the ideal itself. The new regime of self-control provides no guidance of any sort to any dying person, no clue

about the goals toward which any individual might exercise this newly established right to choose.[32] Indeed, the substantive emptiness of the ideal is proudly proclaimed as a supposed strength; it is commanded by the norm of cultural pluralism, by the premise that every individual has a unique set of values which he or she must consult alone, without external regulation—alone and in private. This is, of course, the presentational rhetoric of the ideal. In practice, many patients rely heavily on others in making medical decisions, often simply deferring to their physicians. Nonetheless, the imagery of the self-determination ideal—the isolation of the individual and the utter absence of any substantive guidance about what decision should be made—does convey a sense of the social and psychological aura that surrounds any decisions about death itself, no matter who makes such decisions. The substantive emptiness, this absence of any internally organizing structure, is the intellectual fault line beneath the rationalized pretensions of the self-determination ideal that leaves it—and us—vulnerable to the eruption of the inherently conflicted significations of death.

This condemnatory attitude is not restricted to self-chosen deaths; it is a pervasive characteristic of all chosen inflictions of death, whether to self or to others—in part, because the infliction of death in itself blurs the psychological boundary lines between self and other. We can see condemnatory inhibition in the historical and contemporary data about the willingness of soldiers to kill in combat. Notwithstanding that the socially approved job of soldiers is to kill, careful empirical research has found that the vast majority of soldiers in direct combat engagements have been unwilling to fire their weapons, even in circumstances where their own lives appear imminently threatened. This surprising finding was first documented by a team of U.S. Army historians, led by Brigadier General S. L. A. Marshall, who interviewed thousands of soldiers in more than four hundred infantry companies immediately after they had been in close combat with German or Japanese troops during World War II. Marshall found that of those soldiers along the line of fire during any encounter, whether "spread over a day or two days or three," only 15–20 percent would ever fire their weapons. "Those who would not fire did not run or hide (in many cases they were willing to risk great danger to rescue comrades, get ammunition, or run messages), but they simply would not fire their weapons at the enemy, even when faced with repeated waves of banzai charges."[33] Subsequent research has confirmed this data for soldiers of other nationalities and for previous warfare in the nineteenth and twentieth centuries.[34] Marshall interpreted

his findings as demonstrating the existence in "the average and healthy individual . . . [of] an inner and usually unrealized resistance towards killing a fellow man[,] that he will not of his own volition take life if it is possible to turn away from that responsibility."[35]

Marshall's findings provide confirmation for the proposition that death carries an inescapable connotation of wrongdoing, no matter what the justification for its presence—not just the intentional infliction of death on others (as with physicians or soldiers), or its intentional infliction on oneself, but the very presence of death as an apparently inevitable feature of the human condition. This does not mean, however, that this sense of wrongfulness cannot be overridden, even by "the average and healthy individual." Marshall's research demonstrates this proposition as well.

As might be imagined, American military leaders were not happy with Marshall's findings, whatever comfort many people might take from the conclusion that wellsprings of pacifism run deep in human psychology— from Marshall's observation that "at the vital point [the typical soldier] becomes a conscientious objector." In direct response to Marshall's research, the American military implemented special training programs for combat soldiers designed to overcome these documented inhibitions. Marshall himself researched the results of these programs for combat performance in the Korean War and found that the firing rate had increased to 55 percent of soldiers in combat situations; even more intensified training programs were subsequently adopted and further research found that in the Vietnam War the firing rate had risen to between 90 and 95 percent.[36]

Perhaps the innate reluctance to kill can be overcome among combat soldiers without any adverse psychological consequences to them. Perhaps these inhibitions can be loosened without undermining the possibility that the military hierarchy can contain this violence within socially approved limits. Or perhaps the possibility of adverse impact on combat soldiers and unleashed excessive brutality in the conduct of war should be considered a socially acceptable consequence, a necessary corollary of the proposition that "war is hell." Whatever its justification for warfare, risks of adverse consequences to medical practitioners and patients from implementation of policies overriding the innate sense of death's wrongfulness cannot find equivalent justification.

Medical practice is clearly, though haltingly, changing in response to public and professional advocacy on behalf of this ethos. Physicians' resistance to withdrawing life-prolonging treatment with patient or sur-

rogate consent has markedly diminished in recent years. For example, in 1987–88, 50 percent of deaths in hospital intensive care units (ICUs) occurred notwithstanding the persistent provision of full life support to those patients; 40 percent followed withdrawal of supports while 10 percent involved initial withholding. By contrast, in 1992–93, only 10 percent of ICU deaths involved persistent support while 70 percent of the cases followed withdrawal and 20 percent followed withholding of treatment.[37] Most likely, this new pattern is responsive to the contemporary, widespread public belief that physicians have wrongfully forced aggressive treatment on inevitably dying people. It is not clear, however, whether these changed practices reflect a psychologically satisfying resolution of previous misgivings among most physicians regarding withdrawal or withholding of life-prolonging treatment, or whether the basic reasons for their prior resistance remained untouched.

If my speculation is correct, that this prior resistance is a significant reflection of an underlying aura of wrongdoing surrounding death, we would expect not only persistence but an intensification of some guilt-ridden attitudes among physicians in their more direct engagement in the dispensation of death. The most abusive aspects of physicians' prior conduct toward dying patients—their infliction of suffering through pointlessly aggressive treatment and through disregard of ameliorable pain—can be understood as expressing their underlying convictions about the wrongfulness of death. In its simplest outline, dying patients were being punished because of the immorality implicit in their deaths— a resolution that many physicians would find more comfortable than blaming themselves for this evil outcome. The even more common practice among physicians of abandoning dying patients (avoiding them on hospital rounds or home calls when it became clear that they were dying) can also be understood as responsive to the aura of guilt surrounding death—that is, in simplest outline, physicians were fleeing the scene of the crime.

There is ample opportunity in the new regime of patient self-control for any persistence of these motives among physicians to find equivalently abusive expression. The new regime does not, for the most part, remove physicians from any involvement with dying patients but instead aims at shifting decision-making responsibility to the patients or their surrogates. In matters such as withdrawing life-prolonging treatment, physicians are still actively engaged, notwithstanding that their appointed task is to implement patients' wishes. It is here that new guises for old abuses can arise. For example, a February 2000 article in the

New England Journal of Medicine unequivocally condemned a reported practice among some intensive care physicians of administering neuro-muscular paralyzing drugs to dying patients in the course of withdrawing them from mechanical ventilators. The stated rationale among these physicians for imposing this paralysis was to "guarantee . . . that the patient would not have seizures or make any gasping respiratory efforts after the withdrawal of ventilation," thereby "seeking to relieve the family's suffering" as they stood by the dying patient's bedside. The consequence of this paralysis for the patient was, however, potentially horrific. As the authors of the article observed, the "neuromuscular blocking agents have no analgesic or sedative properties [but they] may mask the signs of acute air hunger associated with the withdrawal of the ventilator, leaving the patient to endure the agony of suffocation in silence and isolation."[38]

The administering physicians were not motivated by purposeful sadism; their consciously beneficent motives to protect family witnesses served, however, to mask even from themselves the abusive implications of their action. Even so, it is difficult to imagine how these physicians could have failed to understand the consequences of paralyzing a dying person, leaving him helpless to express any pain or indicate a need for sedation. This surely represents an abandonment of a dying patient by his physicians. Is it related to the aura of wrongdoing surrounding death, a desire of the physicians to flee the scene? They took flight, moreover, by inflicting suffering—surely a wrongful deed in its own terms, however much they disguised their own motives. Did they impose this suffering because they viewed the dying patient as somehow deserving punishment, because of the wrongfulness of death?

These motives do not neatly parse themselves: all we know for sure is that the moment of death was accompanied by the possible though unacknowledged infliction by physicians of horrific suffering on the dying person. This concatenation of events—death and heedless suffering imposed by physicians—is at least suggestive of a psychological syndrome that Freud observed in some of his patients, a syndrome that he designated "criminality from a sense of guilt." Reflecting on patients he had treated who had confessed to him their participation in criminal activity, Freud stated, "Analytic work brought the surprising discovery that such deeds were done principally because they were forbidden, and because their execution was accompanied by mental relief for their doer. [The patient] was suffering from an oppressive feeling of guilt, of which he did not know the origin, and after he had committed a mis-

deed, this oppression was mitigated. His sense of guilt was at least attached to something. Paradoxical as it may sound, I must maintain that the sense of guilt was present before the misdeed, that it did not arise from it, but conversely—the misdeed arose from the sense of guilt." [39]

If I am correct that in our Western cultural tradition death carries a strong implication of wrongdoing and if this implication persists as a counterpoint to the modern secularized vision of death as a natural process and Nature as an impersonal, amoral force, then it becomes plausible to apply Freud's conception to the abuse of dying patients by their physicians—of misdeeds not causing guilt but arising from a sense of guilt, giving some defined shape to a vague but nagging sense of wrongdoing somewhere in the transactions surrounding death. This conception does not imply that this abuse, this "criminality," is inevitable. The paralyzing of dying patients withdrawn from ventilators, for example, is not a common practice, though its exact current incidence is unknown; and the practice was clearly understood and condemned as abusive by the authors of the *New England Journal* article. But the capacity of even a few physicians to mask this abusive conduct from themselves with self-conscious beneficence should serve as a warning of the likely route by which contemporary reform efforts may fail in their avowed goal of ending past abusive practices toward dying patients.

The greatest risk, as I see it, is in the psychological ease with which beneficent motives, self-proclaimed righteousness, can divert attention from darker, less nobly self-affirming motivations. The unwillingness to acknowledge ambivalently mixed motives—to admit the inclination toward wrongdoing as well as the impulse toward moral virtue—is neither unique to physicians nor restricted to events surrounding death and dying. At least since practitioners of scientific medicine began to seek and were granted primary custody of death and dying in the nineteenth century, however, ambivalence about death and dying has been rigorously suppressed. It may be that prior ritual practices in which clergy took the central role brought this ambivalence into some clearer focus, with the conjoined promise of a comforting afterlife conditioned on personal confession of sinfulness. Thus Peter Brooks has suggested, "crime, guilt, and punishment is effaced in the ancient ritual of deathbed confession, absolution, and reconciliation of the sinner with the human community whose bonds he has so sundered." [40] When scientific medicine took charge, however, ambivalence about death took a different path; death was reconceived as an unforgivable offense which left no room for the transfiguration of the dying person. Contemporary reform efforts, by

contrast, turn the coin: death is imagined as morally neutral and the dying person is seen as the instrument of his own self-controlling absolution. As with the scientific conception that this imagery is intended to displace, there is no room here for contrapuntal acknowledgment of death as both amoral (or even a positive good) and inherently wrong. Though this ambivalence about death can be denied, it cannot reliably be suppressed; like some powerfully surging underground river, it must erupt somewhere.

The warfare between these forces in America today is most intensely fought on the issue of physician-assisted suicide. Jack Kevorkian is at this writing imprisoned in Michigan for his audacity in forcing the issue into public visibility. He was relentless in his campaign for the goodness of death to relieve suffering and the nobility of his motives in inflicting death; there was, nonetheless, something insistently unhinged about his campaign—the publicly flaunted videotapes, the repeated administrations of death in the back of his Volkswagen bus, the blood-drenched ghoulishness of his public art exhibitions. The common reformist view of Kevorkian is that his weird flamboyance was excessive but he served a noble purpose—rather like John Brown's feckless military action to end slavery which, though an apparently quixotic failure at the time and ending in his own execution, nonetheless galvanized respectable but more timid people to take up his moral campaign and bring it to fruition.

Kevorkian's imprisonment has freed the campaign for physician-assisted suicide from the unavoidable acknowledgment of ambivalence publicly provoked by his garish self-presentation; as he receded from center stage, the campaign for legalization moved into respectable company. One state, Oregon, legalized the practice in successive public referenda in 1994 and 1996, after the relatively narrow 1992 defeat of similar measures in Washington and California. According to public opinion polls, legalization is supported in principle by a majority nationwide, though no other state has yet followed Oregon's lead.[41] The current campaigners do not show any sign of ambivalence in their advocacy on behalf of the principle of self-determination, the chosen death as an alternative to hopeless, helpless suffering. Their technique—surely not consciously deceptive, and all the more effective for that—is rigorously to suppress ambivalence about the goodness of death and the virtues of its self-determining embrace.

The Oregon statute epitomizes this approach. To determine eligibility for assisted suicide, two physicians must find that the petitioning individual is "terminally ill" (likely to die in no more than six months) and

"capable" of voluntary decision making. The statute defines the requisite mental capacity in exceedingly minimalist terms ("ability to make and communicate health care decisions");[42] the statute, moreover, does not specify that the evaluating physicians have any special mental health training. The underlying intent of the statute is to discourage any probing inquiry into the motivations of individuals who request physician-assisted suicide; consistent with this goal, the statute requires physicians who approve such requests to report to the state health department only the most minimal information, the patient's name, terminal diagnosis, and a bare certification, without any supporting details, that the physician had found the patient capable and voluntary. The individual's right to choose suicide protected by this statute is based on a plausible conception of "autonomy"—a conception based on considerable psychological distance between individuals and equally sharp boundaries between "rational" and "irrational" thinking within an individual's own mind. Concern about ambivalence is not the hallmark of the Oregon statute.

This bleached view of human motivation is commonplace among advocates for physician-assisted suicide. It is marked, and especially ironic, in the contemporary treatment of Sigmund Freud's death—the way, that is, that he has been enlisted as an exemplar of the virtues of physician-assisted suicide.[43] Here is the account by his official biographer, Ernest Jones:

> He found it hardly possible to eat anything. The last book he was able to read was Balzac's *La Peau de chagrin*, on which he commented wryly: "That is just the book for me. It deals with starvation." He meant rather the gradual shrinking, the becoming less and less, described so poignantly in the book.
>
> But with all this agony there was never the slightest sign of impatience or irritability. The philosophy of resignation and the acceptance of unalterable reality triumphed throughout.
>
> The cancer ate its way through the cheek to the outside and the septic condition was heightened. The exhaustion was extreme and the misery indescribable. . . . On September 21 Freud said to his doctor: "My dear Schur, you remember our first talk. You promised me then you would help me when I could no longer carry on. It is only torture now and it has no longer any sense." Schur pressed his hand and promised he would give him adequate sedation, and Freud thanked him, adding after a moment of hesitation: "Tell Anna about our talk." There was no emotionalism or self-pity, only reality—an impressive and unforgettable scene.
>
> The next morning Schur gave Freud a third of a grain of morphia. For someone at such a point of exhaustion as Freud then was, and so complete

a stranger to opiates, that small dose sufficed. He sighed with relief and sank into a peaceful sleep; he was evidently close to the end of his reserves. He died just before midnight the next day, September 23, 1939. His long and arduous life was at an end and his sufferings over. Freud died as he had lived—a realist.[44]

Jones's account readily fits the contemporary prescription for physician-assisted suicide—heroic suffering by the terminally ill patient until it becomes unendurable, then the patient asks his trusted physician to provide medication to relieve his suffering by hastening the inevitable moment of death. There are, however, other accounts of Freud's death which offer a more complicated scenario. Dr. Schur's own subsequently published version suggests that he did not actually hasten Freud's death, in spite of his apparent prior promise. After recounting Freud's request (virtually verbatim from Jones's version, which itself had relied on Schur's unpublished notes), Schur continues:

> I indicated that I had not forgotten my promise. He sighed with relief, held my hand a moment longer, and said: "Ich danke Ihnen" ("I thank you"), and after a moment of hesitation he added: "Sagen Sie es der Anna" ("Tell Anna about this"). All this was said without a trace of emotionality or self-pity, and with full consciousness of reality.
>
> I informed Anna of our conversation, as Freud had asked. When he was again in agony, I gave him a hypodermic of two centigrams of morphine. He soon felt relief and fell into a peaceful sleep. The expression of pain and suffering was gone. I repeated this dose after about twelve hours. Freud was obviously so close to the end of his reserves that he lapsed into a coma and did not wake up again.[45]

In this account, Schur purposefully understated both the morphine dosage and the number of injections he had administered; as he confessed in a 1954 letter to Anna Freud, the actual dosage was three centigrams, and he "may have administered three rather than two injections." Schur's stated reason for this reticence was that, after Freud's death, "he had consulted a lawyer concerning the question of euthanasia and had, in response, watered down his report."[46] Ironically, however, it is highly unlikely, even in Schur's true version, that his administration of morphine actively hastened death; the physiological effects of morphine in terminally ill patients have not been adequately researched or properly understood until very recently.[47]

It does seem likely that Schur believed he was actually hastening Freud's death; but even on this score, there is some basis for doubt in

the fact that Freud did not die from the first injection, that Schur administered a second and perhaps third injection, and that, according to both his published and his privately amplified accounts, he repeated the same dosages rather than administering an increased dosage in response to the failure of the prior injections to accomplish the apparently desired purpose. Some inhibition obstructed Schur's capacity to draw the obvious empirical lesson that the previous dosage was insufficient to cause death. He may have believed that the repeated dosage would somehow have a cumulative effect, notwithstanding the passage of some twelve hours between them; but if he were truly determined to hasten death, why would he restrain himself from increasing the dosage even if he (erroneously) believed that a repetition of the original dosage was all that was necessary? Why not, that is, add an extra margin for safety's sake—except for the existence of some strong, though unacknowledged, inhibition in his mind regarding the intrinsic wrongfulness of the act?

This inhibition—if I read it right—was, however, only on the physician's part. Freud himself still might shine as the exemplary claimant for the contemporary version of the right to physician-assisted suicide—except for another detail in the transaction which has been bleached away from both Jones's and Schur's accounts. Peter Gay, in his more recent biography of Freud, provides a more extensive reckoning, based on access to previously unpublished letters and an interview with Schur's widow:

> [O]n September 21, as Schur was sitting by Freud's bedside, Freud took his hand and said to him, "Schur, you remember our 'contract' not to leave me in the lurch when the time had come. Now it is nothing but torture and makes no sense." Schur indicated that he had not forgotten. Freud gave a sigh of relief, kept his hand for a moment, and said, "I thank you." Then, after a slight hesitation, he added, "Talk it over with Anna, and if she thinks it's right, then make an end of it." As she had been for years, so at this junction, Freud's Antigone was first in his thoughts. Anna Freud wanted to postpone the fatal moment, but Schur insisted that to keep Freud going was pointless, and she submitted to the inevitable, as had her father.[48]

Gay noted that Schur in his published account had purposefully "distorted" and "minimized" Anna's role and Freud's reliance on her "out of respect for Anna Freud's desire for privacy."[49] But Gay himself distorted the results of his own research. He concluded his account with the observation that Freud "had seen to it that his secret entreaty would be fulfilled. The old stoic had kept control of his life to the end."[50] Ac-

cording to Gay's own version, however, Freud had shared control of his life with his daughter Anna. She, in turn, was reluctant to endorse his death and acceded only after Dr. Schur "insisted" (and Schur then by his account could not bring himself to press the fatal outcome).

Relying on Gay's more complete account (but not on his evaluation of it), where is the heroic individualist who willed Freud's death? Not Freud himself, since he deferred final judgment to his daughter; not Anna, since she only yielded to Dr. Schur's insistence; and not even Freud's physician, since he held himself back from increasing the morphine dosage beyond its obviously self-limiting sedative effect. There is realism and stoicism in this version of Freud's death—but it is not as Ernest Jones, Peter Gay, and even Max Schur imply, in Freud's self-conscious choice for his own death.[51] To the very end, Freud embraced ambivalence about death. As he himself had stated, in the final sentences of his great work *Civilization and Its Discontents:* "it is to be expected that the other of the two 'Heavenly Powers,' eternal Eros, will make an effort to assert himself in the struggle with his equally immortal adversary [the human instinct of aggression and self-destruction]. But who can foresee with what success and with what result?"[52] In his own death, as in his life's work charting the persistent struggle between conscious and unconscious forces both in our individual psyches and in our social lives, Freud profoundly acknowledged these competing forces. He strove to enlarge the domain of conscious self-reflection, but he ultimately acquiesced in his inability to impose rational order on inherently unruly irrational impulses. This is the true measure of Freud's realism and stoicism in facing death. This is the path we ourselves would be best advised to follow.

CHAPTER TWO

HIDDEN DEATH

I Walk through Shadows

In 1947, a three-judge panel of the United States Court of Appeals for the Second Circuit rendered a decision that can be understood as both an early expression and a wise rejection of the reform impulse that was to erupt twenty years later into the dominant contemporary agenda for the dispensing of death. The three judges were Learned Hand, Augustus Hand, and Jerome Frank—today generally considered the most distinguished panel of American judges ever assembled in one courtroom. By my account of this decision, Learned Hand emerges as the role model whom I would commend for avoiding the seductions of triumphalist rationality and working his way toward a solution that gives publicly acknowledged visibility to ambivalence about the moral status of death.

In 1939 Louis Loftus Repouille, a native of the Dutch West Indies living in New York, killed his severely disabled thirteen-year-old son, Raymond. In 1944, Repouille applied for United States citizenship; his application was opposed by the government on the ground that he could not satisfy the naturalization statute's requirement of having been "a person of good moral character" during the preceding five years. When his case came to the Second Circuit Court of Appeals in 1947, the three judges were directly confronted with the task of determining the morality of a death-dispensing decision.

When Raymond was killed in 1939 and when the appellate court was asked to adjudicate his killer's moral stature in 1947, it was unusual that such a child would attract any social attention. According to court records, Raymond had been born with "a brain injury which destined him

27

to be an idiot and a physical monstrosity, . . . blind, mute, and deformed. He had to be fed; the movements of his bladder and bowels were involuntary, and his entire life was spent in a small crib." Most children like Raymond were consigned at an early age to state residential facilities—mammoth institutions located far from populated areas, visited by no outsiders (including most parents of the residents)—and they remained in these institutions until they died, from whatever causes. These warehousing institutions were established following the Civil War and can themselves be understood as yet another expression of the pervasive culture of death's denial—as places, that is, for removing from public visibility people contaminated with the stigma of death. It was not only that retarded children were understood as incurably ill but the very terms of their illness—their incapacity to participate in ordinary social interactions—conveyed a sense of "social death." [1]

Raymond Repouille was unusual in 1939 because he had remained in his parents' home with four younger siblings ("all normal," as the court records said). Because he thus had not been hidden from any contact with ordinary social life, his death attracted more attention than would the unseen deaths typical for his institutionalized counterparts. Here is the public account of Raymond's death that appeared in the *New York Times* on October 13, 1939: [2]

> Louis Repouille, a $25-a-week elevator operator at the Columbia-Presbyterian Medical Center, who had spent his life's earnings trying to cure his incurably imbecile son, Raymond, 13 years old, ended the boy's life yesterday as an "act of mercy."
>
> Frantic with poverty and despair, Repouille, described by Medical Center officials as a "most reliable employee" and by his neighbors as a quiet and respectable man, soaked a rag with chloroform from a one-ounce bottle and applied it several times to the boy's face while he lay awake in a crib in the rear bedroom of a squalid four-room flat at 2071 Amsterdam Avenue. Then he burned the rag.
>
> The boy had been bedridden since infancy. About five years ago he was operated on for a brain tumor at the Broad Street Hospital, according to the police, and had been blind since that time.
>
> "He was just like dead all the time," Repouille told detectives while he was being questioned at the West 152d Street police station on Amsterdam Avenue. "He couldn't walk, he couldn't talk, he couldn't do anything. I spent $500—all the money I had—on an operation, but that didn't do any good. Specialists charged me $25 a visit and told me that there was no hope."
>
> . . . After questioning at the station house, Repouille, who is 40, was led back to the Amsterdam Avenue flat by detectives and Assistant District Attorney James M. Yeargin to re-enact the killing.

For the last three years, Repouille has lived with his wife, Florence, also 40, and four other children—Lillian, 11; Alphonse, 7; Anna, 5; and Jeanette, 2—in the four-room, cold-water flat, for which he pays rental of $14 a month.

The grimness of the gloomy flat was tempered only by the chirping of a number of canaries and love-birds that Repouille keeps in a line of cages in the living room. It was learned later that he supplements his earnings as an elevator man by selling the birds . . .

According to Mrs. Repouille, who, like her husband, was born in the Dutch West Indies, Repouille had talked often of killing the boy to put him out of his misery. For days, apparently, he had been seeking a pretext to get her out of the flat so that he could commit the act.

On Wednesday night, the police learned, he had made a call to Mother Cabrini Hospital in order to summon an ambulance for his wife, who, he said, was intoxicated. When an ambulance surgeon arrived, however, he found her sober and listed the call as "unnecessary."

Yesterday afternoon, however, Repouille found his opportunity. He reported sick at the Medical Center. Later in the day his wife went out shopping, taking her daughter Jeanette. Repouille then sent the other . . . children to the movies.

When Mrs. Repouille returned she found the door locked. Panic-stricken, she remembered her husband's threats to kill the boy and ran screaming out of the house. Outside she encountered John Sullivan, an occupant of the same building, and told him of her fears. Sullivan entered the Repouille apartment through an open window and found the boy with a rag over his face and the father sitting on a bed.

Sullivan told the police he removed the rag and was about to throw it on the floor when Repouille said: "Don't, can't you see I have some birds here." It was then that he burned the rag in the coal stove.

In December 1941, a state court jury, after deliberating "less than an hour,"[3] convicted Repouille of manslaughter and recommended "utmost clemency" in sentencing; the judge imposed a term of five to ten years' probation without imprisonment. Before the sentence was imposed, the assistant district attorney said that the jury verdict had demonstrated that "mercy killings are not countenanced by society," and the defense attorney insisted that Repouille had not engaged in a "mercy killing" but was suffering from "mental aberration at the time." The judge then spoke to Repouille: "This type of killing has become associated in the public mind with the thought that, on certain occasions, it is an act of mercy. The words mercy killing have no sanction in our law. The fact that you were the father of an imbecile did not give you the right to kill him." Nonetheless, the judge continued, he decided for "leniency" because Repouille "never before had run afoul of the law" and

because imprisonment "would greatly affect the lives of your children, who need your support and guidance." The judge concluded, "There is grave danger that the leniency extended to you may encourage others to do what you did. I have taken into consideration that, no matter what punishment I might impose, you will have the burden of remembering for the rest of your life that you killed your child."[4]

The public ritual was thus completed. The killing was neither condemned nor accepted; or, put another way, it was both condemned and accepted in the same gesture. The jury and the judge concurred in this double-dealing, which reflected both a lay and a professional elite understanding of the ritual demands. In proclaiming Repouille guilty of manslaughter rather than murder, the jury found that he had acted involuntarily—though the record, as reflected in the quoted newspaper accounts, unmistakably showed that Repouille had planned and intended to kill his son. Even then, the jury added a recommendation for "utmost clemency" to its already exonerating verdict; but it would not absolve him of guilt. The judge tried to walk this same tangled course, condemning "mercy killing," proclaiming that he had "no right" to kill his son but nonetheless extending "leniency" because Repouille's surviving children needed his "support and guidance"—and insisting that this leniency somehow conveyed a moral reproach, a "burden" of guilt that Repouille would always carry.

Though this disposition by the jury and judge might appear confused, a clear logic lay beneath it—the logic of self-contradiction. Repouille had breached the social norm for dealing with disability and death; he had forced these matters and their reinforcing conjunction into high public visibility. The conventional, publicly acceptable course would have been for Repouille to consign his "imbecile son" to the custody of state authorities, who would have swept him from view to a remote institution where he would remain unseen (even by his family) until he died of "undetermined" causes. Repouille violated this norm of invisibility; and it is not readily apparent how such a norm can be reasserted, how a visible act can be made invisible. This is a paradoxical task; and the best strategy for implementation is, as Repouille's jury and judge understood, to embrace paradox, to engage in a self-contradictory action that "confusingly" cancels itself. Thus invisibility is approximately restored. The killing was neither condemned nor approved; it was neutralized, deprived of cognitively graspable content.

This invisibility is only approximate, the best remedy available for a difficult bind. It was, moreover, not an easy task to reimpose this norm in Repouille's case; his action in fact revealed the vulnerability of the

norm at the time, which was apparent in at least two ways. The first was in the public fascination with the events reflected by its news coverage. I was not able to locate accounts from the tabloid press at the time; but the vivid reportage in the *New York Times* reflected a judgment about the interest of its respectable readership, that this alleged "mercy killing of an imbecile" fit the *Times*'s self-imposed category of "news fit to print." The public appetite in this matter was expressed, moreover, in an even more intense way immediately before Repouille's actions. In May 1939, just four months before Repouille killed his son, a New York city jury had acquitted another man for killing his sixteen-year-old "imbecile" son. This case received extensive publicity. The defendant, a prosperous businessman, testified that "irrepressible voices" came during sleepless nights with the instruction "stop his suffering—stop his suffering";[5] the jury was instructed to acquit if it found the defendant "was suffering from defect of reason"—whether "insanity" or "any cause."[6] The jury's exculpatory verdict had the same contradictory implication as the subsequent disposition of Repouille's case—the killing, that is, was neither directly excused as a "permissible mercy killing" nor condemned as "murder," but effectively negated as a "mentally deranged" act.

This negation could not wholly succeed in undoing the act, in rendering it publicly invisible. Repouille's actions themselves demonstrated this proposition. The news account of Repouille's case reported that a police detective had asked him whether he had known about the earlier killing, and Repouille responded, "I read about it. It made me think about doing the same thing to my boy. I think Mr. Greenfield [the defendant] was justified. They didn't punish him for it. But I'm not looking for sympathy. I don't care what happens to me. My boy is dead and his suffering is over."[7] The reportage of Repouille's case had its direct impact in turn; just three days after that killing, another father drowned his five-year-old stepson and told an arresting officer that "he had read and discussed accounts of recent 'mercy killings.'"[8] The day this killing was made public, a reporter asked Repouille for his response: "The father [Repouille] kept his eyes down and seemed to be groping for the words to express what he felt. Finally he said: 'If the kid was normal, I'd call him a murderer.'"[9] This sudden epidemic of avowed "mercy killings" in New York City was thus highly visible and presented an unavoidable question of social control. The characteristic mode of reimposing control at the time was to combine publicly proclaimed condemnation with publicly averted attention—to disavow killing, but not the killing of "imbeciles" as such.

Repouille himself was not content with this disposition. As he left

the courtroom, free from imprisonment but carrying the sting of a guilty verdict and the judge's reproach, Repouille stated that the jury should not have convicted him and he gave this "penciled statement" to the press: "I am in the market for a job as an apartment house superintendent to support my wife and our other four young children. I love children and am very fond of animals and birds."[10] A few years later, Repouille in effect renewed his quest for explicit public approbation— and it was this revisitation that came before the federal judicial panel of Learned Hand, Augustus Hand, and Jerome Frank. In 1944 Repouille applied to become a citizen of the United States; though he had come to this country in 1922, he had never previously sought citizenship. Repouille filed this application exactly four years, eleven months, and ten days after the date he had killed his son Raymond; and there was the rub. The naturalization statute required Repouille to demonstrate that he "has been . . . a person of good moral character" during the five years preceding his application. Perhaps Repouille intended this, perhaps he did not—but the timing of his application pushed back into public visibility the question of the moral status of his act.

On this occasion, public authorities struggled more visibly than before with this question. In its prior presentation, the central actor in determining moral accountability was the jury; its members' deliberations were conducted in secret; their collective conclusion was expressed without any individualized elaboration; and, as we have seen, it was an essentially inscrutable amalgam of contradictory findings. This time around, the anonymity and public invisibility that surround jury proceedings were not available for disposing of Repouille's uncomfortable claim.[11] Moreover, by 1947, when his claim reached the three judges on the court of appeals, the public commitment to conceal disability and death had itself become somewhat unsettled. The official deliberations on Repouille's claim for naturalization revealed early indications of the public stress and the consequent special judicial role in opening the floodgates on the administration of death twenty-five years later.

Under the statute, citizenship petitions were initially reviewed by an Immigration and Naturalization Service examiner; this bureaucratic official would then recommend a disposition to a United States district judge, but a formal hearing before the judge would occur only when the government examiner recommended against citizenship. In Repouille's case, the examiner made a negative recommendation, and the hearing was held on January 16, 1947, before Judge Robert Inch. Repouille appeared on his own behalf, without a lawyer. In the entire proceeding, ac-

cording to the stenographer's notes, there was only one direct exchange between Repouille and the judge. At the very beginning of the hearing, Judge Inch directed a one-word question to Repouille: "French?"; and Repouille responded, "I am Dutch, but French extraction." Repouille was asked and said nothing else during the rest of the proceeding. The government examiner made a brief statement to the judge about Repouille's conviction and then handed him the report of Repouille's probation officer, dated September 26, 1944. The stenographer noted, "The Court reads the report":

> Louis Repouille, who is on probation to this Department, has requested us to furnish him with this summary of his case so that he may apply for naturalization papers. Repouille was placed on probation in this Court on December 24, 1941, after he had been convicted of Manslaughter in the Second Degree, with a recommendation by the Jury of utmost clemency. He had no previous Court record, and was never arrested before. The offense of which he was convicted involved the slaying of his oldest child, age thirteen, by the use of chloroform. The child in question, according to numerous hospital reports, suffered from birth from a brain injury which destined him to be an idiot and a physical monstrosity, malformed in all four limbs. The child was blind, mute, and deformed. He had to be fed; the movements of his bladder and bowels were involuntary, and his entire life was spent in a small crib. Repouille, however, is the father of four other children, all normal. The care of these additional children, together with the constant attention which the deceased child required, created problems which caused the probationer great mental distress.
>
> Despite the difficulties with which he was burdened, however, considering the entire situation aside from the offense, Repouille was considered a devoted parent whose interests were centered entirely in his children and home. Repouille has established an excellent employment record, and has always contributed his entire earnings toward the upkeep of his home. While on probation during the past three years he has worked with regularity, and his family life has been harmonious in every way. His remaining children have received the best of care, and he has made a good domestic adjustment. Repouille has pursued a socially acceptable manner of living. He has never been given to any personal excesses and his interests have centered in his home and employment. He has been orderly in his personal habits and temperate. If there is any further data desired on this case, do not hesitate to call on us.

An addendum to this report indicated that Repouille had been discharged from probation on December 29, 1945, after only four years of his five-to-ten-year term on the ground that his probation record had been "exceptionally good" and he had been "an honest, orderly, and hardworking man."

After silently reading the report, Judge Inch said, "He suffered terribly. I am going to admit him." According to the stenographer's notes, no one said anything more.

The government subsequently filed an appeal against Judge Inch's ruling. In its appeal brief, the government made only one claim: that Repouille's act, "the chloroforming to death of his invalid son," intrinsically established his absence of "good moral character," regardless of his subsequent "exemplary conduct." [12] Repouille once again had no attorney representing him; but his two-page typed submission in the court of appeals conveyed the clear sense that it was drafted with a lawyer's assistance. Repouille claimed that his application was only "technically . . . placed on the record before 1945" and was "actually intended" to be filed after the expiration of the five-year "good moral character" term; and he tried to back away from demanding a positive finding on this score: "With regard to the argument in the government's brief that I was a person of bad moral character in 1939, I would be reluctant to make an argument on that question. . . . [T]he facts have been reasonably well portrayed in the report of the Probation Department, and I leave it up the Court to say from those facts whether or not it is true, as the Government contends, that I was a person of bad moral character."

The appeals court heard the case on November 12, 1947. It appears from court records that the government's attorney made an oral presentation but that Repouille did not speak; whatever legal assistance he may have gotten in preparing his written submission, he stood alone before this tribunal and was identified in its ultimate opinion as appearing "pro se"—for himself. After the hearing, the judges apparently did not discuss the case but instead—following a frequent practice in appellate courts—deliberated by exchanging memoranda. The first move came from Augustus Hand; on November 19, he sent the following memorandum to his colleagues:

> I am sorry for this poor fellow but am not prepared to say "in spirit or in truth" that there is any wide sentiment in the community that would hold a person of "good moral character" who takes the law into his own hands in a case like this. We may favor "mercy killing" but if sanctioned by law it should have the most careful safeguards to make it accord with social safety.
>
> The appellant . . . has been lucky not to live in Massachusetts where a father living near Pittsfield was convicted last year of murder in the first degree for a mercy killing of an idiot child and finally got off only with a commutation of the sentence to life imprisonment. That disposition was pretty barbarous, yet has a bearing on the sentiment of American communities. There

is before us much more than the question of the subjective morality of the petitioner.[13]

Two days later, Jerome Frank circulated a brief memorandum coming to the opposite position: "To be sure, [Repouille's] crime is a felony. But everyone concerned with this man—the jury, the judge and the probation officer—regarded his offense as one which should be greeted with the 'utmost clemency.' That is a pretty good indication of the 'commonly accepted mores,' the 'prevalent moral feelings.'"[14]

Learned Hand would thus be the deciding vote in adjudicating Repouille's moral status. Hand's prior rulings in naturalization cases clearly inclined him to accept the petition. Just one month earlier, in October 1947, he had rejected the government claim of insufficient moral character in an applicant who had married his niece twenty-two years earlier, raised four children with her, and had the marriage "solemnized" by a Catholic priest with the permission of the local bishop. The government had based its claim on the fact that the marriage was defined as "incestuous" and barred by statute in the state where it had been performed. In his opinion, Hand stated, "Would the moral feelings that are now prevalent generally in this country be outraged because Francioso [the petitioner] continued to live with his wife and four children . . . ? Cato himself would not have demanded that he should turn all five adrift."[15] In his prior conference memorandum to his colleagues on the case, Hand was even more openly scornful of the government's position. He asked rhetorically whether the government might have morally approved of Francioso if he had stayed with his wife and children but relented from incest by remaining celibate; and he continued, "Perhaps not even so low a form of animal life as an examiner in the Naturalization Bureau would go so far as that. Once more I wish to pay my respects to the sanctimonious, hypocritical, illiterate animaleulae who infest and infect the Naturalization Bureau."[16]

Learned Hand thus did not come to naturalization appeals with a deferential posture toward the government. The standard he articulated in this incest case—"whether the moral feelings that are now prevalent generally in this country be outraged"—had been first formulated by Hand himself in a 1929 case where the government had maintained that violation of prohibition laws was an act of "moral turpitude" justifying deportation of a resident alien. Hand rejected this position, and set out the criteria for giving specific content to the "good morals clause" in the congressional act governing both deportation and naturalization:

There are probably many persons in the United States who [would] regard either the possession or sale of liquor [as "shamefully immoral"]; but the question is whether it is so by common conscience, a nebulous matter at best. While we must not, indeed, substitute our personal notions as the standard, it is impossible to decide at all without some estimate, necessarily based on conjecture, as to what people generally feel. We cannot say that among the commonly accepted mores the sale or possession of liquor as yet occupies so grave a place; nor can we close our eyes to the fact that large numbers of persons, otherwise reputable, do not think it so, rightly or wrongly.[17]

Hand was, as his biographer and former law clerk Gerald Gunther observes, a "skeptic, doubtful of any absolute moral standards, [and] he considered it beyond a judge's duty and competence to impose his own moral standards upon the community."[18] In enacting the naturalization and deportation statutes, however, Congress had clearly given federal judges the task of rendering explicit judgments about "moral character." Hand conceived himself, rather like a good soldier, as obliged to accept this assignment; as he put it in the 1929 opinion, "while [the Congress] leaves as the test accepted moral notions, we must be loyal to that, so far as we can ascertain it." Hand obviously struggled to find some formula to avoid a simple conflation of his own moral code and his communal responsibility as a judge applying a congressionally enacted standard. This was the goal of his invocation of the "nebulous" and "conjectural" standard of the "common conscience" and "what people generally feel."

Nonetheless, in his specific judgments in naturalization and deportation cases, it is hard to avoid the conclusion that Hand did elide any distinction between his personal morality and his public responsibility—though perhaps he would have claimed a happy conjunction of these two in the cases that happened to come before him. Thus in the 1929 case he rejected deportation for violation of prohibition laws, and in 1939 he rejected deportation for conviction of possession of burglary tools. (The conviction had come when the alien was "a boy of seventeen and such boys might delight in having jimmies to pry their way into buildings or boxes or barrels merely for curiosity or mischief. Those would be crimes, it is true, but they would not be morally shameful.")[19] In 1947 he approved citizenship over the government's objections, as noted, for a man who had violated incest laws to marry his niece; in 1949 he approved citizenship for a man who, as Hand put it, "in a moment of what may have been unnecessary frankness" admitted to the naturalization examiner that he "now and then" had sexual intercourse with unmarried women, which the examiner saw as disqualifying indication

of bad moral character;[20] in 1961 he approved citizenship over government objections for a man who had lived with and had two children with one woman while remaining married to another[21] and, in another case that same year, for a man who had been convicted as a "scofflaw" by failing to answer twenty-three parking tickets.[22]

Hand thus had a generously forgiving attitude in applying the moral conduct standard for citizenship which was already well developed when he came to judge Louis Loftus Repouille—and this attitude was quite apparent in the memorandum that he circulated on November 21, the same day that Jerome Frank sent out his memorandum voting to approve Repouille's petition. Hand wrote:

> I have been in two minds about this tragic case, and it is particularly trying to be forced to a decision by the fact that, if this unfortunate man had only waited from September 22, 1944, to October 13, 1944, he would have had an absolutely clean slate. However, there is no use in trying to avoid a decision, for it is directly in our path. We have only recently repeated what we said before: i.e. the test in such cases is not how we personally should judge the conduct in question morally, but how it stands in the feelings of people generally. . . . I don't know how we are to apply such a test in a close case. In the case at bar there are probably hundreds of thousands of people in the United States who would think that it was immoral to relieve a family of so terrible a burden; and hundreds of thousands who would not. How are we to say which is the dominant view? And yet that is what we are called upon to do.
>
> On the whole I am disposed to take as a fair sample of what the common man thinks the judgment of the twelve men and women who heard the case and rendered the verdict. It is apparent that they did not morally disapprove of what this man did. That legally he committed murder there is not the faintest doubt; that he did not commit manslaughter in the second degree, there is also not the slightest doubt: that is the crime of killing without meaning to kill. Moreover, even this patent evasion of their strict duty they were unwilling to accept without a recommendation of the "utmost clemency." Thus we have an instance of the deliberate and premeditated killing of a human being without any of the excuses which the law allows, and without the least questions as to all the facts; and in the face of this a jury exercising their power, but contrary to law, finds a verdict which has not a shadow of support in the evidence and which they qualify as much as they can in the aid of mercy. It seems to me that it would be absurd for us to close our eyes to the fact that they did not think that the act was morally reprehensible. Perhaps it adds something that the judge did not punish him.
>
> To hold this is not to say that it should be permissible to kill such a person with governmental authority; obviously, whether it should be permissible or not, the decision cannot be left in the hands of an individual. But that is not inconsistent with saying that the common morals may not condemn such an

act in such a setting, when the law affords no means by which it can be law-fully committed. Not only does the law at times fail to keep pace with current morals; but current morals at times may make the law morally inadequate.[23]

Thus on November 21, the court of appeals stood ready to approve Repouille's citizenship, and his moral character, by a two-to-one vote. The court's decision was announced on December 5. But by that time, Learned Hand had changed his mind; by a two-to-one vote, with Jerome Frank in dissent, the court rejected Repouille's petition. There are no internal court records or diary entries in Hand's private papers that di-rectly record the reasoning process that led him away from his initial in-clination—an inclination so strong that, during his entire thirty-four-year tenure as an appellate judge, from 1924 until 1961, Repouille was the only person whose naturalization Hand was prepared to reject based on flawed moral character.[24] Hand was not himself morally offended by Repouille's murder of his disabled son; this was the clear implication of his concluding observation in his memorandum that "the law affords no means by which [Repouille's act] can be lawfully committed" but that "current morals at times may make the law morally inadequate." But notwithstanding his willingness to give moral approval to—or perhaps more precisely, to withhold moral condemnation from—law violations in other naturalization cases, he held back in Repouille's case, which, unlike the others, involved the intentional infliction of death. Hand's moral struggle—and the complex ambivalence of his resolution—are apparent in his final opinion in the case; and the opinion itself implicitly lays out both the technique and the logic of the dominant ethos at that time of imposing invisibility on death and disability.

Repouille's initial act in 1939 was not simply or even most impor-tantly a violation of law; it was a breach of this specific ethos of invisi-bility regarding death and disability, as was made clear in the internally contradictory official response at the time by both the judge and jury, neither approving nor condemning his action. Repouille's untimely ap-plication for citizenship in 1944 was an even more direct breach of this ethos, in its effectively explicit demand for moral approval of his act. Hand's response to this demand is even more openly revealing of the of-ficial story in these matters—a highly visible public act which paradox-ically tries to impose invisibility on Raymond Repouille's death.

Hand first set out the facts of Repouille's offense, which he adapted and elaborated from the sympathetic account in the probation report. After quoting the description of Repouille's son as "an idiot and a phys-ical monstrosity," Hand observed that Repouille "had four other chil-

dren at the time towards whom he has always been a dutiful and responsible parent; it may be assumed that his act was to help him in their nur-
ture, which was being compromised by the burden imposed upon him
in the care of the fifth."²⁵ Hand then set out the naturalization statute's
standard for judging good moral character by relying on "the generally
accepted moral conventions current at the time"; and he continued,

> [In this] case . . . the answer is not wholly certain; for all we know . . . there
> are great numbers of people of the most unimpeachable virtue, who think it
> morally justifiable to put an end to a life so inexorably destined to be a bur-
> den to others, and—so far as any possible interest of its own is concerned—
> condemned to a brutish existence, lower indeed than all but the lowest forms
> of sentient life. Nor is it inevitably an answer to say that it must be immoral
> to do this, until the law provides security against the abuses which would in-
> evitably follow, unless the practice were regulated. Many people—probably
> most people—do not make it a final ethical test of conduct that it shall not
> violate law; few of us exact of ourselves or of others the unflinching obedi-
> ence of a Socrates. There being no lawful means of accomplishing an end,
> which they believe to be righteous in itself, there have always been consci-
> entious persons who feel no scruple in acting in defiance of a law which is re-
> pugnant to their personal convictions, and who even regard as martyrs those
> who suffer by doing so. In our own history it is only necessary to recall the
> Abolitionists. It is reasonably clear that the jury did not feel any moral re-
> pulsion at his crime. . . . [Their "absurd verdict" and their clemency recom-
> mendation] showed that in substance they wished to exculpate the offender.
> Moreover, it is also plain, from the sentence which he imposed, that the
> judge could not have seriously disagreed with their recommendation.²⁶

To this point in his opinion, Hand seemed on his way toward approving Repouille's petition; but then he swerved aside. "One might be
tempted to seize upon all this as a reliable measure of current morals;
and no doubt it should have its place in the scale; but we should hesi-
tate to accept it as decisive, when, for example, we compare it with the
fate of a similar offender in Massachusetts, who, although he was not
executed, was imprisoned for life." Hand continued:

> Left at large as we are, without means of verifying our conclusion, and with-
> out authority to substitute our individual beliefs, the outcome must needs
> be tentative; and not much is gained by discussion. We can say no more than
> that, quite independently of what may be the current moral feeling as to le-
> gally administered euthanasia, we feel reasonably secure in holding that only
> a minority of virtuous persons would deem the practise morally justifiable,
> while it remains in private hands, even when the provocation is as over-
> whelming as it was in this instance.²⁷

This brief paragraph is all that Hand offers to rebut his more extensive discussion of the high moral status of conscientious law-breaking—his invocation of the Abolitionists' willful disobedience of slavery laws, his comparison of the nullifying purpose of the jury's verdict in Repouille's case, and his dismissal of the moral imperative of "the unflinching obedience of a Socrates." His concluding statement that only "legally administered euthanasia" would be considered "morally justifiable" by more than "a minority of virtuous persons" appears flatly inconsistent with his earlier statement that it was not "inevitably an answer to say that it must be immoral to do this, until the law provides security against the abuses which would inevitably follow, unless the practice were regulated." The two observations stand virtually beside one another in his brief opinion, but he made not even a gesture toward reconciling them. This self-contradiction might satisfy poetic standards, as Walt Whitman famously observed; but Hand's internally inconsistent meandering seems markedly unsatisfactory as a conventional exercise in judicial opinion-writing.

If the inconsistency in his juxtaposition of the moral worthiness of the Abolitionists and the moral imperative of obedience to law were not apparent enough to any reader, Hand made an even more obvious about-face in the final paragraph of his opinion. "We wish to make it plain," he said, that if Repouille filed a new petition for citizenship, there could be no objection to his moral character under the naturalization statute. In effect, Hand said, the statute required a finding of good moral character only during the five years preceding an application; and by 1947, Repouille's 1939 murder of his son was irrelevant: "the pitiable event, now long past, will not prevent Repouille from taking his place among us as a citizen."[28]

Hand's invitation for Repouille to submit a new petition was a debatable legal proposition. The government's brief in Repouille's case had maintained that the five-year time period in the naturalization statute did not exclude consideration of moral taint arising from earlier conduct.[29] (Imagine if Adolf Eichmann had waited until 1950, five years after the concentration camps had been closed down, to file his petition for American citizenship.) There was also precedent that when a naturalization petition had been denied on moral character grounds, the petitioner must wait an additional five years before reapplying.[30] Hand did not acknowledge these difficulties. They would have obstructed his underlying purpose in Repouille's case—neither to approve nor to condemn what he had done, to refuse any judgment of his "moral charac-

ter" notwithstanding the clear requirement of the naturalization statute that some dispositive determination must be made. In this sense, Hand's goal was to throw a shroud over Repouille's act. This was Hand's sense of "the generally accepted moral conventions current at the time" regarding Repouille's murder of his son—to make this administration of death socially invisible.

Hand was virtually explicit about this goal: "the outcome," he said, "must needs be tentative; and not much is gained by discussion." By our contemporary lights, at least, this observation violates ordinary standards of judicial conduct. Judges are supposed to decide disputed issues, not circumnavigate "tentatively" around them; judges are obliged to reveal their reasoning, not decline to engage in discussion. This is the conventional account today of a judge's duty—and this was the basis for Jerome Frank's dissent in the Repouille case.

In his initial memorandum to his colleagues, Frank had stated that he was prepared to accept Repouille's naturalization petition. He took a different tack, however, in his dissent. There is no need, he said, for judgment to remain "tentative"; the "correct statutory test (the test Congress intended)," Frank said, "is the attitude of our ethical leaders [and] that attitude would not be too difficult to learn." Frank concluded that more discussion, not less, would be required for this purpose:

> [C]ourts are not utterly helpless; . . . judicial impotence has its limits. Especially when an issue importantly affecting a man's life is involved, it seems to me that we need not, and ought not, resort to our mere unchecked surmises, remaining wholly (to quote my colleagues' words) "without means of verifying our conclusions." Because court judgments are the most solemn kind of governmental acts . . . they should, I think, have a more solid foundation. I see no good reason why a man's rights should be jeopardized by judges' needless lack of knowledge.[31]

To remedy this deficit, Frank stated that his court should have remanded the case to the district judge with instructions to conduct a public inquiry to ascertain "the attitude of our ethical leaders" about Repouille's actions and, based on this "data," the judge should reconsider his conclusion. "Then," Frank concluded, "if there is another appeal, we can avoid sheer guessing, which alone is now available to us, and can reach something like an informed judgment."

In his majority opinion, Hand did not address Frank's proposal; but he was privately scornful of it. In a letter Hand wrote a week later to Justice Felix Frankfurter, he implied that Frank's suggestion was so out-

landish (he referred to it as an "outré dissent") that it didn't deserve any
response:

> I assume that he expected the district judge, sua sponte [on his own initia-
> tive], to call the Cardinal, Bishop Gilbert, an orthodox and a liberal Rabbi,
> Reinhold Niebuhr, the head of the Ethical Cultural [sic] Society, and Ed-
> mund Wilson; have them all cross-examined; ending in a "survey." Oh, Jesus!
> I don't know how we ought to deal with such cases except by the best guess
> we have.[32]

There was a deep disagreement here between Hand and Frank about the
nature of moral judgment, but this disagreement was obscured by the
way Hand propounded his own position, both in his majority opinion
and in this letter to Frankfurter. In his opinion, Hand justified his conclusion that "the outcome must needs be tentative" on the ground that
the court was "without means of verifying our conclusion, and without
authority to substitute our individual beliefs." This justification virtually invited Frank's riposte that a method of independent verification
was indeed available and that the way to avoid imposition of judges' individual beliefs was to rely on the judicially compiled beliefs of "ethical
leaders" other than judges.

Hand's real reason for insisting on a "tentative" resolution was, however, different and more interesting than absence of verified information; if this were his problem, then his subsequent observation that "not
much is gained by discussion" would be unintelligible. Hand did not
adequately explain himself in this opinion. He did offer his basic rationale in an earlier statement—not in a judicial opinion but, appropriately
enough for Repouille's case, in a 1944 address administering the oath of
allegiance to an assemblage of newly naturalized citizens. The theme of
his address was the meaning of and the proper means for protecting the
"liberty" of Americans. He dismissed the protective value of courts,
laws, and constitutions; "believe me," he said, "these are false hopes.
Liberty lies in the hearts of men and women; when it dies there, no constitution, no law, no court can save it; no constitution, no law, no court
can even do much to help it." Nor is liberty, he said, "the ruthless, the
unbridled will, [the] freedom to do as one likes. . . . [This] freedom soon
becomes a society where freedom is the possession of only a savage few;
as we have learned to our sorrow." Hand then turned to the definition
of liberty: "The spirit of liberty," he said, "is the spirit which is not too
sure that it is right."[33]

This is the core conviction that lay behind Hand's observation that

the outcome in Repouille's case "must needs be tentative." The central focus of his opinion in the case was the same as the theme in this address: the meaning of liberty. His invocation of the Abolitionists' struggle to abolish slavery through civil disobedience, "acting in defiance of a law which is repugnant to their personal convictions," gave a libertarian context and justification for Repouille's lawbreaking. But Hand immediately drew back from characterizing this violation as "morally justifiable," notwithstanding what he saw as the "overwhelming provocation" for it; Repouille's action too much conveyed the negative aspect of liberty as Hand had described it—"the ruthless, the unbridled will, [the] freedom to do as one likes . . . where freedom is the possession of only a savage few."

When Hand spoke of this savagery in 1944, the war against Nazi Germany was in full force; his insistence that liberty at its core is "the spirit which is not too sure that it is right" clearly conveyed a contrast with the totalitarian mindset. His discomfort with the task of determining "moral character" imposed on judges by the naturalization statute was of a piece with his disdain for judges and constitutional adjudication as the protectors of fundamental moral values; and from this attitude of pervasive moral skepticism, it is not surprising that he dismissed Frank's proposal for a fact-based inquiry into the opinions of ethical leaders. The underlying premise of Frank's proposal was that Repouille's action could be definitively characterized by some authoritative source as either morally justified or not. Hand denied that this was desirable or, indeed, that it was a coherent possibility.

Hand could not consistently hold to his posture of moral skepticism without falling into a paradoxical conviction of moral certainty about the value of skepticism; but whatever his inconsistencies as a systematic philosopher, he did not flee from the imposition of moral judgment as a judge. In this role, he was prepared to render definitive judgments about the moral character of applicants for citizenship (though his forgiving attitude carried a strong flavor of condemnation toward the moral absolutism of the naturalization officials who were routinely prepared to find evil in any lawbreaker). Repouille was an exceptional case for Hand; and that is why it is instructive for our purposes. Hand self-consciously saw himself acting in the "expert" role that Jerome Frank envisioned for the panel of ethical leaders that he would have convened before the district court. Hand made his "best guess," as he put it in his letter to Felix Frankfurter, about the dominant moral evaluation in American society at that moment regarding Repouille's act. His esti-

mation was that it could neither be approved nor condemned; it could not be acknowledged.

There was a terrible cost to this practice. The cost was implicitly revealed, though unacknowledged, by the fact that neither Hand nor Frank referred in their opinions to Louis Repouille's murdered son by his given name. Raymond Repouille was anonymous, faceless, nothing but "an imbecile and an idiot"—not only in the judges' rendering but in the government's brief, in the probation officer's report before the district court, in all of the papers regarded as officially relevant to reaching a judgment about the father's moral character, except for the formal indictment in the original murder charge against him. If the father had surrendered custody of his son to public officials, they would have effectively erased his identity; they would have hidden him in a remote institution until he died and kept him in such brutal custodial conditions as to hasten that death. Repouille's real offense was in taking direct, visible responsibility for his son's death—as Learned Hand implied in his refusal to approve "euthanasia . . . while it remains in private hands." The accepted official response was concealment, death accomplished by burial while alive.

Judge Frank's dissenting proposal for a judicial inquiry about the moral status of Raymond Repouille's murder did not envision that the court would investigate this official policy of live burials in state retardation institutions. But the hypocrisy involved in state prohibition of private murder would most likely play some role in the deliberation of "ethical leaders" about the father's action. Indeed, no less an ethical leader than Justice Oliver Wendell Holmes had stated just twenty years earlier that "it is better for all the world, if instead of waiting to execute degenerate offspring for crime, or to let them starve for their imbecility, society can prevent those who are manifestly unfit from continuing their kind." This was not a private communication by Holmes, but a public proclamation in a Supreme Court opinion upholding state-compelled sterilization of "mental defectives." [34] In his unpublished memorandum to his colleagues, Frank had already indicated his willingness to endorse Repouille's moral character notwithstanding the killing; and it seems likely that he anticipated endorsement of this position in the public hearing he proposed.

Learned Hand's initial instinct had also been to forgive Repouille's act, and it is not clear what constrained him from publicly acting on this inclination. It seems clear in retrospect that public endorsement of these murderous impulses toward retarded people carried consequences be-

yond unacknowledged, hypocritical acceptance. The avowed public policy of sterilization in this country was later cited by German physicians and officials as part of their justification for similar policies in the late 1920s, which had led them to avowed euthanasia of institutionalized retarded people in the succeeding decade; and this acknowledged policy seemed to serve as a justificatory prelude to the mass killings of other social undesirables (as Holmes had put it, "those who already sap the strength of the State") in the concentration camps.[35] By 1947, when Repouille's case was decided, this was public knowledge; the Holocaust had been revealed, and the German physicians tried at the Nuremberg tribunal for "medical experiments" that involved killing the experimental subjects had justified their conduct in part by invoking American sterilization practice and Justice Holmes's encomium specifically.[36]

Hand knew about the Holocaust, of course; he had been outspoken in his concerns before and during the war about the brutality and wrongfulness of Nazi racial policies.[37] It is not clear, however, that he saw any strong link between these events and the possible consequences of official endorsement of Repouille's act; he did, after all, speak sympathetically about Repouille's act and motives in his opinion. Nor does it appear that any of the judges were aware of the connections between Repouille's action in 1939 and the immediately preceding jury acquittal of another father who had murdered his "imbecile" son, or of the subsequent paternal infanticide reportedly prompted by the publicity about Repouille's act. Even if the judges did not know about the expansive consequences of publicly justified killings that had been specific to Repouille's case, it seems more than plausible that the possibility of such consequences would have worried them, and that this concern played some role in Learned Hand's decision to join the disposition initially urged by Augustus Hand based on the need for "most careful safeguards" necessary to make so-called " 'mercy killing' . . . accord with social safety." [38] The safeguard that these two judges ultimately agreed upon was in one sense to embrace the dominant social policy of their day—to rebury the entire transaction away from public view.

This reassertion of social invisibility—this ratification of the cultural "denial of death"—is not, however, the basis for my embrace of Hand's position as a model for social regulation of death-dispensing actions. He might have wished that the "mercy killing" could be concealed from public view—as he somewhat plaintively envisioned in his parting observation that if Repouille submitted a new citizenship application "the pitiable event [would be] now long past." But Hand's invitation was an

inescapably public act, as were the criminal prosecution and the disputed naturalization proceedings leading up to this wistful hope for forgetting. He could not succeed in suppressing any public knowledge of Repouille's murderous act; all that he truly could accomplish was to enact a resolution that visibly faced in opposite directions at the same time—to disapprove and approve of Repouille's moral standing in the same gesture. Perhaps he imagined that this resolution, like a double negative, would somehow cancel itself, leaving no residue for public attention.

In fact Hand's double negative was a precise and very public expression of ambivalence toward the death of Raymond Repouille. He could not succeed in burying the event; and this was not his fundamental goal. Hand's fundamental goal was to oppose Jerome Frank's insistence that ambivalence was the wrong response. Frank asserted that, once the question had become a matter of public attention, judges should definitively proclaim whether Raymond's death was a moral good or a moral evil. His position anticipates the post-1960s willingness of judges, who found themselves confronted with the sudden public visibility of death-dispensing decisions regarding terminal illness, abortion, and capital punishment, to issue definitive proclamations about their moral status. In rendering such proclamations, moreover, these judges were models for a more generalized social ambition for everyone to impose rational order on the administration of death.

Hand stood against this impulse. His openly avowed ambivalence arose from many possible sources—perhaps from his conception of the democratic ethos as "the spirit which is not too sure that it is right"; perhaps too from an unwillingness to imagine a profoundly impaired person like Raymond Repouille as a full-fledged member of the common moral community. Whatever the full meaning of this studied irresolution for Hand, his articulation of his conclusion points in the direction that I would commend. As he put it, in determining the "moral feeling as to legally administered euthanasia, . . . the outcome must needs be tentative." As I would reformulate this conclusion, social arrangements for death-dispensing decisions must be visibly tentative. The arrangements must not simply be motivated by ambivalence—for that is inevitable, whatever our contrary wishes for univalent, definitive dispositions; the arrangement must demonstrably express and thereby effectively acknowledge ambivalence regarding the basic question whether death is a moral good or a moral evil.

CHAPTER THREE

DEATH AT WAR

In the Presence of My Enemies

From the end of the Civil War until the mid-twentieth century, an undeclared state of warfare existed between the "mentally normal" community and people with mental retardation or mental illness, between Whites and Blacks, and between the "living" and the "dying." These hostilities were masked, and open aggression thereby somewhat contained, by increasingly rigid social and geographic segregation restricting or even (beginning in the nineteenth century for the "mentally abnormal" and in the twentieth century for the "dying") entirely eliminating face-to-face interactions. In all of these relations, the dominant party was clear; yet those who were "normal / White / not dying" nonetheless often imagined themselves intensely threatened by those who were "abnormal/Black/dying," and accordingly their aggressions against these enemies intensified.

We can see increased techniques of isolation and surveillance of mentally disabled people in the enactment of sterilization statutes in the early twentieth century, which followed the late-nineteenth-century confinement of increasingly large numbers of such people in geographically remote institutions. We can see the "normal majority" fears in Justice Holmes's embattled approbation of the sterilization statutes "in order to prevent our being swamped with incompetence" by "those who already sap the strength of the State."[1] We can see similar techniques in the increasingly rigid and pervasive patterns of social segregation and enforced rituals of deference imposed on Blacks from the latter part of the nineteenth century. Fears among Whites were expressed in celebratory accounts of the Ku Klux Klan (as in D. W. Griffiths's film, *Birth of*

a Nation) and, without pretense of restraint, in the lynchings and vigilante patrols by the Klan.[2] We can see the intensified social containment and fear of the "dying" in the transfer of their custody from family and clergy to physicians, in the increasingly relentless warfare by physicians against death and, by easy extension, against the dying patient subjected to endlessly aggressive treatment, and in the culmination by the mid-twentieth century of the shift from home to hospital as the socially preferred, segregated locus for dying.

Today we are in a new era in all of these social relations. We must, however, try to understand the social dynamics underlying the change in relationships, the reasons why the old battle lines drawn against mentally disabled people, African Americans, and the dying were replaced by the 1970s with promises of peace and hopes of reconciliation. These promises and hopes have not been fully implemented by the "normal/White/living" majority; but the old vocabulary and specific forms of containment and surveillance have clearly changed. Unless we understand the dynamics driving these changes, we run a significant risk of recreating the old oppressions in new, and newly disguised, forms.

The central focus of this book is social treatment of death and dying; and I intend only briefly, and in a drastically abbreviated way, to allude to an equivalent social treatment of mentally disabled people and African Americans. I do so because of the striking parallels I see among these three social contexts: warfare waged by the dominant majority, driven by exaggerated fears of counteraggression or contamination; techniques of social isolation as the preferred instrument of aggression (typically masked by professions of beneficent motives toward the subjugated group, but often erupting into murderous violence); and a roughly similar time frame for the establishment and then the abandonment of these overtly hostile terms of social relations.

In order to understand the future implications of the contemporary abandonment of this hostility, the most important question to pursue through these parallels is why the old terms of battle were changed. The change occurred in a kind of nested progression among these three groups: beginning with the suddenly visible claims of African Americans in the 1950s,[3] the new visibility of claims in the 1960s by and on behalf of mentally disabled people (self-consciously using the vocabulary of Black civil rights, seeking the same substantive remedies of "integrated communal participation and acknowledgment," and pursuing these remedies initially and primarily through the federal courts),[4] and then the visibility of claims in the 1970s by and on behalf of dying people

(also claiming liberation through a judicially recognized "right to self-determination" against physicians' domination and abuse). The crucial factor for change was not in the awareness of abuse by the scorned groups, of the falsehoods behind the masks of majority beneficence; critiques of the terms of subjugation had always been available from the experience of the oppressed. The key was instead a sudden new willingness, and even a new capacity, among the oppressors to hear this critique and to acknowledge its correctness.

Where did this sudden new willingness and capacity come from? One view is that the pathway to moral enlightenment was revealed by the newly insistent complaints of the oppressed and that this revelation suddenly fell into the hearts of the oppressors as if from heaven. This view implies that our forebears were blind but we now see, and will thus avoid, the evil that they inflicted. This is a falsely comforting view. The oppressed "suddenly" spoke for themselves because the oppressors were ready to hear them; and, in my view, this readiness came because the old terms of battle no longer satisfied the oppressors. The old terms did not fit a new regime; the apparent victory imposed by the oppressors on the subjugated groups was no longer convincing (on either side of the battle lines); the oppressors' fears were no longer adequately appeased by the apparent surrender and subordination of the rigidly segregated prisoners of war.

What was this new—this newly unsettled and unsatisfying—regime? I believe we can locate the novelty and the urgent, unaccustomed fearfulness it provoked by focusing attention on the social treatment of dying people and by applying a psychosocial analysis that Freud offered in 1915, explaining why the terrible experience of World War I would lead to a new comprehension of death for Europeans. Freud's analysis can help us understand why our Civil War precipitated a new understanding, new fears, and new social subjugations regarding dying people (and, for the same underlying reasons, regarding the newly freed Black slaves and mentally disabled people), and why American experiences following World War II, which were climactically felt during the Vietnam War, ultimately unsettled these post–Civil War arrangements.

In the midst of the European experience of World War I, Freud saw a new "sense of estrangement in this once lovely and congenial world." In 1915 he published an essay entitled "Thoughts for the Times on War and Death." Though the full horrors of extended trench warfare were yet to come and the heroic trumpeting from the home fronts had not yet faded away, Freud spoke of a sudden distance that had opened from

a "once lovely" world.[5] He identified two bases for this estrangement. The first was "disillusion" prompted by the "low morality shown externally by states which in their internal relations pose as the guardians of moral standards, and the brutality shown by individuals whom, as participants in the highest human civilization, one would not have thought capable of such behavior."[6] By disillusion, Freud meant literally "the destruction of an illusion" about the moral reliability of states and individuals—the destruction, as I would put it, of accustomed confidence in the caretaking character of social life. The second source of estrangement, which Freud viewed through his unique psychoanalytic perspective, was "the disturbance that has taken place in the attitude which we have hitherto adopted towards death."[7]

In elucidating this second source, Freud began with a premise that became the most frequently cited proposition from this essay—"the assertion that, at bottom, no one believes in his own death, or, to put the same thing in another way, that in the unconscious every one of us is convinced of his own immortality."[8] Freud's treatment of this assertion in the body of his essay is, however, more complicated (even contradictory) than the conventional citations of it acknowledge. Freud first suggested how fictionalized presentations of death are truly in the service of denial, of maintaining our unconscious belief in immortality: "In the realm of fiction we find the plurality of lives which we need. We die with the hero with whom we have identified ourselves; yet we survive him, and are ready to die again just as safely with another hero." (This could explain how our contemporary inundation with violence and death in the mass media is in the service of denying rather than acknowledging mortality.) But Freud then continued, "It is evident that war is bound to sweep away this conventional treatment of death. Death will no longer be denied; we are forced to believe in it. People really die; and no longer one by one, but many, often tens of thousands, in a single day." Freud thus basically appears to claim, notwithstanding his initial assertion, that denial of death is not an unconscious inevitability but a psychologically defensive maneuver that external events can overwhelm. Freud offered this diagnosis: "in my opinion the bewilderment and the paralysis of capacity, from which we [now] suffer, are essentially determined . . . by the circumstance that we are unable to maintain our former attitude towards death, and have not yet found a new one."[9]

We can use Freud's insight to account for two turns in American social patterns—the late-nineteenth-century extrusion of dying people and the mid- to late-twentieth-century "rediscovery" of dying people.

For the first turn, the American experience of the Civil War appears amply to confirm Freud's observation about the impact of large-scale warfare on general social attitudes toward death. In the direct aftermath of that war, a new constellation of attitudes took hold—most saliently, the bestowal of exclusive custody over dying to the newly organized medical profession and the social commitment to render death "invisible"; the grip of this postbellum conception remained firm until the 1970s.

The devastation of the Civil War was beyond any prior experience of warfare; the number of lives lost still exceeds the total of all other American casualties from the Revolutionary War through the Vietnam War. When the Battle of Shiloh was fought in April 1862, it was the bloodiest battle ever to take place in the Western Hemisphere; by the end of the war the deaths at Shiloh ranked only seventh among Civil War battles. On a single day, September 17, 1862, some 4,800 soldiers were killed at Antietam. In the entire Revolutionary War, only about 4,000 had died. In just two months in 1864, 65,000 northern and 35,000 southern soldiers were killed or wounded. This amounted to three-fifths of the total number of combat casualties suffered by the Union army and the smaller Confederate army during the entire previous three years. At the end of the war, slightly more than 2 percent of the American population had died (1.6 percent of the more populous North and 2.8 percent of the South); in World War II, by contrast, 0.28 percent of the American population was killed. There were 384,000 American war-related deaths in World War II. If the World War II ratio had equaled the northern proportion in the Civil War, some 2.5 million would have died; if the ratio had equaled southern proportions, the total would have been almost 5 million.[10]

In his Second Inaugural Address on March 4, 1865—little more than a month before the end of the war and, three days after that, his own assassination—Abraham Lincoln gave public testimony to the desolation of the war:

> Neither party expected for the war the magnitude or the duration which it has already attained. Neither anticipated that the *cause* of the conflict [slavery] might cease with or even before the conflict itself should cease. . . . If we shall suppose that American slavery is one of those offenses which, in the providence of God, must needs come, but which, having continued through His appointed time, He now wills to remove, and that He gives to both North and South this terrible war as the woe due to those by whom the offense came, shall we discern therein any departure from those divine attributes which the believers in a living God always ascribe to Him? Fondly do we hope, fervently

do we pray, that this mighty scourge of war may speedily pass away. Yet, if God wills that it continue until all the wealth piled by the bondsman's two hundred and fifty years of unrequited toil shall be sunk, and until every drop of blood drawn with the lash shall be paid by another drawn with the sword, as was said three thousand years ago, so still it must be said "the judgments of the Lord are true and righteous altogether."

This passage, which occupies almost one-fourth of Lincoln's entire address, is the most extraordinary public statement made by any president in our history. Here was the commander in chief of the nation's forces, then still engaged in battle, openly acknowledging the possibility that the entire nation itself was so deeply stained by wrongdoing—by the maintenance of "American slavery," not Southern slavery—that God had decreed a war that would only end when all the nation's wealth "shall be sunk" and "every drop of blood" drawn from a slave shall be repaid in blood "both North and South [in] this terrible war as the woe due to those by whom the offense came."

Two years earlier, in his address at the consecration of the Gettysburg battlefield cemetery, Lincoln had spoken in a different register—insisting that the lives lost there would lead to "a new birth of freedom," that the war deaths had a redemptive implication for "those who here gave their lives that [this] nation might live." [11] In his private correspondence in 1863, Lincoln had confided more despairing thoughts; [12] but it is hard to conceive greater sorrow than his public utterance two years later.

The most dramatic implication of the war on the public experience of death, beyond the sheer impact of the unprecedented numbers of war dead, was the geographic remoteness of those dying on the battlefield from family and communal witness and from involvement in ritual practices that had traditionally provided structure and comfort in the experience of dying. In practical terms, this distance shattered those practices and led to a new social arrangement, the development of undertaking as a distinctive professional service and a new respectability for the practice of embalming corpses. Before the war, embalming itself was "almost exclusively" performed by the newly emerging group of professional medical researchers, and undertaking as a profession was socially "peripheral"; from the practical imperative of the war, because bodies had to be shipped long distances from the battlefield to home, embalming by professional undertakers became "an accepted, highly visible, and desired treatment for the dead." [13]

The war was also instrumental in transforming social attitudes toward the status of dead bodies. Before the war, the use of cadavers for

medical research and education had been advocated by physicians and endorsed by some state legislation, but the practice remained well outside general public tolerance, and was even regarded as scandalous. The establishment of the Army Medical Museum in 1862 for the systematic collection of "specimens of morbid anatomy" from battlefield corpses was an early ratification of the changing attitude that acknowledged a socially sanctioned custodial relationship between the medical profession and the dead.[14]

There was also a significant change regarding the physician's role in certifying death. For about a century before the Civil War, there had been widespread public concern, if not hysteria, about the possibility of premature burials. This concern had grown from the discoveries of eighteenth-century physicians about techniques for resuscitating apparently dead people, through such means as artificial respiration and electrical cardiac stimulation. These medical advances did not inspire public confidence; to the contrary, they fueled a "public panic" because they undermined lay and professional confidence that death could be definitively diagnosed.[15] Before the eighteenth century—indeed, for the entire previous history of Western medicine—physicians played no role in certifying death. Hippocratic medical ethics explicitly prohibited physicians from treating terminally ill people; "the doctor's duty was to forecast an impending demise and then withdraw from the case, not to remain in attendance long enough to diagnose or certify actual death."[16]

Following the Civil War, however, physicians took on the exclusive social (and increasingly state-mandated) role of certifying death. Physicians held themselves out to the public as entirely confident in their technological capacities to identify death and thus to dispel any public concern about premature burial; by the end of the nineteenth century, this concern had virtually faded away. "Although innovations in diagnostic technology played a role, the new medical self-assurance owed more to social forces than to technical discoveries. . . . [P]rofessional and public confidence in [the scientific basis of the new death tests] derived far more from the new deference to technical expertise, than from a careful analysis of the underlying evidence."[17]

This post–Civil War public bestowal of custody over death to physicians did not occur because of the high social status of the medical profession or because of the demonstrated capacities of medical science to cure disease. For most of the nineteenth century, "the medical profession was generally weak, divided, insecure in its status and income, unable to control entry into practice or to raise the standards of medical

education."[18] By the end of the century, however, the social stature of the profession had been considerably enhanced; most notably, between 1870 and 1900 state legislatures across the country had required licenses for medical practice and given licensing authority to organized representatives of the profession itself.[19] In the late nineteenth and early twentieth centuries, medical science was indeed responsible for significant health improvements, not only in general public health measures but in new treatments provided in individual encounters between physicians and patients.[20] These demonstrable medical successes did significantly affect public eagerness to rely on and defer to physicians. But these successes came after—and thereby both ratified and intensified—the public's prior, war-driven wish to turn toward this source of caretaking authority, to find new meanings for death.

The most dramatic expression of this search for new meanings and the newly central role played by the medical profession was in the changed social attitude toward abortion immediately following the war. This change was accompanied, moreover, by the same sense of unmasked wrongdoing regarding prior practice and self-righteous proclamations of moral progress that have characterized the post-1960s reform charges regarding the medical abuse of dying people.

Abortion was the first place where American society self-consciously and explicitly turned to physicians both to combat death and to take exclusive custody of its occurrence. During the first half of the nineteenth century, American physicians had experienced a sharp decline in public favor. A democratic ethos swept the country that debunked all sorts of claims for professional expertise, not only among physicians.[21] By the mid-nineteenth century, stimulated by concerns about public support for unsubstantiated health claims of various "folk" practitioners and by concerns for their own social prestige and economic status, physicians who regarded themselves as "regular" or "scientific" practitioners banded together, founding the American Medical Association (AMA) in 1849. Holding fast to the teachings of scientific medicine presented something of a dilemma to these newly organized professionals, however, since the mid-century advances in empirical scientific investigation recurrently led to the conclusion that the remedies available to medical practitioners were as demonstrably ineffective as the cures promoted by their unscientific competitors. The best guide that could emerge in these early moments of scientific research was for practitioners to provide precise diagnoses of illness and then do nothing to interfere with the body's own restorative capacities. However much wisdom might rest behind their cautious empiricism, physicians' primary insistence on do-

ing no harm—their new professional ethos of "therapeutic nihilism"—was not exactly a strong rallying cry for attracting the confidence or the fees of prospective patients.

Scientific-minded physicians could, however, unite on action campaigns to expose the false claims of their competitors; and early in its organizational existence, just ten years after its founding, the American Medical Association resolved to embark on a national campaign to change public tolerance for abortions. There had been an apparent consensus in American society that a fetus was not alive until the pregnant woman could feel its movement in her womb, the moment of "quickening" around the end of the first trimester. Until this moment, the fetus was regarded as inert, and there were no legal restrictions on abortions, which were regularly and openly performed by various folk practitioners as well as through self-devised home remedies. At its 1859 convention, the AMA formally challenged this consensus and seized on abortion as a focal issue for its public self-presentation as a profession. These physicians claimed that scientific evidence clearly established the fetus was alive from the first moment of conception and therefore that any abortion was a killing. Like any killing, it could only be justified as an act of self-defense, that is, to save the mother's life; this justification, moreover, could be determined only as a scientific proposition by a scientific physician.[22]

Unlike other items on their professional agenda, such as licensing of medical schools and restrictions on unqualified practitioners, the AMA campaign against abortion achieved stunning and relatively rapid public success. Between 1860 and 1880, some forty state and territorial legislatures made abortion criminal at any stage of pregnancy, except where a physician decreed its life-saving necessity (the so-called "therapeutic exception").[23] This dramatic shift in public attitudes and legal policy was the first expression of the approach toward death that by 1950 had become dominant throughout American culture—that the entire subject was the exclusive preserve of scientific medicine.

There is a considerable irony that this medical colonization should have begun with abortion, since the initial problem for imperialistic physicians was to persuade the public that abortion involved death. Indeed, as the leading scholar of the nineteenth-century legal change observed, "the vigorous efforts of America's regular physicians [were] the single most important factor in altering the legal policies toward abortion . . . [and the] origins and evolution of anti-abortion attitudes in the United States owe relatively little to the influence or the activities of organized religion."[24]

The ultimate expression of the medical custody of death and its con-sequent social invisibility was the changed location of dying from home to hospital. This shift did not occur, however, until long after the Civil War. It was only in the 1930s that hospital confinements were provided for people who were obviously beyond any medical curative possibilities; this was when, as Philippe Aries classically described it, "hidden death in the hospital . . . began very discreetly" and then "became widespread after 1950" so that "the dying man's bedroom . . . passed from the home to the hospital."[25] This considerable intervening time does not neces-sarily break any causal connection with the Civil War experience. The hospital as an institution was simply unavailable in the nineteenth cen-tury as a place for general medical custody of dying. As late as 1870, the exclusive social role of hospitals was to serve as almshouses for the poor; their modern institutional conception as indispensable adjuncts to the ordinary practice of medicine first took hold between 1890 and 1920, and they subsequently became the virtually exclusive sites for the provi-sion of medical care for all seriously ill people.[26]

This institutional transformation in the social role of hospital as a preferred locus for medical curative efforts did not necessarily dictate that hospitals would become the place of choice for dying. (The estab-lishment of the modern hospice movement demonstrates that this link-age need not follow; its organizational premise is that hospitals should be reserved for curative efforts and that dying patients should be cared for at home with the assistance of hospice personnel or, though only in particularly difficult cases, in special hospice facilities.) By the 1930s, however, the institutional transformation of hospitals during the pre-ceding half-century made it plausible to use them for carrying out the social role regarding death that had been bestowed on physicians in the wake of the Civil War.

By the 1950s the public grief and disorientation of the Civil War ex-perience was no longer a direct impetus for the massively expanded use of the hospital as the locus for dying. As the sociologist Paul Starr has ob-served, the growth of industrialization and urbanization after the mid-nineteenth century "meant less labor power and physical space at home to handle the acutely ill"; changes in hospital hygiene and antiseptic surgery made hospitals less dangerous places at the same time that the moral taint associating them with impoverishment faded; changes in lo-cal transportation networks made specialized hospitals more accessible for use by families and physicians; these factors in turn created new op-portunities for specialization among physicians and an impetus to base

their practices in offices and hospitals rather than traveling to the homes of their middle- and upper-class patients.[27] Nonetheless, the public turn toward physicians following the Civil War had established a pathway which, to use a rough metaphor, expanded over time to a superhighway. With careful archeological excavation, we can see how the initial direction chosen for the pathway remained a hidden but nonetheless persistent influence in the mapping of the larger and now exclusively visible thoroughfare.

The wounded distress to which Lincoln had testified at the end of the Civil War was salved in the succeeding generations by the general public turn toward medical authority. This custodial role for medicine was expanded exponentially during the late nineteenth and early twentieth centuries from death as such to all manner of disorder, to both physical and social disabilities and deviancies. Medicine kept confident hold of this custodial enterprise until the mid-1960s, the moment when unaccustomed public questions were raised and charges of medical abuse and betrayal of trust were suddenly given wide public currency. This was the beginning of a precipitous decline in the prestige of medicine, in its capacity to inspire social confidence in its discharge of caretaking custodial functions.

To understand this second turn in American treatment of death and dying people—from the nineteenth-century extrusion to the mid-twentieth-century "rediscovery" of dying people—we must understand important parallels in our experience of the Civil War and the Vietnam War. Unlike American participation in the European-based world wars, both the Civil War and the Vietnam War were widely unpopular in this country while they were being fought.[28] Both wars ended in defeat for American forces; this was clearly so for Vietnam, and it was also obviously true for the Southerners in the Civil War, who were forced to rejoin the American Union as a result of their defeat. More fundamentally, both wars were quickly followed by a pervasive public conviction that they had been pointless enterprises—unnecessary and even foolish in their inception, excessively and uncontrollably destructive in their execution, and irredeemably wasteful in their consequences.[29] In these three characteristics, the wars were unique in American experience—uniquely unsettling for public confidence in the reliability and nurturant quality of American social institutions, and uniquely pressing into unaccustomed public visibility questions specifically about death, its social meanings, and the possibility of adequate social reassurances. The stripping away of illusions about the civilized character of our own country and

the reliability of our social caretaking, coupled with an unprecedented intimacy with death on a massive scale, thus first occurred for us in the mid-1860s and then again in the late 1960s.

The dramatic rise in public deference to medical authority between the end of the Civil War and the decade of the Vietnam War has been ascribed by Starr to late-nineteenth-century and early-twentieth-century "revolutions in technology and social organization [which] altered perceptions of the value of specialized knowledge. The new order of urban life and industrial capitalism generally required people to rely more on the complementary skills of others and less on their own unspecialized talents."[30] The consolidation of professional control in highly articulated organizational formats, based on claims to special expertise, was not unique to medicine during this time; it was the common pattern in a broad range of social and economic enterprises.[31] As Starr concludes, "on the shoulders of broad historical forces, private judgment retreated along a wide frontier of human choice."[32]

The 1960s surely saw no diminution in the complexity and vast scale of American social and economic organization and the consequent need for specialized knowledge, both generally and for medical matters specifically. Nonetheless, in medicine most notably, this long-standing "retreat" of the ethos of "private judgment" was dramatically reversed. Individual self-determination, consumer control in the deployment of medical technology, became the order of the day, beginning in the mid-1960s. One might say that this was a reaction against technical complexity and organizational scale; but if, as Starr suggests, these societal characteristics were important causal agents in originally producing deference to medical and other experts, it is at least puzzling to understand why the deference should reverse itself though the characteristics remained equally salient. It is more plausible that the technical and organizational complexities had been widely prized because they offered apparent order and comfort, and that public deference to the experts, the high priests of this complexity, exploded into charges of purposeful abuse and betrayal when the promised order and comfort were no longer apparent.

The Vietnam War was the immediate precipitant for this sense of lost order and comfort, our "estrangement," as Freud put it, "in this once lovely and congenial world." American deaths in the Vietnam War did not come close in raw numbers or in proportion of the population to the losses of the Civil War. But the Vietnam War experience was equally disillusioning—in the sense of shattering the prior illusion of social

safety—for a different reason. Since the end of the Second World War, American society had been struggling—with some apparent success—to stave off the sense of social devastation and betrayal that had flooded across Europe through the combined experiences of the two world wars. After the First World War, this country had quickly retreated from acknowledged engagement in European affairs; our late and relatively limited involvement in the war itself permitted this distancing maneuver. We did not retreat in the same way after the Second World War, but we nonetheless magnified every opportunity to differentiate our experience from their obvious physical and moral devastation.

Our economic strength and our bountiful gifts for European reconstruction were one clear basis from which to maintain differentiation. In another register, the sudden surge of attention to the oppressed status of American Blacks—the new public receptiveness for their complaints and the growing commitment for remedial action, climaxed by the civil rights legislation of the mid-1960s, the so-called Second Reconstruction—was precipitated by the felt need to differentiate this country from the racist practices of Nazi Germany, our enemy. It was a source of considerable embarrassment that the Nazis could claim support for at least their initial impositions of segregation and humiliation on Jews from our state policies toward Blacks, and could even find support for their extermination of Jews in our state policies of sterilization and life-term confinement of retarded people.[33] This embarrassment had pragmatic implications for international relations with newly independent African and Asian nations, especially as Cold War competition for their allegiance emerged with the Soviet Union.[34] More fundamentally, however, the clear similarities between the racist impulses underlying the American Jim Crow and Nazi regimes and the exterminative impulses evident in our treatment of retarded people and their treatment of Jews pressed forward the intensely uncomfortable question whether "it could happen here"—the *it* of the Holocaust.[35]

More than a half-century has passed since the German concentration camps were opened to full public view. We are no closer today than in the immediate shock of 1945 in our understanding how the governmental machinery of an entire nation could embrace a purposeful policy of murdering an entire vulnerable minority group. The depth of betrayal—for ordinary standards of morality, for any sense of sympathetic connection with fellow-citizens, with neighbors or remote acquaintances, with fellow human beings—is still staggering to contemplate, still virtually beyond comprehension, no matter how deeply we dig into

the historic record of who did what to whom, who actively collaborated, who knew but remained indifferent.

For some twenty years after 1945, no one did dig deeply into this record. In particular, the criminal prosecutions of Nazi leaders at Nuremberg could not find a conceptual framework to address the Holocaust. The basic prosecutorial claim was that the Nazi leaders were guilty of waging wrongful aggressive warfare against other nations. Evidence was introduced at the trials of the mass killings in the concentration camps, but this evidence was not clearly linked to the explicit charges of criminal conduct. It was as if this purposeful killing of an entire group of helpless people by their own government was so unimaginable, so incomprehensible that it could not be fit into any ordinarily recognized category of wrongdoing.[36]

Though we have by now devised a vocabulary for this wrongdoing (genocide, or crimes against humanity) and even begun to establish regularized institutional structures for adjudicating and punishing such wrongdoing, this has not been the most consequential reexamining of the Holocaust that has occurred following the first wave of disbelief and denial. The most striking change in this country, at least, has been the shift from the question "could it happen here" to the widespread assertion that "it *has* happened here." The initial discomfort about parallels in American and Nazi racial policies gave impetus to the civil rights movement in order to prove that we were fundamentally different.[37] This discomfort was not, however, fully appeased by the limited though tangible successes of that movement; the unease persisted and led over time to a reexamination of our history and our contemporary social life in order to prove that we were not so different. The American embrace and expansion of slavery before the Civil War and the betrayal of Black Emancipation after that war, the physical annihilation of Native Americans in the nineteenth century and their cultural obliteration in the twentieth, the expropriation and confinement of Japanese citizens during World War II—all of these race-based group injuries became much more salient elements of American historic self-understanding by the mid-1960s than in the preceding postwar years.

Charges of parallels between Nazi and American conduct were not restricted, moreover, to domestic uses of race. The first condemnation of the American use of the atomic bomb in Japan to receive widespread public attention was published in 1965—a condemnation not simply based on racism but on the criterion of waging aggressive warfare against innocent civilian populations by which the Nazi leaders had been found

guilty at Nuremberg.[38] At this same time, moreover, the Nuremberg charges against German doctors were directly applied to the conduct of American medical researchers. In 1966, Henry Beecher, a professor at the Harvard Medical School, published an article in the *New England Journal of Medicine* demonstrating that research subjects were routinely subjected to risky experiments without their prior consent[39]—thus corroborating a claim that the German physicians had originally put forward in their defense at Nuremberg.[40]

These various charges of direct similarities between Nazi and American conduct were not universally admitted; they were heatedly disputed by many people and substantially discounted by most. But their currency in public debate, their attainment of sufficient public plausibility to require some response and refutation rather than casual dismissal, was testimony to some persistent discomfort on the topic. Between 1967 and 1975, the Vietnam War brought this discomfort into sharp and painful public focus.

Direct accusations of Nazi parallels became commonplace among opponents of the war in charges of racial genocide against innocent noncombatants or the disproportionate use of Black American soldiers in the war ("Black men killing Yellow men in a White Man's war to protect the land stolen from the Red Man" was the catch phrase for this charge). These charges were passionately contested by supporters of the war and resisted by some of its less agitated opponents. Beneath this noisy confrontation of opposed views, however, there was a shared—though unacknowledged—common complaint. The opponents of the war believed that they had been betrayed by their government—that basic virtues of honesty and morality were being utterly and surprisingly dishonored. Supporters of the war believed that they too were being betrayed—not by their government but by their fellow citizens who opposed the war in a way that dishonored basic virtues of patriotism and social solidarity with American soldiers whose lives were at risk. On both sides, there was a deep sense of betrayal, of broken trust in values that had been understood as the elemental bond of social life.

This was the same common theme that characterized the abortion debate which erupted following the Supreme Court's 1973 decision in *Roe v. Wade*—the belief on both sides that traditional caretakers had betrayed their most fundamental obligations to protect helpless dependents. For pro-life advocates, the betrayal came from mothers intent on killing their helpless fetuses—and, even worse, not restrained but abetted by Supreme Court Justices. For pro-choice advocates, the betrayal

of adequate caretaking came from physicians, abetted by state legislators, forcing vulnerable women to bear unwanted children. In the depth
of feeling that characterized the conflicts over the Vietnam War and
abortion—the shared sense of betrayal, of imminently threatened social
isolation and consequent vulnerability—there is a reverberation from
the impact of the Holocaust in shattering assumptions about the reliable safety of social life.

The betrayal enacted by the Holocaust on German citizens of Jewish
descent—the betrayal by government, by fellow citizens, by neighbors
and acquaintances—was complete, sudden, and unexpectedly murderous. Strenuous efforts were made in this country after the war to "ex-
ceptionalize" this betrayal—only Nazi "barbarians" or "madmen," only
Germans with their long history of militaristic cruelty or their long
history of "exterminative antisemitism" would ever behave this way.
Not normal people. Not my government, not my fellow citizens. And
certainly not against me, because I am not a member of any vulnerable
minority. I am invulnerable, unlike the victims of the Holocaust, because . . . because . . . or *can* I trust my neighbors and acquaintances, my
fellow citizens and my government not to decide, arbitrarily and un-
predictably, that I am expendable and easily disposed of, like the victims
of the Holocaust?

This is the underlying question raised by the most publicly insistent
complaints about American life following the Second World War—the
complaints raised by proponents of Black civil rights, of mentally disabled people's rights, of women's rights, of fetal rights, of the rights of
American soldiers sent to die in Vietnam's rice fields. Even the immediate postwar accusations of Communist conspiracies at the highest levels
of American government conveyed this same underlying theme of betrayal and infliction of terrible harm on vulnerable subordinates. The
public force of these complaints—their power to attract widespread
empathic identification and passionate support among people who
were not themselves members of one or another of these categorical
groupings—is testimony to the applicability to American society after
World War II of Freud's diagnosis: "a present sense of estrangement in
this once lovely and congenial world" that we resisted for some twenty
years but that finally erupted in the waging of the Vietnam War.

In one way, at least, the Vietnam War was a more shattering public
experience than any other event in our history, including the vastly destructive Civil War. This was not simply in its unprecedented conclusion
as a complete defeat; it was because this ending only confirmed the

worst forebodings implied by the public discord that had accompanied the entire war—the belief that the American deaths were meaningless, without any comforting redemptive value. Even Lincoln's terrible summation in his Second Inaugural Address offered a meaning for the war deaths, of suffering incurred as the cost of past sins. No public figure, no president or other acknowledged representative, gave public voice to any characterization of the Vietnam War directly comparable to Lincoln's stark accounting. But there was one event that did publicly and officially present this latter war in its most desolate terms: the construction of the Vietnam War Memorial on a site adjacent to the Lincoln Memorial in Washington, D.C. In the same way that Lincoln's Second Inaugural Address broke with any prior public memorializations of a national war, so the Vietnam War Memorial was unlike any other public monument to war dead in American history. In Freud's terms, moreover, the design of the memorial spoke to "the disturbance that [had] taken place in the attitude which we [had] hitherto adopted towards death."

The design chosen in a national competition for the memorial was the work of Maya Lin, then a graduate student in the school of art and architecture at Yale University. Her design had a stark simplicity: a black marble wall with the names of the American war dead inscribed in the chronological order of their deaths, cut into the earth so that the memorial was invisible from a distance and could be fully seen only by walking down into it. Lin later recounted that the initial inspiration for her design came from the Yale University war memorial; located in one of the most heavily traveled corridors in the university grounds, at the entrance hallway of its largest auditorium, this memorial has etched in white marble the name of every graduate who died in all American wars, beginning with the "War of the Revolution."[41]

There are, however, striking differences between the Yale memorial and what Lin took from it for our own time. The only words on the Vietnam Memorial are the names of the war dead. The Yale memorial also lists each individual's graduating class year, armed service branch and rank, and specific date and place of death. The Yale memorial thus inscribes a network of social affiliations for each of its dead that is absent from the Vietnam Memorial wall.

Each of the Vietnam War dead seems more alone, more isolated from social involvements. At each end of the wall, there are thick books that visitors can consult with a more detailed network of identifications for each name, along with a map location of the name on the wall; but these

books stand apart from the memorial itself, whereas the dense affiliations listed in the Yale memorial are intrinsic to it. Even more revealing, the Yale memorial is studded with captions above the lists of names: "Peace Crowns Their Act of Sacrifice"; "Devotion Gives a Sanctity to Strife"; "Memory Here Guards Ennobled Names"; "Courage Disdains Fame and Wins It." Above the passageway from the memorial corridor to an exterior rotunda is the motto, "We who must live salute you / who have found strength to die." There are no such homilies, no such noble sentiments, engraved anywhere on the Vietnam Memorial wall. Whatever meaning its visitors ascribe to the listing of Vietnam War deaths, no communal formulation is provided.[42]

Maya Lin took very little in fact from the Yale war memorial. Its pervasive assertions of social affiliations and assigned meanings were out of place in 1981 when the Vietnam War memorial was commissioned. One difference between the two memorials, however, ultimately points to a deeper commonality. The Yale memorial was first proposed in June 1865, immediately at the end of the Civil War; no plan was adopted, however, until some thirty years later and, even then, the actual construction was delayed for almost twenty more years. When the memorial was finally dedicated in 1915, it addressed only the Civil War dead. Five years later, a listing of the graduates killed in World War I was added, and it was not until the late 1920s that Yale deaths from earlier wars were inscribed.[43] The Yale memorial, like the Vietnam War memorial, was thus originally conceived and executed in reference to a single war experience—the trauma of the Civil War. The Yale tribute, however, was not completed until fifty years after the end of its memorialized war; even the initial planning for it had stalled for some thirty years. One reason for this long delay is apparent on the face of the lists of the Civil War dead: Yale graduates had fought on both sides of the Civil War; and it was not easy to decide how the Union and Confederate dead should be treated— whether they should be listed "separate but equal" (to borrow a formula from another aspect of the Civil War aftermath), whether the defenders of the Union and of Emancipation should be treated differently from their adversaries, or whether no distinctions at all should be drawn among any Yale graduates killed in the war.

The course ultimately chosen was to visibly identify whether the dead had served in the Union or Confederate forces but to intermix the names with no discernible pattern based on that specific affiliation. The inscription on the floor beneath the flanking wall tablets testifies to the basic tenet adopted: "To the Men of Yale who gave their lives in the Civil War

the University has dedicated this memorial that their high devotion may live in all her sons and that the bonds which now unite the land may endure." It had taken a half-century before Yale University could find the words to give communal meaning to the Civil War, before Lincoln's prescription could be fulfilled "to bind up the nation's wounds." The Vietnam War memorial could follow so much closer to the conclusion of this divisive conflict only by withholding any ascription of meaning to its deaths. The absence of this ascription did, however, in itself convey a distressing implication—that the deaths suffered in that war were without communal meaning, that each combatant died alone.

This deepened sense of the loneliness of death and the consequent necessity for each individual to devise meaning for his own death was not restricted to these memorialized few. This was the common response to "the disturbance that [had] taken place in the attitude which we [had] hitherto adopted towards death," not only in warfare but generally. As the Vietnam War precipitated the abandonment of medicine as death's custodian—the post–Civil War reparative effort—so the national memorial to the Vietnam War spoke to the impetus for, as well as the pathos of, the new model, the self-determination ideal.

Social changes in deep-seated assumptions about possibilities for comfort in the face of death do not occur quickly. The unsettling experiences of warfare prompt many people to reassert traditional conceptions, to hold ever more tightly to their promise for salve and salvation in response to these new events. Thus the full depths of the challenge presented by World War II to Americans' sense of social safety was kept at bay through complacent insistence that *It* could never happen here— that the transformation of a civilized, highly cultivated nation into barbaric tyranny, marked by the genocide of a vulnerable minority among fellow citizens had no possible relevance to past historical practices or future prospects in American life. Even when the Vietnam War exploded this complacent self-differentiation, many Americans still clung to the prior sources of social comfort. Thus, as Robert Putnam has observed, "In April 1966, with the Vietnam War raging and race riots in Cleveland, Chicago, and Atlanta, 66 percent of Americans *rejected* the view that 'the people running the country don't really care what happens to you.' In December 1997, in the midst of the longest period of peace and prosperity in more than two generations, 57 percent of Americans *endorsed* that same view." [44]

In retrospect, we can now see how profoundly the experience of the Vietnam War, both in its own terms and as an amplification of the most

distressing implications of World War II, undermined the belief in the promise of American institutions for protecting against social vulnerability generally and for providing comfort against the wrongfulness inherent in death specifically.

The 1970s were a watershed moment, just as the 1860s had been. As Andrew Delbanco has elegantly portrayed the shifting locus of American emblems of "hope," the Civil War marked a turning away from principal reliance on God, on the comforting standard of organized religion, toward a new idealization of the Nation, the Union as redemptive (given public expression by Lincoln's eloquence and powerful symbolization by his martyrdom). This cultural construct, as Delbanco sees it, remained salient until the 1970s, when the Self displaced the Nation as the symbolic repository of our "hope" for ourselves, of the "story that leads somewhere and thereby helps us navigate through life to its inevitable terminus in death."[45]

In retrospect, the cult of the Nation provided its comfort in substantial part through the subordination—the social degradation and physical annihilation—of vast numbers of people, of "resident aliens," one might say, such as African Americans, mentally disabled people, dying people, and others similarly vulnerable to imposed invisibility. Will there be an equivalent list of victims sacrificed on the alter of the Self, and specifically of self-determination in death and dying? Does the contemporary shift in the symbolic locus of comforting hope in the face of death represent moral progress, a break in the prior cycle of triumphalist self-righteousness masking terrible abuses of vulnerable people—or is this contemporary movement only another turn of the wheel?

CHAPTER FOUR

JUDGES AND DEATH

Lead Me in Paths of Righteousness

The underlying elements in our shifting cultural attitude toward death—the loss of faith in traditional caretakers and the emergence of individual self-control as a preferred alternative to the old ethos—were revealed with special vividness in two court cases in the 1970s: the *Quinlan* decision in the New Jersey state courts and the U.S. Supreme Court's decision in *Roe v. Wade.* Closer attention to the decision-making process in those two cases will illuminate these elements and point us toward an appreciation of the essential weakness, the pathos, of the self-determination ideal as an adequate alternative, as an imagined antidote to the lost faith.

The trial judge in the *Quinlan* case was determined to rely on the old faith, the century-long tradition that death and dying were the exclusive province of physicians. In his final opinion, Judge Robert Muir stated, "The nature, extent and duration of [medical] care is the responsibility of the physician. The morality and conscience of our society places this responsibility in the hands of the physician. What justification is there to remove it from the control of the medical profession and place it in the hands of the courts?"[1] Judge Muir was not accurate in his sweeping assertion that courts always deferred to physicians regarding medical care; he ignored the well-established use of malpractice suits, and even of possible criminal prosecutions, against physicians regarding the "nature, extent, and duration" of medical care. But Muir was not thinking about these after-the-fact judicial controls. He did not want to decide whether to remove the mechanical ventilator that appeared to be prolonging Karen Ann's life; he did not want to decide whether Karen Ann should live or die. He wanted doctors to decide.

In particular, the judge showed his reliance on medicine's territorial imperative by refusing to enter Karen Ann's hospital room. Her parents' attorney formally requested that the judge go to Karen Ann's bedside so that he could see her condition and her suffering for himself. Muir responded, "I'm an ordinary human being, with ordinary thoughts, ordinary emotions. . . . I have the right to go and see Karen, if I think it is appropriate. However, given all of the considerations and recognizing that emotion is an aspect that I cannot decide a case on, I do not think it's appropriate for me to go see her. So I'll deny the motion."[2] Judge Muir's reticence was, however, out of step with the times. The new imperative was apparent before the state supreme court unanimously reversed him, in the very fact that the case had been brought into the judge's courtroom.

The initial, and the most puzzling, question about Karen Ann's case is why a court proceeding ever occurred, why the time-honored process for non-public decision making by her physicians and family was superseded. The first step toward answering this question is provided by an account of the case subsequently published by Karen Ann's parents; they recounted that after they had concurred in the attending physician's recommendation to discontinue treatment, he unexpectedly called them to report that the hospital administrator and attorney had vetoed this course and insisted on obtaining a prior court order before proceeding.[3] The hospital was run by a Catholic order of nuns, but this religious affiliation provides no obvious explanation for the administrator's resistance; Catholic doctrine approving the discontinuance of "extraordinary" treatment had been propounded in a 1957 papal encyclical, and Karen Ann's hopeless diagnosis, coupled with her apparent dependence on a mechanical respirator, clearly fit the application of this doctrine (as the family priest had found).[4]

There was, however, an intervening event since the promulgation of this encyclical that might have changed the context of this decision for some American Catholics, at least within the upper reaches of the church hierarchy. The Supreme Court's 1973 decision in *Roe v. Wade* had profoundly offended Catholic religious sensibilities and ultimately provoked reexamination within the American church of attitudes toward withholding medical treatment from anyone; the hospital bureaucracy's unexpected action may have reflected an early instance of this. The bureaucrats did not, however, adamantly refuse to remove their patient from the respirator; they instead insisted on judicial authorization. The hospital attorney undoubtedly had some role in suggesting this novel require-

ment; and he was most likely influenced by another legal development that was apparently unrelated to *Roe v. Wade*.

By 1975, the medical profession felt itself embattled, to an unprecedented degree, by courtroom challenges in malpractice litigation. In previous years, physicians and their attorney-advisors confidently relied on the awed deference of judges and lay juries to protect them from litigative complaints by dissatisfied patients; but this deference seemed less automatic by 1975. Fear of subsequent liability might have seemed outlandish in Karen Ann's case; her family was prepared to sign any release from liability that the hospital attorney might have drafted, and there was simply no prospect that the local district attorney would initiate a criminal prosecution for discontinuing the respirator. Nonetheless, physicians and their attorney-advisors were in the grip of fantastic imaginings on this score. A 1973 report by a federal commission, convened by the Secretary of Health, Education, and Welfare to investigate the "malpractice crisis," conveys the professional paranoia of the time in its opening observation:

> Even the doctor who has never been sued is ever conscious of the sword of Damocles hanging over his head. As one member of the Commission put it, "As a physician, I live in an aura of fear—fear of suit. . . . It may be hard to believe but we are a frightened profession. The doctor feels put upon. He feels nude on the corner of the Main Street of life. He often tries to cover himself with pride, and even occasionally arrogance, only to find himself being castrated. He really doesn't want to believe the hostility he feels."[5]

Whatever the full basis for these imaginings, opinion polls at the time did indeed confirm that physicians had experienced a sharp drop in public favor. In 1966, 73 percent expressed "great confidence" in the profession while in 1973, this number had dropped to 44 percent; by 1993, it was only 22 percent. During this interval, moreover, physicians' status had diminished in an even more hurtful way. In 1966, public confidence in physicians had been considerably higher than for all other professional groups, including lawyers and political leaders; by 1973, confidence in the other groups had also fallen, though by a somewhat smaller margin than for physicians—from 40 percent with "great confidence" in 1966 to 25 percent in 1973. Whatever comfort physicians could take in their relatively higher status vanished, however, by 1993. Between 1973 and 1993, the opinion poll measures regarding other professions remained almost the same while confidence in physicians crept downward; and in 1993 itself, for the first time the ratings for physicians dipped below the

others—22 percent to 23 percent.[6] This may or may not be castration; it was certainly an unkind cut for the medical profession.

Quinlan's transformed status from a medical to a legal case can thus be understood as a kind of preemptive strike initiated by the hospital attorney against the possibility that some legal retribution might somehow, someday fall on the hospital unless they obtained advance judicial exculpation before following the wishes of her physicians and family to disconnect the respirator. The hospital attorney in the Quinlan case now believed, as others in the medical and legal professions were coming to believe, that physicians could no longer confidently act on their own authority but must turn to judges to rehabilitate their authority.

This rehabilitative imperative is also the key to understanding *Roe v. Wade*. It has become conventional in retrospect to cite *Roe* as a triumphant proclamation of the principle that every woman has sovereign autonomy over her own body; this was the proposition that the New Jersey Supreme Court distilled from *Roe* to find a constitutional right in *Quinlan* for every person to control the provision of life-prolonging medical treatment. *Roe* was not, however, originally conceived in this framework; the justices in that case were centrally concerned with protecting the authority of physicians rather than the autonomy of their women patients. It is important to recapture this original meaning of *Roe* to show how the initial impulses that prompted judges to reassert medical custody remained powerful even as their rhetoric transmuted into a celebration of individual autonomy in death-dispensing choices.

Though organized medicine had succeeded after the Civil War in persuading the American public that all abortions were murderous acts, the newly restrictive laws were not an absolute prohibition but a virtually explicit license to physicians to engage in killing as they alone saw fit, through application of the statutory permission to abort fetuses in order to protect the mother's life. If one accepted at face value the premise strenuously advocated by postbellum organized medicine about the homicidal character of abortion, then by 1900 the practical application of the "therapeutic exception" by individual physicians had become so varied and flexible as to suggest a medical practice of widespread murder.

There was, moreover, hardly a conspiracy of silence within the medical profession on this matter. In fact, physicians regularly and publicly admitted that the seemingly narrow therapeutic exception was given quite expansive and also quite discrepant application by individual practitioners. Numerous articles were published in medical journals between 1900 and 1950 debating the merits of varying interpretations of this ex-

ception—whether "protecting the mother's life" meant only her physical survival or whether it meant "preserving the quality of life in the broader, more social sense of the word."[7] The articles made clear that these variant definitions reflected actual differences in practice among large numbers of physicians who were quite unembarrassed by this disclosure. In published surveys, respectable physicians acknowledged that they were performing abortions—that is to say, murdering human beings in both its "scientific" and "legal" meanings—simply to protect the mother's "mental health," or for "fetal deformity," or for "social reasons to prevent disgrace," or for "economic reasons [of] poverty." Kristin Luker, the leading scholar of twentieth-century changes in abortion policy, has observed that these publications were "debates physicians held among themselves"; between 1890 and the late 1950s, "neither the public nor individual physicians appear to have been very troubled by the discrepancies."[8]

Death by abortion was thus openly occurring but was nonetheless rendered invisible because physicians had exclusive custody of the enterprise. Borrowing from Edgar Allan Poe, this might be called the strategy of the purloined letter: evidence of the crime was hidden in plain view, and no one—neither state legislators nor prosecuting attorneys nor the general public—noticed it. This was the same social format for the dispensation of death by physicians prior to the *Quinlan* case—the format of "don't ask and we won't tell." The abortion regime established immediately after the Civil War at the instigation of the medical profession was indeed the precursor for this general pattern of regulating death. The public face of the abortion statutes embodied a clarion commitment to protect "the sanctity of life"; but buried in the interstices of these statutes was a grant of virtually complete discretion to the medical profession to perform abortions—that is, to commit "murder" as depicted within the logic of the abortion restrictions—whenever an individual physician deemed it "necessary." As with the general medical dispensation of death, this "open secrecy" of the abortion regime implicitly acknowledged the shamefulness of the act at the same time that it enabled its commission.[9]

During the 1950s, however, this social strategy began to unravel for abortion. At first the uneasiness was palpable only among physicians themselves. During this decade, medical professionals promoted a new institutional mechanism to transfer administration of the "therapeutic exception" from individual, unsupervised physicians to therapeutic abortion boards within hospitals, consisting of internists, obstetrician-

gynecologists, and psychiatrists, to provide advance review of proposed hospital-based abortions.[10] Approval by these new abortion boards was not required by any state statutes at the time; individual physicians remained free to perform abortions in their own offices or, if they were still practitioners of the fast-disappearing traditional style of "house call" medicine, in the woman's own home. But hospital-based practice was becoming common, and Luker suggests many physicians were quite willing to submit their abortion practices to the oversight of hospital boards, in order to secure "institutional support so that opponents of any given abortion decision would have to challenge an entire hospital rather than a single doctor."[11]

It is important to underscore that the newly anticipated challenges in the 1950s were seen as coming from within, not outside, the medical profession. Luker's survey of newspapers, periodicals, and other mass media as late as 1960 indicates such a dearth of public discussion as to suggest a virtual absence of any "formal 'public opinion' on abortion."[12] During the 1950s, discomfort about past abortion practice was essentially restricted to physicians, and the new establishment of hospital boards was intended to appease this discomfort. In the early 1960s, however, this uneasiness erupted into public view.[13] By the end of this decade some sixteen states had amended their abortion laws, supplanting the single prior life-saving justification with explicitly liberalized standards—primarily to protect pregnant women's mental as well as general physical health—and requiring approval of any abortion by a hospital board.[14] These new statutes were, as it turned out, only way stations toward the complete elimination of abortion restrictions; in 1970 four states—New York, Washington, Hawaii, and Alaska—ended all restrictions for first-trimester pregnancies, and *Roe v. Wade* effectively nationalized this abrogation just three years later.

The rapid emergence in public debate of this more thoroughgoing critique of restrictive abortion laws—the rejection of liberalized availability and insistence on nothing less than free choice for abortion—came from the sudden appearance of the "women's liberation" movement in the mid-1960s. The central premise of this new movement—or, more precisely, of this resurgence of feminist thinking that had been eclipsed since the 1920s—was that traditional social caretaking arrangements were fundamentally flawed, were masks for the infliction of constraint and degradation. Feminist advocates insisted that the dominant social image of women as caretakers—as wives and mothers principally committed to the nurturance of their husbands and children—was an instrument of assaultive domination at the hands of male authority.

In one sense this critique embodied the same perception of American society that was contemporaneously expressed in charges against the social treatment of people with mental disabilities—that supposedly caretaking institutions were masks for the exercise of abusive social subjugation. The feminist movement, however, added a distinctive twist to this indictment: that the traditional caretaking role itself was a form of social subjugation in its restrictive application to the lives of women. The critique of social caretaking was thus extended beyond most denunciations of the "rehabilitative ideal" in prisons and mental institutions—not simply that the promises of benevolent treatment made in the alliance between physicians or behavioral professionals and state officials were betrayed in practice but that the very idea of social caretaking was tainted and even false in its entirety.[15]

The apparent stridency of these charges provoked great controversy—but nonetheless the underlying criticism of the reliability of traditional caretaking arrangements soon became an accepted proposition by all sides in this new debate. Abortion was the context in which this ironic (and unacknowledged) agreement emerged. In the unmasking of social mistreatment of mentally disabled people, it was relatively easy to characterize the vulnerable and the powerful parties, the abusers and the abused. For abortion, however, these categories imploded. Who is more oppressed, more subjugated, more vulnerable: (a) a woman whose body is occupied by a biological organism, put there by a man who may or may not disclaim responsibility and kept there against the woman's wishes by patriarchal legal authority; or (b) a fetus whose growth to maturity is wholly dependent on a mother intent on its destruction, assisted by doctors who are supposed to protect life but have allied themselves with death and abetted by judges who are supposed to guard the public welfare but instead obstruct the rescue efforts of aroused public guardians?

The protagonists in the contemporary abortion dispute were quick to provide definitive (though conflicting) answers to this question, but each could do so only by obliterating the claim to human status for the other side. The most adamant pro-choice forces opted for the oppressed woman by insisting that the fetus is nothing but biological protoplasm, not a recognizable being; the most adamant pro-lifer forces opted for the oppressed fetus by reducing the unwillingly pregnant woman to nothing but a biological container.

The noisy certitude of these conflicting positions obscured the underlying agreement of the two sides, their shared conviction that the old promises of nurturant caretaking had been betrayed in contemporary

American society. The protagonists differed in their blame for that betrayal: the pro-choice forces indicted doctors, legislators, and patriarchal authority for subjugating women; the pro-life forces indicted mothers, doctors, and Supreme Court justices for killing fetuses. Whatever the differences in their list of traitors, the combatants had a common, and equally grim, conception of the contemporary social reality, that those who occupy the formal social roles of caretaker—doctors, mothers, judges, legislators—do not deserve confidence. Specific individuals in those roles may be trustworthy; but this determination must be made person by person, individual encounter by encounter. Occupancy of the role itself no longer provided even a presumption of reliable nurturance.

This assessment was especially grim because it ran exactly contrary to the dominant organizational characteristic of contemporary social life. Caretaking relationships that had been centered in tight-knit networks of personal ties—the family doctor, the multigenerational family itself—are increasingly gone. The bureaucratic organizations supplanting these networks offer no individualized personal assurances but only promises of role compliance; and paradoxically enough, these are the promises that the protagonists in the abortion debate understand to be utterly worthless. These protagonists are noisier in their denunciations of these promises than the rest of the population; but they also believe that they have the one clear answer to the problem that afflicts everyone but confuses most. The problem is the demonstrated unreliability of traditionally trusted caretakers.

The abortion debate has assumed such large dimensions in our public life because it vividly articulates this problem and, at the same time, vividly implies that the problem is insoluble. This is because each of the protagonists in the dispute itself has a plausible claim of abuse by traditional caretakers and each claim can only be solved at the expense of the other. The majority of the population who watch this combat from ringside sense a proposition that the combatants furiously deny—that the inevitability of loss is the true lesson in this dispute. This is not, however, a comfortable lesson. It is more comforting to hear confident prescriptions for victory, even if the prescribers disagree with one another. This is the persistent public attraction of the endlessly circular abortion dispute.

The Supreme Court's decision in *Roe v. Wade* can itself best be explained as the justices' response—their imagined solution—to this problem of lost faith in traditional caretaking. The implicit strategy of the Court majority in *Roe* was essentially the same wish that Judge Learned

Hand had pursued in *Repouille:* to rebury a question about the administration of death that had unexpectedly and uncomfortably pushed itself into public visibility. The *Roe* justices were less self-conscious than Hand in devising this strategy, and they were much less successful, but they failed only because confidence in traditional caretakers had fallen with increasing speed between 1947 and 1973, reaching a cascading pace in the years immediately before 1973.

Roe tried to hold back this deluge by demanding renewed faith in traditional caretakers—ironically enough, by indicting the existing abortion restrictions for insufficient deference to physicians. *Roe* today is conventionally understood as demanding legislative respect for each woman's personal choice; the decision has indeed come to stand for this proposition. But that was not its meaning when the case was decided in 1973. The ruling looked like a revolutionary act because it struck down the restrictive abortion statutes in forty-six states. The Court did not intend, however, to foment a revolution; its ruling was in fact deeply conservative in its motivation, even counterrevolutionary—at least in the minds of four justices: Harry Blackmun, who wrote the Court's opinion, Warren Burger, Lewis Powell, and Potter Stewart.

In his concurring opinion in the companion case to *Roe,* Chief Justice Burger stated, "Plainly, the Court today rejects any claim that the Constitution requires abortion on demand." [16] Set against the currently dominant view of *Roe,* this seems an inexplicable observation—but Burger had it right. He was refuting the dissenting claim of Justices Byron White and William Rehnquist that the Court's ruling meant that a pregnant woman could obtain an abortion for any reason that she might choose—"convenience, family planning, economics, dislike of children, the embarrassment of illegitimacy, etc." without any proof of a "threat to life or health." [17] Burger's full counterstatement was that "the dissenting views discount the reality that the vast majority of physicians observe the standards of their profession, and act only on the basis of carefully deliberated medical judgments relating to life and health. Plainly, the Court today rejects any claim that the Constitution requires abortions on demand." Burger thus assumed that the medical profession would itself impose on women the same kinds of restrictive criteria on the availability of abortion as did the state laws invalidated in *Roe.*

On its face, this appears to be a patently inadequate response to the dissenters' claim. Even if the "vast majority of physicians" accepted these restrictions, state laws might still be needed to regulate the practice of the "small minority" of "excessively liberal" physicians—unless,

of course, the Constitution prohibited any such state regulation. But this proviso simply restates the question. If the Constitution forbids such state regulation because a woman has a right to choose her own reasons for an abortion—whether she wants to protect her "life and health" or because, as the dissenters observed, she cannot afford or just "dislikes" children—then Burger's rejoinder seems to miss the point. In fact, Burger's rejoinder identified, though only implicitly, the basic underlying premise of the Court's holding in *Roe*—that the restrictive state abortion laws violated the Constitution, not because they interfered with a woman's privacy right, but because they infringed on physicians' rights to practice medicine, including the provision of abortions, as they saw fit. This was the relevance of Burger's response to the dissenters that the "vast majority of physicians . . . act only on the basis of carefully deliberated medical judgments relating to life and health." Even if there is a miscreant minority, he implied, this is no justification for state regulation.

Justice William O. Douglas also wrote a concurring opinion in *Roe*, and he did explicitly base his concurrence on the existence of a woman's "privacy right" derived from the Court's prior decision in *Griswold v. Connecticut*,[18] which overturned a state prohibition on the use of contraceptives by married couples. This was also the basis for Douglas's dissent in a case decided only two years before *Roe* where the Court majority dismissed, almost cavalierly, a constitutional challenge to abortion restrictions in the District of Columbia.[19] But in *Roe*, as in this earlier ruling, Douglas was alone in giving primacy to a woman's right to choose abortion. Justice Stewart had been the other substantive dissenter in this earlier case, but he had a very different basis for his dissent. Stewart asserted that the criminal conviction under the District of Columbia statute was invalid on the ground that "the question of whether the performance of an abortion is 'necessary for the . . . mother's life or health' is entrusted under the statute exclusively to those licensed to practice medicine, without the overhanging risk of incurring criminal liability at the hands of a second-guessing lay jury. I would hold, therefore, that a 'competent licensed practitioner of medicine' is wholly immune from being charged with the commission of a criminal offense under this law."[20]

There is some ambiguity in Stewart's position in the earlier case about whether he found physician immunity based on his reading of the D.C. statute or on his construction of a constitutional right to physician immunity. But there is no such ambiguity in Justice Blackmun's opinion for the Court in *Roe*. At the end of his lengthy and somewhat rambling

exposition, Blackmun stated this conclusion: "[F]or the period of pregnancy prior to this 'compelling' point [that is, until the end of the first trimester], the attending physician, in consultation with his patient, is free to determine, without regulation by the State, that, in his medical judgment, the patient's pregnancy should be terminated." Though earlier in his opinion Blackmun had referred in general terms to a "right of privacy" as "broad enough to encompass a woman's decision whether or not to terminate her pregnancy,"[21] he clearly emphasized by the end of his opinion that this was not the central justification for invalidating the state abortion restrictions.

Thus, immediately after his endorsement of the (presumptively male) attending physician's freedom to choose, Blackmun reiterated: "To summarize and to repeat: A state criminal statute of the current Texas type, that excepts from criminality only a life-saving procedure on behalf of the mother, without regard to pregnancy stage and without recognition of the other interests involved, is violative of the Due Process Clause of the Fourteenth Amendment: (a) For the stage prior to approximately the end of the first trimester, the abortion decision and its effectuation must be left to the medical judgment of the pregnant woman's attending physician."[22] After listing the permissible range of state regulations in the second and third trimesters, Blackmun returned to his central premise:

[Our] decision vindicates the right of the physician to administer medical treatment according to his professional judgment up to the points where important state interests provide compelling justification for intervention. *Up to those points, the abortion decision in all its aspects is inherently, and primarily, a medical decision, and basic responsibility for it must rest with the physician.* If an individual physician abuses the privilege of exercising proper medical judgment, the usual remedies, judicial and intra-professional, are available.[23]

With this stirring endorsement of "the right of the physician," Blackmun concluded his opinion; he immediately proceeded to the formal declaration that "the Texas abortion statutes, as a unit, must fall" and remanded the case to the lower court for enforcement proceedings. The pro-choice celebrators of *Roe v. Wade* focus exclusively on Blackmun's earlier reference to the "woman's decision whether or not to terminate her pregnancy"; they ignore the clear structure and repeated emphasis in his opinion that the physician's right, not the woman's, was at the center of the Court's holding.

In the companion case to *Roe*, involving a recently enacted, liberal-

ized Georgia statute which permitted abortions to protect the mother's physical and mental health, as well as her life, the Court was equally explicit in placing physicians' rights at the center of its reasoning. The Georgia statute required individual physicians to obtain approval of any abortion from two additional practitioners and then by a three-member hospital committee. The Court held that this procedural requirement had

> no rational connection with a patient's needs and unduly infringes on the physician's right to practice. The attending physician will know when a consultation is advisable—the doubtful situation, the need for assurance when the medical decision is a delicate one, and the like. Physicians have followed this routine historically and know its usefulness and benefit for all concerned. It is still true today that "reliance must be placed upon the assurance given by [the physician's medical] license, issued by an authority competent to judge in that respect, that he possesses the requisite qualifications." *Dent v. West Virginia*, 129 U.S. 114, 122–123 (1889).[24]

This citation of an 1889 Supreme Court precedent is quite revealing of the *Roe* Court's essential mindset. The late nineteenth century was the time when a visible alliance was forged between medical authority and state power in taking custody of all sorts of dependents—mentally ill and retarded people, juvenile delinquents, mentally disordered adult criminal offenders. In *Dent v. West Virginia* itself, the Court unanimously upheld a criminal conviction under a recently enacted state medical licensure law against a practitioner "publicly professing to be a physician" but without having graduated from "a reputable medical college." In this struggle between folk practice and the organized proponents of scientific medicine, the Court clearly sided with Science: "[Medicine] has to deal with all those subtle and mysterious influences upon which health and life depend. . . . Every one may have occasion to consult him, but comparatively few can judge of the qualifications of learning and skill which he possesses."[25] This was the same premise enacted by state legislatures between 1860 and 1880 in taking abortions away from pregnant women and folk practitioners and placing control in the hands of physicians.

As Paul Starr observes in his excellent study *The Social Transformation of American Medicine,* it was only in the late nineteenth century that dependence on professional authority became the dominant cultural response to public concerns about health and life. The relatively low status (and incomes) of American physicians before the Civil War

"stemmed partly from Americans' ingrained self-reliance, their disbelief in the value of professional medicine, and the ease with which competitors entered the field." [26] By the end of the nineteenth century, however, this ethos of democratic individualism had been fundamentally displaced: "Americans became willing to acknowledge and institutionalize their dependence on the professions" as, "[o]n the shoulders of broad historical forces, private judgment retreated along a wide frontier of human choice." [27] In *Roe v. Wade,* the Supreme Court struck down state licensing restrictions regarding abortion—but not in order to vindicate "private judgment," not to unravel Americans' "dependence on the professions." The explicitly avowed goal of the Court majority was to strike down state laws in order to enhance professional authority— to immunize medical practitioners, as Justice Stewart had put it two years earlier, from any "risk of incurring criminal liability at the hands of a second-guessing lay jury." As Justice Blackmun stated at the end of his opinion in *Roe,* "[Our] decision vindicates the right of the physician to administer medical treatment according to his professional judgment." The underlying impetus for *Roe* was thus deeply conservative— to reassert the traditional dominance of professional judgment in the face of challenges to their caretaking authority.

By 1973, however, this restorative effort was doomed to fail. The very terms of the effort revealed its intrinsic weakness. The physician portrayed in *Roe* was dramatically different from the physician as he appeared in his traditional caretaking role regarding abortion. In the traditional role, the physician was not acting on the basis of his independent judgment. He was exercising explicitly delegated authority on behalf of the state (which legally enacted the "therapeutic exception") and his fellow professionals (who presented a uniform face to the nonprofessional public, notwithstanding their internal disagreements about the proper standards for adjudicating the content of the "therapeutic exception"). By contrast, *Roe's* physician stands alone, on his own authority. Neither the state nor his fellow professionals (through such instruments as hospital boards) are permitted even the pretense of regulation.

The justices in *Roe* may have thought that this kind of independence, this "rugged individualism," was at the core of the physician's caretaking role; but it was not so. The core characteristic of this role was its expression of social solidarity, of a seamless concordance between corporate entities—the State and the Profession—and the individual embodiment of these entities, the Physician. This appearance of solidarity was the basic reason why the role could provide caretaking comfort for the

laity. To break this solidarity was to undermine the caretaking role itself. In the supposed service of supporting the physician's traditional role, *Roe* visibly isolated him from the sources of his social strength. *Roe* itself thus gave both unwitting testimony and unintended impetus to a general loss of confidence in the caretaking role and the nurturant qualities of our social life.

Within three years after *Roe* was decided, the Supreme Court dramatically recast the rhetorical trappings of its ruling—though without any acknowledgment that a shift had occurred.[28] The Court itself thus virtually acknowledged the emptiness of its effort to bolster physicians' authority in *Roe* by embracing the right of individual women to control the abortion decision and repudiating its explicit holding that "the abortion decision . . . must rest with the physician." The shift came so quickly, moreover, that it was almost unnoticed as such; almost all of the initial commentators on *Roe* itself, whether for or against, had construed that ruling as fundamentally grounded in the privacy rights of individual women.

The rapid disappearance of the Court's endorsement of physicians' professional authority was testimony to a dramatic shift in cultural attitudes. At this same time, the principle of individual patient choice emerged center stage in judicial rhetoric about the provision of life-prolonging medical treatment generally. The background impetus for this movement was the same as for abortion; and even more powerfully than for abortion, the underlying loss of faith in traditional caretakers revealed itself in the almost transparent insufficiency—the weakness, even the pathos—of the patient self-determination principle in accomplishing the task assigned to it. The magnitude and virtual impossibility of that task become apparent if, as we have done for *Roe*, we retrace the halting steps by which the patient self-determination principle came into its current rhetorical prominence.

The role that the Nuremberg Code has played in the evolution of the self-determination principle in American jurisprudence is the key to our understanding. The code was originally formulated as the basis for condemning medical experimentation in Nazi concentration camps; as it was translated into the basic foundation for the regulation of American physicians in the provision of ordinary medical care, its horrendous origins receded—but never wholly disappeared. This horrific provenance for the self-determination principle reveals both the significance of the memory traces of World War II in the 1970s shift in American cultural attitudes toward death and the inherent weakness of the self-determination

principle for which the Nuremberg Code is now recurrently and ritually invoked.

The Nuremberg Code was originally promulgated by the tribunal convened in that German city by the victors immediately following the Second World War. This tribunal was a legal innovation pressed by the United States on its reluctant allies, who had been initially inclined to follow past wartime practices of summary executions for defeated enemies; we were intent, however, on creating a new regime of international law to establish principles of wrongful aggressive warfare and inhumane conduct during war, as part of a new world order represented by the establishment of the United Nations. The defendants in the first Nuremberg trials, held in 1945 and 1946, were high officials of the Nazi government and military command and leading industrialists. By 1947, American officials pressed for the extension of the trials to lower echelon officials; our former allies, for various reasons, were content to leave this extended adjudicatory enterprise to us.

The so-called Nuremberg Code was formulated in 1947 by a war crimes tribunal composed entirely of American judges, to adjudicate the guilt of German doctors for experiments conducted on concentration camp prisoners. The code consisted of ten principles identified by the judges as accepted tenets for the conduct of medical research which the defendant physicians had violated in their experiments. The first of these principles, according to the tribunal, was that "the voluntary consent of the human subject is absolutely essential." This statement of priority became the basis for the subsequent invocations of the Nuremberg Code in American jurisprudence to establish the principle of patient self-determination in medical care generally.

A *New England Journal of Medicine* article published in 1997, to mark the fiftieth anniversary of the code, declared in its opening sentences, "The Nuremberg Code is the most important document in the history of the ethics of medical research. . . . It served as a blueprint for today's principles that ensure the rights of subjects in medical research."[29] Yet for the first twenty years after its formulation, this observation would have been unintelligible. It was only in the late 1960s that the code was, in effect, uncovered or rediscovered.[30] Whatever the deepest reasons for this long amnesic interval—perhaps some general inability to acknowledge the full horror of the Holocaust's occurrence[31]—there is one clearly apparent reason that the Nuremberg Code was ignored for so long in the United States. This was because American physicians specifically, and the American public generally, believed that the conduct of

the German doctors in concentration camps had no relevance to the practice of medicine, that these were Nazi zealots—sadists not scientists—who simply happened to have M.D. degrees.

This was not, in fact, an accurate account of the German experience. The physicians who conducted the concentration camp experiments were respected members of the German medical profession—many with prominent medical school affiliations and even prestigious university chairs. After World War II, for obvious reasons, the German medical profession adamantly denied this fact; but recent historical scholarship documents the high professional status of the perpetrators beyond any doubt.[32] These revelations did not, however, necessarily speak to any attributes of American medical practice. The Nuremberg Code might conceivably remain linked only to Germany, necessitated by whatever special vulnerabilities in German society led to its embrace of Nazism— a rule required "for barbarians but an unnecessary code for ordinary doctors."[33]

So it seemed until the late 1960s—but not afterward. The Nuremberg Code was then embraced as directly relevant to American medicine, but still embedded in its Nazi significations. The code, that is, was not reconceived as applicable to ordinary doctors rather than barbarians; instead ordinary American doctors suddenly seemed to have close resemblances to barbarians.

This new equation took several public forms. One was the vocabulary invoked for criticisms of medical care. Karen Ann Quinlan was characterized not simply as subject to excessive life-saving zeal by her physicians and their high-technology interventions; she was portrayed as the victim of "imprisonment" and "torture"—a portrayal that quickly spread from her case to a general public critique of medical treatment for seriously ill people.[34] Another form was in prominent public accusations that American physicians were currently engaged in research activities that directly paralleled the Nazi experiments—most notably, the Tuskegee syphilis experiment (conducted from the mid-1930s until 1973, when it was publicly exposed) where effective treatment was purposefully withheld from unsuspecting Black men in order to trace the "natural history" of the untreated illness, and the intentional infection with hepatitis of mentally retarded children for research on a possible vaccine in Willowbrook, a New York state residential institution (conducted from 1956 through 1971, and publicly exposed in 1978).[35] This purposeful infliction of harm without consent on members of vulnerable minority groups for avowed medical research purposes was, of course,

the essence of the German concentration camp experiments. Public revelations of these and similar medical experiments by reputable American physicians led to congressional hearings and the creation in 1974 of a commission to formulate protective regulatory measures, the National Commission for the Protection of Human Subjects of Biomedical and Behavioral Research.[36]

The central regulatory principle endorsed by this commission was patient autonomy, and the Nuremberg Code was prominently displayed to underwrite the proposition—as the Nuremberg tribunal judges had initially insisted—that in the conduct of the human research, "the voluntary consent of the human subject is absolutely essential." This was not, however, the only regulatory standard that the code endorsed. Of the tribunal's additional nine criteria, only one dealt with self-determination— the ninth, which specified that the subject must be free to discontinue the experiment at any time. The remaining eight criteria all relied, more or less explicitly, on the application of reasonable professional judgment—the second, for example, provided that "the experiment should be such as to yield fruitful results for the good of society, unprocurable by other methods"; the sixth stated that "the degree of risk to be taken should never exceed that determined by the humanitarian importance of the problem to be solved." The National Commission followed the Nuremberg Code in endorsing these additional criteria as well and recommended the creation of review boards within every federally funded medical research institution to assure compliance with their standards. This recommendation was the basis for the statutory requirement of Institutional Review Boards to oversee all human experimentation in institutions receiving any federal funds—in effect, covering all human research conducted in the United States.[37]

There was an internal tension in the substantive criteria of the Nuremberg Code, however, that neither the original tribunal nor the commission acknowledged. The standard demanding respect for individual consent and the criteria depending on reasonable professional judgment face in very different directions. We have become so accustomed today to the consent norm that we easily overlook the disturbing implications of this difference in direction. At the moment that the Nuremberg tribunal promulgated these standards, the tension was impossible to ignore. We must recapture that disturbing difference in order to grasp the full implications—the implicitly conveyed message—that follow from the fact that the Nuremberg judgment against Nazi concentration camp experimenters was resurrected in the 1970s to serve as the central

guide for regulating (as well as the central indictment against) the conduct of American medicine generally.

The disturbing implications can be seen if we cast ourselves back to the time of the Nuremberg judgment itself—if we imagine ourselves to be the judges in that tribunal who had presided over 133 days of testimony about the concentration camp experiments before we wrote the ten standards in our formal judgment, before we carved the stone tablets that have come to command ritualistic deference as the Nuremberg Code. During the 133 days of testimony, we judges would have heard about camp inmates placed in pressure chambers where the simulated altitude was increased until their lungs and other body organs exploded; we would have heard about inmates plunged into ice water clothed in heavy military uniforms, or stripped naked and thrown outdoors in winter temperatures, where they remained (clothed or naked) until they had frozen to death; we would have heard about inmates purposefully burnt or cut by ground glass and left untreated until they died from the infection of their wounds; we would have heard about inmates whose healthy arms or legs were severed simply to test various surgical techniques for amputations.

After hearing all of this, during more than four months of testimony, imagine that we judges adjourned to our conference room and talked among ourselves to arrive at a verdict regarding the physicians who carried out these experiments. How plausible is it, in these discussions, that any of us would say: "The basic problem with these experiments is that the subjects did not agree to participate"?

To insist on the importance, or even the relevance, of consent in these matters is surely peculiar. But the Nuremberg tribunal judges did indulge in this seemingly fantastic imagining. How could they have come to this? After hearing about these barbaric experiments for 133 days, how could they begin their judgment by proclaiming that their primary standard of moral evaluation was, "The voluntary consent of the human subject is absolutely essential"?

There is a plausible answer to this question, but it is disturbing. The answer is that no other imaginable criteria offered any comfort for the future. The fact was, as the months of testimony clearly demonstrated, that these experiments had been approved and carried out by recognized leaders of the German medical profession, by respected teachers and researchers of worldwide reputation. In the face of this social reality, other more apparently plausible condemnatory criteria—in particular, the criteria subsequently set out in the tribunal's judgment that

good physicians never purposefully inflict death or disabling injury on anyone—lacked convincing effective force.

The Nuremberg judges did not pursue the chimera that many people, including the organized German medical profession, later embraced—that the concentration camp experiments were not "good science" because they had not been carried out by reputable scientists. The judges followed a different strategy. They refused to put their trust in the existence of "civilized standards" among future professionals—neither in doctors who might consider whether to perform experiments nor in government officials who might prospectively or retrospectively judge the propriety of those experiments. The Nuremberg judges established, as their first line of defense against recurrence of these barbarities, the individual subject-patient armed with the principle of self-determination.

The implicit lesson that the Nuremberg judges drew from the trial testimony was that they could not place principal reliance on the self-restraining decency of traditional embodiments of social authority. This was the lesson taught not only by the doctors' trial but by the preceding war crimes trials of high government officials. The judges were led to their reliance on the protection of individual self-determination by the same route that had conveyed Thomas Hobbes to this conclusion three centuries earlier. Sitting in Nuremberg in 1947—surrounded by the physical wreckage of war and confronted by a human spiritual degradation beyond any previous experience—the judges could readily have imagined themselves plunged into Hobbes's state of nature where no one could trust another for protection or comfort; a time without social bonds, a "war of all against all," where everyone was at the mercy of others' unconstrained avarice and aggression. As Hobbes had seen in the aftermath of the seventeenth-century English civil war, the only predictable source for human protection in such a world was each individual's solitary instinct for self-preservation.

Hobbes also saw that perpetual warfare, where each individual could rely only on himself, was an intolerable state for human affairs, since life would necessarily be without valued meaning, would be "nasty, brutish, and short." We need not endorse Hobbes's proposed solution, that each of us should enter a social contract surrendering personal authority to one absolute sovereign, to understand the powerful truth in his diagnosis that this endless sense of personal vulnerability and consequent perpetual wariness in all human relations is unbearable. But this unendurable world is precisely what the judges at Nuremberg glimpsed—and then tried strenuously to avoid.

The contemporary invocations in American life, beginning in the 1970s, of the self-determination ideal in physician-patient relations and the self-conscious reliance on the Nuremberg Code as the source of that ideal embody the same underlying sense of betrayal and helpless vulnerability that framed the deliberations of the Nuremberg judges. The shadow of the Nazi experiments hovers in the background of our contemporary images of Karen Ann Quinlan, of the Tuskegee syphilis and Willowbrook hepatitis experiments—the images of vulnerable people subjected by predatory doctors to inhumane scientific procedures in order to benefit some dogmatic social policy unrelated to the individual welfare of the patient-subjects.

In our contemporary invocations, as in the Nuremberg judgment itself, the triumphalist recitation of the self-determination ideal masks several nagging background questions: How did these once-trusted caretakers become transformed into heartless predators? If they no longer can be trusted to protect vulnerable people, who can be trusted? Can I trust no one but myself when I am helplessly vulnerable? And even more poignantly, is it enough to trust myself when I am helplessly vulnerable?

To understand the self-determination ideal not as a trans-historical postulate but as the answer offered to these questions, questions that erupted urgently in a specific cultural and historical context, does not necessarily impeach its abstract principled justification. The constantly recited linkage between this ideal and Nuremberg, however, reveals its internal weakness—its fragility and pathos. In its ritualized contemporary invocations, the ten standards enunciated in the Nuremberg Code seem to have biblical authority and solidity, with their descending order of importance from the first commandment that "the voluntary consent of the human subject is absolutely essential." Fully understood, however, the Nuremberg Code is an emblem of war—a memorial to betrayal, disillusion, and irretrievable loss. The self-determination ideal conveys this understanding in spite of itself.

In this emblematic status, the code speaks to deeper characteristics of the self-determination ideal—that is, as I set out in the first chapter, its underlying philosophic origins in our culture and the psychological processes by which individuals in our culture come to see themselves as self-controlling Selves. Betrayal, disillusion, and irretrievable loss are at the core in both the phylogeny—that is, the cultural history—and the ontogeny—that is, individual developmental histories—of the ideal of the self-controlling Self. The weakness of the self-determination ideal is magnified in confronting the inevitability of death.

CHAPTER FIVE

DOCTORS AND DEATH

They Comfort Me

If it is true that an underlying cultural attitude about death's inherent wrongfulness has fueled past medical abuses against dying patients, the reformist move to patient self-determination would not be a reliable corrective, because dying people themselves would be prone to mirror the relentless hostility of their physicians. The stage would thus be set for reiteration of past abuses, embraced by patients in collaboration with physicians. There is, moreover, a further element in medical practice that gives added impetus to this malign possibility. Physicians' mistreatment of dying patients has arisen not simply from their condemnatory attitudes toward death but also as an expression of misgivings, of deep-rooted but ordinarily denied ambivalence, about the moral status of medical practice itself.

On its face, this observation may seem utterly implausible. Medical practice has bestowed great advantages on vast numbers of people; the physician's office is still a prized place of benevolence in our society. But this benevolence has the same status as the secularized rational conception of death: it is a clear truth widely understood as such; and yet, at the same time, there is a strong undercurrent of disbelief, a powerful contrary attitude, that remains in persistent contrapuntal tension with these rationally apprehended truths. As with the claims for patient self-determination, the existence of this ambivalence is not a reason to reject belief in the virtues of medicine or its professional practitioners. It is, however, a reason for caution, and for especially intense skepticism where some medical practice is ostentatiously dependent for its acceptability on unalloyed good motives among physicians.

The goal of this chapter is to set out grounds for ambivalence among physicians about the moral status of their professional enterprise and to identify the potentially malign consequences of this ambivalence for their patients. I mean by this ambivalence much more than the familiar complaints about greed or incompetence among physicians, which are really about some disputable number of proverbial "bad apples" in a fundamentally well-cultivated estate. I mean deeper misgivings about the moral worth of the entire enterprise of medicine—misgivings that are often glimpsed by the general public but that are felt with special intensity, and frequently denied with great adamancy precisely because of this intensity, by physicians themselves. From the discussion of the sources of this fundamental ambivalence in medical practice, we can then turn in the next chapter to consider the claims for—and the special vulnerabilities for abuse of—physician-assisted suicide, where the interlocking themes of patient self-determination and physician benevolence have come together most powerfully in the contemporary reform agenda.

In his classic observational study of surgical practice, the medical sociologist Charles Bosk was impressed and "surprised" at the ambivalence of surgeons who worked in elite hospitals on the most difficult cases with a correspondingly high fatal outcome. Bosk reported:

> I was surprised at the degree that informants sought me out to relate stories of practice that they disagreed with. . . . I knew that observers were often sought by organizational malcontents; what surprised me was that all my informants were at one time or another malcontents. . . . Disfiguring palliative operations, patient discomfort, and the openness of communications among the [surgical] ranks were the most common complaints. As a "sounding board," I was implicitly asked to play a quasi-therapeutic role: to listen without judging and to understand. The fact that I was asked to play this role so often by so many speaks . . . to the deep feelings that physicians repress as a matter of course. As a rule, we, as medical sociologists, have not concentrated enough on how fragile physician defenses are, what events disturb them, and how primal the existential material they are dealing with is. Birth, life, death are not questions that one works through definitively. We need to pay more attention to the provisional nature of the resolution physicians make to the conflicts such subjects present. . . . Like house officers (although the opportunity arose less frequently), [senior] attending [surgeons] unloaded themselves on me. It is worth noting here that I was ten years younger than the youngest attending, so the fact that they used me as a "sounding board" points to ways in which the surgeon's role remains disturbing even to those who have practiced it all of their adult lives.[1]

One of the ways that this disturbance expressed itself was in the surgeons' difficulties in distinguishing between personal and official or im-

personal dimensions of their involvement. This is apparent in Bosk's account of the professional value system that governs surgeons' response to
operating errors. He identified a descending hierarchy of values which
he called "normative," "quasi-normative," and "technical." Errors in
the technical category—that is, failures in surgical technique—were
quickly forgiven, so long as they were openly confessed. The normative
category referred to "standards of dedication, interest, and thorough-
ness"[2]—one might say, the degree of wholehearted personal engagement and even obsessive perfectionism that the surgeon displayed in his
work. Breaches in this category are essentially unforgivable—so much
so that senior attending surgeons are expected to accept personal responsibility for failures by any of their subordinates, to "wear the hair-
shirt" and openly acknowledge guilt by association, in the so-called
morbidity and mortality conferences that are regularly convened to discuss unfavorable surgical outcomes.

Bosk's intermediate category of quasi-normative breaches is even
more intensely personalized. This category refers to surgical practices
that are idiosyncratic to specific senior attending surgeons—practices
where the scientific data for preferring one approach over another are
uncertain but each senior attending has his own, typically dogmatically
held, preference. In Bosk's study, house staff rotated among various senior surgeons' teams; and on each team, these subordinates were expected to adhere to the personal dogma espoused by the team's leader,
notwithstanding that an equally senior colleague on another team would
consider a variant practice not only acceptable but imperative. In collective decisions by senior attending surgeons evaluating subordinates,
the technical merits of the conduct were essentially irrelevant; all of the
seniors agreed that subordinates were obliged to acquiesce in the personal authority of the particular team leader, even though that leader
demanded compliance in technical practices that the others adamantly
rejected. As Bosk noted, in accounting for the intensely personalized
ethic thus imposed on subordinates' conduct: "For the attending, more
than professional pride is involved in quasi-normative errors: housestaff
using their own independent judgment appear insubordinate to him.
Compliance with attending dictates, however open to debate they are,
is an indicator that a subordinate is a responsible member of the team
who can be trusted. Attendings feel that the subordinate who makes
quasi-normative errors is also likely to make normative errors: his behavior does not inspire trust."[3]

This intense personalization of surgical practice is one measure of
difficulty in distinguishing between personal and impersonal roles, lead-

ing to an exaggerated sense of personal responsibility that gives no room for subordinates to engage in scientifically supportable individual conduct. This difficulty in finding a comfortable balance between personal and impersonal also occurs in another dimension of surgical practice—a dimension that extends throughout medicine but is especially intense in surgery—the fact that bodily invasion and implicit violence are at the core of the surgeon's enterprise.

Surgeons address this fact by depersonalizing the drugged body of the patient lying on the operating table—by reimagining this person as a collection of organs, muscle tissue, and the like. This scientific conceptualization may seem easy and unremarkable in its own terms; but it has not been an automatic or easy attainment, either in the historical development of the profession or in the individual development of typical physicians. The historical difficulty is amply illustrated in the resistance of the profession to engage in open-heart surgery for some time after it had become technically feasible and therapeutically desirable to do so. The profession had to break itself loose from the mystique that surrounded the heart as the locus of each individual's "soul"—a mystique that remained unchallenged so long as invasive surgery was not feasible—and to reconceive the heart as simply another impersonal biological organ.[4] Once the personalized taboo was overcome, this historical difficulty seems easy to dismiss as a residue of superstition and magical thinking from which all of us modern rationalists have been happily liberated. But there is a close analogy to this difficulty that still intrudes in contemporary medical practice—a taboo that all physicians must confront and somehow overcome in their individual developmental pathway from lay to professional identities.

The existence and impact of this anathema are apparent in the encounter with the so-called first patient of every medical student—the dead body confronted and dissected in the first-year anatomy laboratory. As a historical proposition, medical professionals and the lay public engaged in a prolonged struggle before the use of human corpses for medical education and research was accepted by the mid-nineteenth century—before the practice could be scrubbed of its "ghoulish" personalization. In contemporary medical education, this purging is still discernible in various ritual practices that routinely frame medical students' encounter with their cadavers.

It is especially notable that no medical student is ever told the actual name of the cadaver. Virtually no more information than the individual's age at death is provided; anything else is revealed by the corpse it-

self and whatever well-grounded or fanciful deductions medical students might draw from it. In a study of a typical group of first-year medical students, Frederic Hafferty reported that, notwithstanding the official depersonalization of the cadaver and "in contrast to the initial pronouncements of many of the students . . . , it turned out that only a small minority . . . consistently and singularly viewed their cadaver as a biological specimen / learning tool. Virtually all students at some point ruminated about who their cadaver was, what kind of a life he or she had led, and what might have been the cause of death." [5] The difficulties that the students experienced in navigating their course between seeing the cadaver as specimen and as person were apparent in the students' observance of the official etiquette that their cadaver's face be covered during dissection work and the corresponding difficulties that arose for many students when they came to dissecting the head and neck, as well as the hand, arm, and pelvic areas. [6]

These difficulties were most powerfully revealed in two related reactions by the students to questions that Hafferty posed. The first was a fanciful though demonstrably erroneous deduction that most students made about whether their cadaver "had been an unclaimed body." Hafferty reports: "Most students preferred to believe that their cadaver was donated rather than unclaimed, taking obvious refuge in the fantasy that their cadaver had 'given permission' for them to do the dissection work they were performing. Perhaps reflecting the importance of this issue for students, it apparently mattered little to them that the clues they used to establish their cadaver's former status were shaky at best." [7] The actual fact was, as Hafferty reports, that "most of the cadavers . . . were purchased from another state or were unclaimed bodies" and that most students knew this fact but exempted their cadavers from it. [8] The second—and directly contradictory—reaction was revealed when Hafferty asked students, toward the conclusion of their first-year laboratory experience, whether they would donate their own bodies to medical schools for educational purposes.

> This question was asked of ninety-nine students, always near the end of an interview. Eighty-two students replied in the negative, eleven in the affirmative; six maintained that they were unsure of their position. Even more striking than the numbers were the tone and phrasing of the answers. In response to this question, the students abandoned their customary calm. Their answers became abrupt, tension-laden, and filled with emotion. Often responses were accompanied by an unsolicited confession that the students had thought about this issue before and had shared their decision not to donate with other

students, usually during a period of peak emotional stress in lab. For example, during the face or perineal dissection, many students were overheard making remarks like these to their table-mates: "There's no way you would ever get me to be in his [the cadaver's] shoes," or "I wonder if when she was a little girl, she ever thought she was going to end up like this. I could never do it." . . . The most striking feature [of the responses] is the language the students used in verbalizing their decision not to donate. One cannot help but be struck by the symbols of violence and destruction. Answers rarely contained such scientifically neutral terms as dissection, probe, and pick. In their place emerged more physical, graphic terms: slash, rip, pull apart, hack. For virtually all of the students interviewed, this question and its underlying issue were unrestrained by feeling rules [regarding the required etiquette of neutrality and scientific detachment that the students had quickly absorbed in their first-year curricular experience].[9]

Hafferty notes that the contradiction between the students' assumptions about their cadaver's voluntary presence in the laboratory and their unwillingness to donate their own bodies was noticed as such only by two of the eighty-eight refusers, and he speculates that this unacknowledged contradiction was an initial and powerfully formative step in their socialization as medical professionals—a step away from empathic identification with their patients, a willingness to set aside the Golden Rule in medical practice by doing "unto others as one would not have done unto oneself."[10] I would frame this observation somewhat differently, and without the pejorative implication that accompanies it. The refusing medical students were able to acknowledge to themselves the violence endemic to ordinary medical practice—the transgression of deep taboos about respect for bodily integrity—only when they thought of themselves as the targets of violation. In order, however, for them to engage in this violence—to be the instruments of violation—they had to reimagine, to depersonalize, the encounter. In one sense this can be understood as a failure in empathic identification; but in another sense, equally plausible but normatively praiseworthy, this is a necessary step for any physician toward developing the capacity to invade another person's body in order to help him, to do good works.

Anna Freud made a similar observation in an address to medical students in 1964. Invoking her experience and authority as a psychoanalyst of children (and as the founder's child), she identified underlying motives that inclined many young children toward adult careers in medicine. "Curiosity, the wish to know" was an important motivation, she said, and this impulse merged into the wish to help and to cure; and for nursery school children, she reported, these wishes often found expression in the establishment of "a hospital for insects, frogs, or lizards."

And these small animals will be tended carefully in boxes, fed and looked after and, as the child says, cured. Sometimes, especially when it is an insect, legs will be pulled off beforehand so that a patient is produced, and the patient is cured afterwards. Which means that the child's wish to help and to cure [as well as to satisfy his curiosity] is still very close to the wish to hurt and to maim. The younger the child, the stronger his wish to hurt. The older and more socially adapted he becomes, the more this aggressive wish can be submerged under a strong urge to help. Both wishes can lead the growing individual straight into medicine. Naturally, no need for the doctor anymore to provide his own patients by harming them. Fate does that for him. He only needs to cure them. But this wish to deal with those who are hurt, in pain, maimed, has to be there, and probably always underlies, even though hidden in the unconscious, the wish to cure and to help.[11]

If we focus attention on surgeons specifically, this formulation is not quite right. While Fate does indeed produce surgical patients, it is still nonetheless necessary for the surgeons intentionally to maim and to inflict pain on patients as an essential intertwined motive toward satisfying their wish (and their patients') to cure and to help. This is not condemnatory but merely descriptive. But, just as with attitudes toward death, a morally neutral characterization does not arise automatically; some cognitive and emotional effort is required to banish a sense of wrongdoing in the infliction of violence, no matter how admirable the ultimate goal of the infliction might be. With repeated practice, this sense of guilty infringement might seem utterly vanquished; but there is a danger, a hidden cost, in this triumphant posture.

This issue is not restricted to surgery but pervades medical practice. Physicians routinely engage in conduct with their patients that transgresses deep-seated social inhibitions, that would be morally questionable but for the fact that the acts occur between physician and patient. The ordinary social etiquette that regulates the touching of body parts or viewing the body disrobed is routinely set aside in physician-patient relations. In some medical specialties, penetrations into bodily orifices are regularly performed that many people would not tolerate even in their most intimate physical relationships; in all medical practice, even in psychiatry where physical contact with patients rarely occurs, intrusions into socially sacrosanct spaces are routine events. Moreover, as Anna Freud observed, the idea that the physician's role permits indulgence of guilty pleasures has roots in the explicitly denominated "doctor play" of young children—frequently conducted, as she says, "in secret, because it doesn't always respect the bounds set by the adult world, but it combines curiosity about the other child's body with the wish to interfere with that body."[12]

How do these explorations become both legitimate and routine in adults' medical practice? Here is an account by one physician of his professional exposure to this question:

> At the end of that first year [of medical school], we were . . . taught physical examination and diagnosis. In order to learn the technical skills of examination, we practiced initially on each other. In our group of five students, there were three men and two women. This quite naturally caused some embarrassment as we came closer to the days when we would practice breast exams, genital exams, and rectal exams. I remember asking the question of our instructor, "How does one handle one's own feelings of sexual arousal when examining someone of the opposite sex?" His answer was essentially that those feelings should not arise, that they should be suppressed as completely as possible.[13]

In one sense, the instructor's answer was clearly correct. Feelings of sexual arousal should not be indulged by physicians in performing physical examinations on their patients. There is even a commonsense correctness in the instructor's evasive refusal to specify how those feelings could in fact be banished. With repeated practice, with increasing desensitization of the sexualized charge in these contexts and an increasingly assured self-definition in the social role of physician, the suppression of sexual arousal "just happens"—in the same way that the violent feelings about cutting into bodies "just go away" in the routine practice of surgery.

The psychological processes of suppression have some hidden traps, however, that must be scrutinized. Though these processes are necessary means toward producing great personal and social benefits, they are also steps toward the infliction of terrible suffering and injustice. These two radically divergent outcomes are intricately intertwined. The weakened ethos of caretaking that characterizes our times requires closer attention to this intertwining, and a more self-conscious effort at unraveling these contradictory impulses. At times when this ethos seemed more solidly rooted, it was more plausible to believe that caretakers' "natural" beneficence would "automatically" displace self-aggrandizing or predatory motives. Perhaps the social supports at those times effectively worked to this end—though it is more likely that there never was such a time, and that predatory motives were never fully suppressed but emerged in the various abuses of medical authoritarianism that now seem so patent but then remained socially invisible. Whatever the truth about past times, it is clear for our times that we cannot rely on the automatic dominance of beneficence in social caretaking relations.

This lesson was powerfully taught by one of the most important and disturbing social science experiments ever conducted—a study carried out in the mid-1960s by Stanley Milgram, a psychologist at Yale University. Milgram designed his study in the immediate wake of Adolf Eichmann's trial in Jerusalem in order to test the willingness of ordinary people to "obey malevolent authority" by inflicting terrible suffering on innocent victims.[14] The results he obtained speak to a much broader issue—not simply to the dynamics of obedience to authority but more generally to the way in which people who are themselves in positions of authority readily persuade themselves to inflict unjust abuse. By exploring Milgram's experiment, we will see the underlying mechanisms in the contemporary Supreme Court's self-blinding response to the persistent and escalating abuses in the administration of the death penalty and the cruelties inflicted in modern medical practice on many vulnerable people, and especially on terminally ill patients. Milgram's results make clear that these abuses do not arise from active malevolence but paradoxically from an intense commitment to "do good," to pursue justice in social settings where wrongdoing seems pervasive and virtually unavoidable. Through Milgram's experiment, we can see the way in which the background misgivings—the unavoidable subliminal suspicions that I have identified—about the inherent wrongfulness of death press judges engaged in the administration of capital punishment and physicians engaged in treating people with fatal illnesses onto a "slippery slope" toward wrongdoing.

This was the experiment. Milgram advertised in local New Haven newspapers for participants in a psychological experiment about learning techniques.[15] He obtained volunteers from a virtual cross-section of the community; and when each one arrived at his laboratory, Milgram arranged through a rigged drawing of lots that the volunteer would be designated the "teacher" and an associate posing as another volunteer would be designated the "learner." The so-called learner was then strapped into a formidable-looking machine and the teacher—the volunteer experimental subject—was told that he should administer electrical shocks from this machine each time the learner made a mistake in recalling a list of word associations. The electrical shocks were marked on the front panel of the machine with indications of escalating intensity from 15 volts to 450 volts; and labels appeared above the voltage markings that ranged from "slight shock" to "danger: severe shock" at 375 volts to only a chilling "XXX" at 435 volts. At the beginning of the experiment, the teacher-subject was himself subjected to an actual shock from the machine at a 45 volt level, which most described as somewhat painful.[16]

The experiment then proceeded. In its basic format, a grey-coated laboratory technician who described himself as "the experimenter" stood by the side of the teacher-subject and the learner was in an adjoining room, able to be heard but not seen; as the shocks escalated in intensity, the learner cried out with escalating intensity. At 150 volts, the learner complained that he had previously suffered from a "heart condition" and that his heart was "bothering" him, and demanded that the experiment be ended; at 270 volts, the learner let out what Milgram described as "an agonized scream"; at 300 volts, the learner refused to say another word, and thereafter remained utterly silent.[17] Whenever the teacher-subject hesitated or outright refused to administer a further electrical shock, the experimenter coolly instructed him that the "experiment required that he continue," or that he "had no choice" and he "must go on." If asked whether the shocks were truly dangerous for the learner, the experimenter would respond with a bland assurance, "although the shocks may be painful, there is no permanent tissue damage, so please go on."[18]

In fact, the machine was rigged so that no shocks were actually administered; but the illusion of real-life shocks was utterly convincing to all of the teacher-subjects. As Milgram noted, and as the film he made of the experiment amply confirmed, the teacher-subjects show such distress as they administer these shocks that it is clear they believed in the reality of their painful and even life-threatening consequences.[19] Indeed, at the end of the sequential administration of shocks, several of the teacher-subjects stated that they believed the learner had actually died.[20] In this basic format of the experiment, almost two-thirds of the teacher-subjects administered the electric shocks up to 450 volts, "XXX," the highest level possible.[21]

After the conclusion of the experiments, many of the teacher-subjects justified their actions in various ways—that they were "just following orders" or that they trusted that the experimenter would not really let anything bad happen, notwithstanding the overwhelmingly contrary evidence of their senses during the experiment. Not all of them, however, engaged in this post-hoc justification; some were openly condemnatory of their own conduct—including one man who said that when he told his wife of the experiment, she responded, "You can call yourself Eichmann."[22]

In attempting to explain the experiment's results, Milgram claimed that they showed that most people are willing to obey authority rather than question its moral standing.[23] This may be a true observation but,

in the context of his experiment, it is a misleading truth. This explanation contains a background assumption that the commission of evil requires the presence of active malevolence somewhere—in Milgram's paradigm, there is active malevolence in the person giving orders, though the agent is dumbly willing to obey whether or not his leader is purposefully evil.

This is too glib as a way of understanding the essential dynamics involved in Milgram's experiment; there was in fact no clear division between "blind agents" and "evil principals" in it. Consider, in particular, the role that Milgram himself played in this experiment. Like the teacher-subjects, he was inflicting escalating pain on helpless, unwilling victims; he, that is, was putting the teacher-subjects in his experiment at considerable risk, without their consent, for lifelong future suffering when they confronted the personal implications of their own moral weakness, their own willingness to injure an innocent person. Moreover, Milgram persisted in this enterprise long after it became evident to him that many of his experimental subjects were experiencing great pain. Milgram reported that 15 of the first 160 subjects experienced "full-blown uncontrollable seizures" in the course of administering the escalating shocks;[24] and many more showed stress through "trembling, anxious laughter, acute embarrassment."[25] But notwithstanding these early indications of the subjects' suffering, Milgram persisted in conducting his experiments for several years, placing more than a thousand subjects at considerable apparent risk of immediate and longer-term injury.

Unlike the teacher-subjects in his experiments, however, no one directly ordered Milgram to inflict pain. Does this mean that Milgram himself was the evil instigator of this unjustified infliction? Or does it mean (as I would say) that Milgram's own role in blinding himself to the unjustified pain he was inflicting points to the deeper significance of his own experiment—that obedience to authority is not its key, that something more pervasive and important is at work in explaining why so many people (including Milgram) set aside their ordinary moral intuitions against harming obviously innocent, unwilling, and helpless human beings.

I believe we can come toward a deeper understanding of the Milgram experiment—and the general phenomenon of self-deluded commission of evil—in two steps. The first step is provided in a recent essay by David Luban, who maintains that the results of the Milgram experiment can be explained by the seductive force of the "slippery slope."[26] Luban suggested that the teacher-subjects never asked themselves, "Should I in-

flict intolerable pain on this helpless person?" This is the question that appears salient to us as outside observers, but from the perspective of the participating teacher-subject, the relevant question was much narrower; it was, "I have already inflicted x volts on this person. Should I now inflict x plus a small added increment?" The addition of each of these small increments ultimately amounted to apparently lethal force in almost two-thirds of the cases; but the teacher-subjects never directly confronted this ultimate result. Instead, when the actual decision presented itself about whether to escalate by a small increment, the teacher-subject could acknowledge the destructive and immoral implication only by admitting that his immediately preceding act of adding a small increment was itself destructive and immoral in retrospect. The teacher-subject, that is, was so intent on justifying his prior action—in holding to a conception of himself as a decent, moral person—that he could not acknowledge that he was precipitously sliding into ever more destructive inflictions of evil.

An outsider might think that a decent, moral person would have refused to participate in the experiment from the outset, that its potential for terrible inflictions should have been apparent to all of the teacher-subjects from the first moment that they saw the voltage panel with its explicitly threatening escalations up to "danger: severe shock" and "XXX." But the teacher-subjects walked into the Yale laboratory carrying with them the assumption not only that they were decent, moral people but that these strangers whom they were meeting for the first time—the Yale experimenter and the other apparent volunteer—were also decent and moral; and that they were all engaged in pursuing an obviously moral result, to increase scientific knowledge. This is also the best explanation and even justification for Milgram's own conduct in initiating the experiment in the first place and even in deceiving the experimental subjects. Milgram could reasonably have concluded that the scientific study of obedience to authority, of the Eichmann paradigm, was socially important, and that it could only be studied by withholding information from experimental subjects, but that almost no one would escalate the shocks after the moment of the learner's protests. This was the advance assurance that Milgram obtained from a panel of psychiatrists before launching the experiment; and, at the time, this assurance seemed plausible.[27] Even if, however, the initiation of the experiments was a reasonable and decent act, their continuation after the first few escalations—accompanied by enormous emotional upheavals on the part of the teacher-subjects—should have alerted Milgram to

the transformed and now monstrous implications of what he was doing. But he was blinded by his own good intentions, and by the evident reasonableness of his first step onto what became a slippery slope into wrongdoing.

This explanation, however, is itself only a first step toward fully understanding the brutal transformation of the enterprise by the teacher-subjects and by Milgram himself. Luban is correct that the incremental shocks on the voltage meter appeared quite small; but this overlooks the immediate events that surrounded the teacher-subjects' decisions to increase from one increment to the next. There were no sharp distinctions between 15 and 120 volts; but at 120 volts, the learner shouted in pain for the first time. There was another novel break at 150 volts, when the learner for the first time tried to withdraw from the experiment, and (even if we ignore the novelty conveyed by the obviously increasing agony of the learner's screams of pain) there was another break at 300 volts when the learner for the first time announced that he would no longer speak. The increment beyond, say, 150 volts was not simply another 25 volts but 25 volts plus for the first time overriding the learner's protests; and it is difficult to see how the teacher-subject would view this as an insignificant and merely incremental addition.

The crucial question, then, is what led the teacher-subjects to ignore anything that the learner said—to treat not only his protests but his agonized screams of pain as if they had no relevance, as if they didn't exist. I believe the answer to this question can be found in Luban's observation about the blinding force of the teacher-subjects' commitment to think of themselves as decent, moral people; but the observation requires some elaboration before we can see its full significance.

We can provide this elaboration by returning to the questions raised earlier in this chapter about the violence embedded in the practice of medicine. I have suggested that the purposeful infliction of injury is an inescapable aspect of medical practice, not only in surgical interventions but in other painful bodily intrusions by physicians; that the process by which physicians come to a neutralized or positive professional attitude toward these interventions involves some relearning, some suppression, of the contrary, socially condemned meanings attached to the infliction of violent injuries; and that this suppression of old moral lessons is never complete but must be reworked at various times, particularly in response to some special stress. To grasp the significance of the Milgram experiments for medical practice generally, we should consider one additional aspect of this suppressive dynamic—that patients are never as

successful as their physicians in suppressing the sense of violence and terror inherent in medical interventions. This disjunction is obviously true in a direct sense when the patients experience pain and accompanying terror; but even when patients anticipate the possibility of pain and terror, they are less practiced than their physicians in suppressing this concern and redefining the interaction as neutral or beneficial to them. This disjunction thus means that physicians, however adept they have become in suppressing their own sense of violence and breach of ordinary social norms in their daily professional activities, must recurrently respond to their patients' contrary (unprofessionalized) views.

There is one obvious—one sensible, rational—path for physicians' response to their patients' actual or anticipated pain: that is to provide medical treatment specifically for it, if such treatment is available. It is, however, a well-documented fact about contemporary medical practice that most physicians ignore their patients' pain and fail to offer readily available palliative treatments; this inattention, moreover, reaches a peak of intensity for life-threatening and irreversibly terminal illnesses. The most extensive research ever conducted into the treatment of dying people in the United States, published in 1995, found that "the last few days" of half the patients "were spent in moderate or severe pain" without adequate provision of palliative care.[28]

Many different explanations have been offered for this pervasive medical misfeasance: physicians' ignorance about pain treatment, legal constraints on use of pain-relieving narcotics, physicians' fears about causing addiction or hastening death, physicians' aversion to dying patients.[29] All of these are plausible, though only partial, explanations. The inattentive physicians do not, however, have evil motivations, they are not purposefully taking pleasure in their patients' suffering; something more difficult to grasp is at work here. In effect, these physicians are engaged in a quite common maneuver of turning away from victims, of refusing to listen to their pain, of imposing a regime of silence on them so powerful that even their agonized cries cannot be heard. This is the same self-deafening that occurred in the Milgram experiments— imposed by the lay subject-teachers on themselves and by Milgram, the scientist, on himself.

Marguerite Lederberg, an attending psychiatrist at Memorial Sloan-Kettering Cancer Center in New York, offers a profoundly illuminating account of the underlying reasons that well-meaning physicians, as well as family members, are inclined to "silence the victims" of life-threatening illnesses—an account that can equally explain the results of the Milgram

experiments. This imposed silence, Lederberg suggests, is part of a fundamental dynamic of scapegoating, of blaming the victim for his own suffering; and the underlying cause of this scapegoating is not evil motivation but, ironically enough, quite the contrary. As she put it, speaking of cancer patients, their physicians and family are inclined to tacitly blame them "for their own afflictions as an inadvertent side effect of desperate compassion." Those, that is, who love the patients "cannot tolerate [their] undeserved and incurable suffering." [30]

Lederberg illustrates this proposition with a case where parents asked her to evaluate their twenty-year-old terminally ill son for what they believed was a psychologically based eating disorder. On interviewing the young man, she found that he—like his parents—was blaming himself, that he was "letting his family down by not eating and not having 'a better attitude.'" Lederberg concluded that the young man's failure to eat was not psychological in origin but was biologically based in his illness, a "terminal anorexia"; but the interesting phenomenon for her— and for us—is the reason that the parents in particular were so eager to ascribe their son's anorexia to psychological causes:

> In reality, his parents loved him passionately and were desperate with grief at seeing their child becoming more and more wasted. At some level, they felt they had failed their child in having been unable to protect him against this catastrophe. Racked by their helplessness, they would feel moments of emotional exhaustion and a desire to flee, as well as moments of resentment and rage about their own suffering, all of which led to irrational guilt and anxiety. Yet they were determined to stand by him and function supportively at the hospital bedside even in the face of their looming loss. It was too much to bear without seeking some relief. So, like him, like all of us, they searched for a way out of meaninglessness. The current excitement about the role of mind in altering the course of cancer provided them with a ready-made framework. It gave meaning and it dictated a course of action. If their son could harness the power of his mind, that, at least, would be a possible intervention in the face of intolerable helplessness. Thus, focusing not on the sick body but on the allegedly underutilized mind, they had made their son responsible for his terminal anorexia rather than confronting and enduring the injustice and tragedy of their situation.

The young man's own response, of blaming himself for his "poor attitude," had a similar impetus; as Lederberg puts it, "the need to seek for explanations that give meaning to toxic events is universal, and self-blame is often preferable to betrayal or random tragedy when the reward is a sense of control, illusory though it is." [31]

I believe that this analysis gives us the key to understanding the Milgram experiments. The teacher-subjects who ignored the agonized screams of the learner were not, of course, motivated by the kind of desperate, passionate grief felt by the parents of Dr. Lederberg's cancer patient. But Milgram's experimental subjects, like the parents and the patient himself, were "search[ing] for a way out of meaninglessness," they were struggling to find some "sense of control" in a situation that seemed suddenly and inexplicably to have spiraled out of control.

Put yourself in their shoes, into their own sense of their immediate experience. The teacher-subjects had come to a laboratory at Yale University in response to a public advertisement to participate in a scientific enterprise; all of this seemed benign, respectable, and predictable. The subjects at first encountered exactly what they had expected: a well-spoken, properly attired experimental scientist, an array of scientific-looking equipment, another pleasant-looking volunteer, also apparently eager to do his bit for the advancement of scientific knowledge. But suddenly this prosaic, seemingly benign enterprise appeared to be transformed into something completely different, completely unexpected: agonized screams from the learner, bland assurances from the experimenter that there would be "no permanent tissue damage" coupled with an adamant insistence that the experiment must continue.[32] The situation simply made no sense, so far as the teacher-subjects could fathom it. Was the learner truly in pain? But how could this be, given the assurances and demands of the experimenter. Was the experimenter lying? But why would he want to have the learner not only hurt but possibly even killed—which was the inescapable implication of the learner's anguished shouts?

There were, of course, many different ways for the teacher-subjects to make sense of this incredible situation. Most of them followed the path that Lederberg identified; they refused to admit the existence of injustice. If the learner were truly suffering pain, that would be unjust; he was an apparently decent, innocent man who did not deserve to suffer. If the experimenter were lying to them about the harmless consequences of the shocks, that would also be unjust; he would be betraying his obligation to be decent and honest toward them and the learner. The teacher-subjects were thus caught in a bind; no matter which way they turned, toward the learner's version that he was suffering intolerable pain or the experimenter's version that any pain should be ignored, something or someone would be unjust, something or someone would be wildly wrong here.

This is more than injustice. These utterly contradictory accounts of

what is going on—the contradiction between the learner's version and the experimenter's version—undermine the teacher-subjects' ordinary ways of making sense of the world. In a word, Milgram's experiment had created a world of meaninglessness. In order to restore meaning to their world, the teacher-subjects were obliged to ignore either the learner's version or the experimenter's; most subjects, when forced to choose, opted for the correctness of recognized authority, the Yale-affiliated scientific experimenter. This bias toward constituted authority is the conventional understanding of the experiment's result—though it is likely that the teacher-subjects were more inclined toward this bias than the general population, based on their willingness to volunteer as participants in scientific experiments. Whatever the soundness of Milgram's hypothesis that most people are inclined to obey constituted authority, the more interesting finding—and the more universal characteristic to which it testifies—is the dynamic that pushed his subjects to look toward constituted authority. That dynamic was the teacher-subjects' underlying conviction that the world cannot be a meaningless place, that there must be a coherent explanation for anything that happens.[33] This is obviously not an objective reality but only a wish, a hope, a normative belief; and there is a kind of desperation behind this belief, because if it is not true, then the world is a random and unsafe place.

Some people may pride themselves in their capacity to acknowledge this existential reality, that the world truly *is* a random and unsafe place. But none of us really live out our daily lives based on that belief. Who would dare get out of bed in the morning, if this were really true? But then, who would dare stay in bed? Paralysis, craziness—this is what would follow from really, truly believing that the world has no reliable structures of meaning. Or—to put the matter in other, equivalent words—this is what follows from believing that the world is an unjust place.

The Milgram experiments demonstrate the close correspondence between injustice and social incoherence, between the conceptions of wrongfulness and of meaninglessness. The experiments demonstrate how much the conventional conceptions of "self" and its ideological companion "self-determination" are dependent on stable referents of social coherence; for it was precisely the confusion, the meaninglessness, of the social context in which the experimental subjects found themselves that prompted most of them to deny personal responsibility and assign their ordinary capacity for self-control to another. And the experiments also show how the subjects, shaken loose from their customary

conceptions of self, readily expressed this unhinged state by acquiescing in conduct which they knew to be wrongful. The Milgram experiments thus encapsulate the dynamic by which self-determination in the imminent face of death can readily become an instrument for wrongdoing implicitly understood as such by its self-punitive purveyor.

The readiness with which the Milgram subjects' confusion found expression in their willing participation in wrongdoing might be explained by the observation Freud made about patients of his who were impelled to commit crimes to mitigate an "oppressive feeling of guilt" which was "present before the misdeed and . . . did not arise from it." [34] For the Milgram subjects, we can surmise that the equation between the incoherence of their social circumstances and a corresponding aura of injustice led them, just as Freud's patients were pressed by a prior sense of guilt, into wrongful conduct.

None of this is, however, readily accessible to conscious deliberation for most people. Indeed, for most people, their needed belief in the predictability, the safety, the meaningfulness, the justice of the world requires continuous, rigorous denial of much regularly repeated and convincing evidence to the contrary. And when some especially disturbing evidence of meaninglessness and injustice forces itself on our attention—when our son is struck with terminal cancer, when our fellow volunteer in the Milgram experiment screams in pain—the first impulse for most of us is to deny this plain evidence of our senses. It requires an act of will to acknowledge this injustice; denial is the path of least resistance, the easy and tempting path.

This is the path, the slippery slope, toward escalating evil. As the evidence of innocent suffering increases, the initial commitment to denying this evidence mounts—it even races ahead as a kind of preemptive strike against the looming, fearful prospect of even more convincing evidence that might, unless fiercely and relentlessly opposed, break down our walls of resistance. This is not an inevitable dynamic; it is possible to interrupt it as a conscious act of will in response to clear evidence— but surrendering to this dynamic is the easy and always tempting path. Contrary to Milgram's suggestion, this is not obedience to some external authority; more fundamentally, it is obedience to a voice within, obedience to an internal commitment to maintain one's belief in the goodness and justice of the world.

Physicians encounter difficulty in maintaining their belief in the goodness and justice of their professional enterprise on a more recurrent basis than do people engaged in most other endeavors. This is

partly because violent intrusions into other people's bodies are intrinsic to the medical enterprise; and the goodness and justice of these interventions must continually be reasserted. Even more powerfully, this is because death has a more palpable presence in the enterprise of medicine than in most other endeavors and—no matter how biologically natural or inevitable it is, no matter how skillfully or responsibly individual physicians acquit themselves in postponing the inevitable—the presence of death always conveys some sense of evil and injustice. Physicians' fierce commitment to reclaim goodness and justice in the face of these recurrent challenges, the pervasive sense of lawlessness in their daily work, is the impetus for escalating inflictions of evil. Milgram's own injurious conduct toward his experimental subjects, which he proudly justified by the norms of scientific inquiry, provides sobering confirmation of this dynamic. This escalating evil is not an unavoidable imperative, but interrupting it requires careful attention. If left unattended, the impulse takes on a life of its own.

There is a special warning here for those who claim that the afflictions of dying people—including the abuses inflicted on them by physicians' warfare against death—can be ameliorated by authorizing physicians to hasten death for their patients, and that rationality and justice can be assured in this enterprise.

CHAPTER SIX

CHOOSING DEATH

He Makes Me Lie Down

Dying people, their families, and their physicians are all vulnerable to unruly psychological forces unleashed by the imminent prospect of death. The success of the contemporary reformist claim that death can be subject to rational control depends on the capacity of vulnerable people to tame these unruly forces. The reformist claim, moreover, rests not simply on the possibility of individual self-control by dying people and their families and physicians but also on the capacity of formal institutional actors—judicial or administrative agency regulators—to exert rationalized bureaucratic control to protect dying people against previous patterns of social and medical abuse. The reformist claims, however, have rested essentially on the assertions that rationality is good and that most people are fundamentally rational in this as in all matters. (Judge Richard Posner, for example, has formulated a complex calculus purporting to demonstrate the rationality of deliberations about suicide—concluding "that the availability of physician-assisted suicide increases the option value of continued living"—in a way that unintentionally and even comically illustrates the psychological implausibility of this ratiocination.)[1] The ideals of scientific rationalism themselves would seem to require some empirical validation of this claim; but almost no systematic research has been carried out.[2]

There is, however, evidence that casts indirect light on the question. The most illuminating recently accumulated data are from a research project carried out between 1989 and 1994, known by the acronym SUPPORT (Study to Understand Prognoses and Preferences for Outcomes and Risks of Treatments), the most extensive study ever done of

hospitalized dying patients and their professional caretakers. The goal of this project was to test the possibility of improved implementation of the first phases of the reformist efforts regarding end-of-life care, that is, the right of dying people or their surrogates to refuse life-prolonging medical treatment and the campaign to popularize advance directives— so-called "living wills" and appointment of health care proxies by mentally competent individuals to specify their future wishes regarding medical treatment, against the possibility that they might become unable to exercise those choices.[3] Generously funded by a $30 million foundation grant, the SUPPORT researchers closely monitored some nine thousand patients in two separate phases, so as to obtain a controlled study of the extent to which informed, collaborative choices could be facilitated for patients and physicians about end-of-life treatments. The first phase was a so-called naturalistic study of the current use of DNR ("do not resuscitate") orders, provision of pain palliation, and explicit discussion and shared decision making about treatment alternatives between professionals and terminally ill patients or their families. At the conclusion of this phase, the researchers found that "physicians did not know what patients wanted with regard to resuscitation, even though these patients were at high risk of cardiac arrest. Orders against resuscitation were written in the last few days of life. Most patients who died in the hospital spent most of their last days on ventilators in intensive care. . . . Except for the comatose, more than half of the patients . . . were reported (by the patient or a family member) to have substantial pain" in the last days of their lives.[4]

The researchers then convened focus groups to explore the reasons for these results and to identify possible correctives that would enhance the possibilities of patient self-determination. In these focus groups, a rationalistic explanation was most prominently offered: "many physicians claimed to be eager to improve care and decision making for the seriously ill, but they maintained that improvements took too much time and they often did not have the needed information about prognosis and patient preferences." The SUPPORT researchers accordingly designed the second phase of their study "to reduce those time-and-information barriers."[5] For this phase, the researchers implemented an intensive intervention for one group of patients—"frequent reports" entered in the patients' records from a sophisticated computer model of prognoses for survival and from interviews with patients and their families "anchored . . . by specially trained and committed nurses who spent all their time counseling patients and families, convening meetings with

physicians and others, eliciting preferences, making plans for future contingencies, and ensuring that the best possible information about prognosis and preferences was available to the care team."[6] For a concurrent control group, no new interventions were provided but, as in the first naturalistic phase, treatment provision and decision making were closely monitored.

The results of this second phase were stunning: the intensive intervention changed almost nothing. The extensive provision of information about prognoses and patient preferences, the counseling of patients and their families to elicit preferences and engage in future planning, and the continuous communication by specially trained nurses with the professional care team about these matters—that is, implementation of the most intensive mechanisms imaginable to the researchers to promote rational decision making based on accurate prognoses and to actively elicit patient choices to guide professional treatment—had *zero* impact on the provision of end-of-life medical care. Between the first and second phase of the SUPPORT study, and between the experimental and control groups in the second phase, there was essentially no difference regarding the timing of DNR orders, the accord between physicians and patients regarding DNR, the time spent in an intensive care unit or on a ventilator before death, the extent of untreated pain in the last days before death, and the resource use for dying patients.

The existence of an advance directive, moreover, made no difference regarding the medical treatment actually provided at the end of life. The SUPPORT intervention succeeded in ensuring that every advance directive completed by a patient was entered in the patient's medical record, but the directives "had no effect on decision making."[7] In particular, physicians were no more likely to enter DNR orders for patients who had expressed this preference in their advance directives than for others who had not indicated any advance preference.

When the results of the SUPPORT study were first reported and received widespread publicity, the commonly offered explanation for this disregard of advance directives was that physicians, through neglectful inattention or willful arrogance, were ignoring the wishes of their patients. Even the press release issued by the American Medical Association—not an organization likely to be attracted to physician bashing—gave this characterization to the research results as initially published in its journal. This was not, however, what the SUPPORT data demonstrated. The fact was that most patients were reluctant to discuss advance directives with their physicians, even when they themselves had completed the directives; and physicians did not initiate conversation

about them. (Only 12 percent of the patients had discussed the directives with their physicians in the course of writing them, and only 42 percent had mentioned them at any time thereafter.)[8] For patients who had completed advance directives (even in response to the intensive counseling provided by the special-duty SUPPORT nurse), it seemed as if they had participated in an empty ritual—a gesture performed because it seemed "the thing to do" when asked, but which they themselves ignored in actual practice.

As Dr. Joanne Lynn, one of the principal SUPPORT researchers, subsequently observed: "As we worked with the press, over and over we explained that the problem was much more difficult than that doctors did not hear their patients' requests; it was that no one involved was talking about these subjects. This was clearly not as good a story, and it was often not written. What showed up was the mistaken notion that patients could not get a hearing."[9] To portray physicians as ignoring the demands and pleadings of their patients was a "better story," I believe, because it was more comforting to believe in the thwarted possibility of self-control than to acknowledge helpless passivity in the face of the looming injustice of death. News reporters and the general public—those who viewed the SUPPORT data at a safe distance themselves from death—held fast to the comforting image of terminally ill people determined to take control of their own destiny and wrongfully obstructed by resistant physicians (a more plausible target for sustaining the belief that evil can be corrected than to castigate death itself). Yet for those people in the SUPPORT study who were close to death—the actually dying patients and their attending physicians—this image of self-control offered no comfort; it perhaps even seemed irrelevant. If the patients and physicians were intent on holding to their wish for self-control in the imminent presence of death, the preferred strategy appears to have been silence, a mutual refusal to talk about its possibility.[10]

The SUPPORT data do not demonstrate that end-of-life care satisfied the preferences of patients or their families; in particular, it is hard to imagine that the documented existence of untreated and unnecessary pain during the last few days of life was consistent with patient or family wishes. What the data do suggest is the weakness of the self-determination principle as a protection for terminally ill patients. Even with the continuous assistance of trained counselors and the provision of extensive information, only the paper formalities of patient self-determination were affected; as the reality of death came closer, choice was an ineffective instrument to protect patients against unnecessary suffering, This was not because patients' attempts to exercise choice were

thwarted by resistant medical professionals; the resistance to exercise choice came from the patients and their families themselves.

The SUPPORT data do not, of course, demonstrate that no terminally ill patient wants to exercise choice to dictate the terms of his death or that no patient is capable of effective self-protection by this means. They indicate only a general characteristic among most terminally ill people; but the documented existence of this general characteristic raises a systemic question which had been obscured by the individualistic, anecdotal focus on the normative importance of patient self-determination. The systemic question is: What would be the impact on terminally ill people who are reluctant to exercise choice if our system for end-of-life care placed substantial reliance on individual choice making?

This question raises essentially the same issue as the empirical data about physician resistance to withdrawal of life-prolonging medical treatment, their nagging suspicion that this action directly implicates them in their patients' deaths and that the withdrawal is somehow "murderous" in its implications.[11] On both sides of the transaction—for patients and for physicians—we can design a system that ignores this resistance, even disfavors it by explicitly or implicitly portraying it as irrational and therefore an intellectual if not moral failure.[12] Or we can anticipate that this resistance is likely to persist, whatever our systemic efforts to the contrary; and that this persistent sense of "wrongness" among substantial numbers of patients and physicians regarding the choice-making enterprise will have unfortunate and uncontrollable impact in practice.

The willful disregard of this possibility was palpable in recent judicial decisions by the United States Courts of Appeals for the Second and Ninth Circuits, upholding claimed constitutional rights to legalized physician-assisted suicide. These circuit court rulings were unanimously reversed by the Supreme Court;[13] but though they are no longer "good law," the appellate judges' opinions in these cases are worth close exploration because they typify the reasoning offered by advocates for legalization, and they illustrate in particular how strenuously these advocates look away from the unruly psychological forces precipitated by death's imminence. These judicial opinions, that is, provide some additional empirical support for the proposition suggested by the SUPPORT study, that most people avert their gaze from the imminent prospect of death (whether, as in the SUPPORT study itself, by refusing to discuss it when it realistically looms, or as in the appellate judges' opinions, by pretending that their ordinary reasoning processes are essentially unaffected).

The Second Circuit Court of Appeals held that it was irrational and therefore unconstitutional for New York state to forbid physician-assisted suicide while it permitted patients to direct their physicians to withdraw life-prolonging treatment. In his opinion for the court, Judge Roger Miner stated,

> Physicians do not fulfill the role of "killer" by prescribing drugs to hasten death any more than they do by disconnecting life-support systems. Likewise, "psychological pressure" can be applied just as much upon the elderly and infirm to consent to withdrawal of life-sustaining equipment as to take drugs to hasten death. There is no clear indication that there has been any problem in regard to the former, and there should be none as to the latter.[14]

Judge Miner thus ignored the extensively available empirical evidence that many physicians view their actions as somehow "murderous" in disconnecting life-support systems;[15] and he ignored the inadequacy of any systematic data exploring beliefs among "the elderly and infirm" about whether they felt "psychological pressure."[16]

Recent research about use of medical resources for end-of-life care has demonstrated that age alone appears to be a significant determinant, with much fewer high technology expenditures for people over eighty than for younger people with the same specific disease diagnoses.[17] This age differential may reflect patients' wishes or sensible medical determinations that the greater frailty of elderly patients warrants less aggressive interventions than for younger patients—or it may result from inappropriate "psychological pressure" and discriminatory attitudes toward elderly people. Judge Miner's airy dismissal of any concerns on this score—any worry, in particular, that elderly disabled people would be specially vulnerable targets for physician-assisted suicide or would have difficulty resisting pressures to volunteer for it—has no adequate empirical basis.

There is another kind of psychological pressure which some advocates invoke as a basis for opposing legalized physician-assisted suicide— not pressure on dying individuals as such but on others, such as physicians, judges, legislators, and the general public, to expand the reach of such statutes beyond the apparently narrow category of "voluntary, imminently dying people." This is the fear of the "slippery slope"—the inclination of a previously resisted social practice to expand beyond its proclaimed target once the initial resistance has been breached. The conjunctive disregard of this possibility and its unintended confirmation was revealed by Judge Stephen Reinhardt in his opinion for the Ninth

Circuit Court of Appeals, overturning a Washington state law that prohibited physician-assisted suicide.

Judge Reinhardt did not base his conclusion on the irrationality of
the Washington statute but rather on the ground that it unduly interfered with the constitutional rights of terminally ill people to make autonomous choices about the valued duration of their lives. In the course
of claiming that the state had insufficient basis for overriding an individual's choice to hasten death, Reinhardt recited this historical account:

> Step by step, the state has acknowledged that terminally ill persons are enti-
> tled in a whole variety of circumstances to hasten their deaths, and that in such
> cases their physicians may assist in the process. Until relatively recently, while
> physicians routinely helped patients to hasten their deaths, they did so dis-
> creetly because almost all such assistance was illegal. However, beginning
> about twenty years ago a series of dramatic changes took place. Each pro-
> voked the type of division and debate that surrounds the issue before us to-
> day. Each time the state's interests were ultimately subordinated to the lib-
> erty interests of the individual, in part as a result of legal actions and in part
> as a result of a growing recognition by the medical community and society
> at large that a more enlightened approach was essential.
>
> The first major breakthrough occurred when the terminally ill were permit-
> ted to reject medical treatment. The line was drawn initially at extraordinary
> medical treatment because the distinction between ordinary and extraor-
> dinary treatment appeared to some to offer the courts an objective, scientific
> standard that would enable them to recognize the right to refuse certain
> medical treatment without also recognizing a right to suicide or euthanasia.
> That distinction, however, quickly proved unworkable, and after a while, ter-
> minally ill patients were allowed to reject *both* extraordinary and ordinary
> treatment. For a while, *rejection* of treatment, often through "do not resus-
> citate" orders, was permitted, but *termination* was not. This dividing line,
> which rested on the illusory distinction between commission and omission
> (or active and passive), also appeared for a short time to offer a natural point
> of repose for doctors, patients and the law. However, it, too, quickly proved
> untenable, and ultimately patients were allowed both to *refuse* and to *ter-
> minate* medical treatment, ordinary as well as extraordinary. Today, many
> states also allow the terminally ill to order their physicians to discontinue not
> just traditional medical treatment but the artificial provision of life-sustain-
> ing food and water, thus permitting the patients to die by self-starvation.
> Equally important, today, doctors are generally permitted to administer
> death-inducing medication, as long as they can point to a concomitant pain-
> relieving purpose.[18]

Judge Reinhardt offered no causal explanation for this "step by step"
progression, only noting that each step "provoked . . . division and
debate" and that "the liberty interests of the individual" repeatedly pre-

vailed over "the state's interests," which signified "growing recognition" of a "more enlightened approach." Reinhardt was clear, moreover, that the progression he discerned in this historical unfolding had not yet reached a stopping point, even with the vindication his court was awarding the plaintiffs in overturning the state statute that prohibited physician-assisted suicide.

The plaintiffs in the Ninth Circuit case had sought authorization for physicians to prescribe lethal medication to terminally ill, mentally competent patients; they did not demand that physicians be permitted directly to administer the medication. There were both principled and tactical reasons for this limitation of the plaintiffs' claim. The principled reason was that patient self-administration of lethal medication is an added protection to assure the voluntariness of the act and to provide clear opportunity for patients to have second thoughts.[19] The tactical consideration was that voters in both Washington and California had defeated a referendum proposal in 1992, by a margin of 55 to 45 percent, that would have authorized direct physician administration of lethal medication, so-called "voluntary euthanasia"; though contemporaneous voter disapproval would not logically bar a court from declaring a contrary constitutional entitlement, most judges would be more hesitant.[20] (This shift among advocates of physician-assisted suicide toward the more modest version was not limited to litigation; the 1994 referendum proposal put forward in Oregon was itself limited to physician prescriptions, and this proposal was popularly approved by the slim margin of 51 to 49 percent.)[21] But Judge Reinhardt was not content simply to approve physician-assisted suicide, as the plaintiffs in the case had requested. He unmistakably signaled his court's willingness to take a next step:

> [I]t may be difficult to make a principled distinction between physician-assisted suicide and the provision to terminally ill patients of other forms of life-ending medical assistance, such as the administration of drugs by a physician. We recognize that in some instances, the patient may be unable to self-administer the drugs and that administration by the physician, or a person acting under his direction or control, may be the only way the patient may be able to receive them. The question whether that type of physician conduct may be constitutionally prohibited must be answered directly in future cases, and not in this one. We would be less than candid, however, if we did not acknowledge that for present purposes we view the critical line in right-to-die cases as the one between the voluntary and involuntary termination of an individual's life. In the first case—volitional death—the physician is aiding or assisting a patient who wishes to exercise a liberty interest, and in the other—involuntary death—another person acting on his own behalf, or, in some instances society's, is determining that an individual's life

should not continue. We consider it less important who administers the medication than who determines whether the terminally ill person's life shall end.[22]

Reinhardt's candor is unusual in judicial opinion writing; the more typical course is for a judge to restrict his attention to the specific claim in the case at hand rather than reaching out (though not "directly," as Reinhardt teasingly observed) to decide an anticipated next case. But his candor does illuminate how public debate about physician-assisted suicide is likely to proceed, and specifically how the autonomy principle will expand according to its internal logic in this procession. Reinhardt's application of the autonomy principle to justify not only physician prescription but also the "next step" of direct physician administration of lethal drugs demonstrates the underlying mechanism of the historical progression of the "right to die" during the past twenty years which he described in his opinion. His reasoning exemplifies how the "division and debate" about this issue repeatedly paused at an apparently "natural point of repose"—for example, the distinction between terminating "ordinary" and "extraordinary" care or between withholding and withdrawing treatment—but then broke loose again, driven by "the liberty interests of the individual."

Each of these distinctions was originally intended to diminish the discomfort—and more specifically, the aggressive implication—invoked by the disputed action. Thus although professional and popular resistance to withdrawing life-prolonging treatment faded, nonetheless withholding food and water seemed somehow "murderous"—until the perception of a technological administration of "nutrition and hydration" through a nasogastric tube displaced the initial imagery of providing food and water to a helplessly starving person. Withdrawing "artificial feeding" no longer had an assaultive implication; the key transformation was not, however, in the conception of the technological character of the feeding but in the conception of the recipient of the food. The recipient was no longer a helpless starving person but an inert body "unnaturally" invaded by liquids poured through the nose rather than sustained by food entering "naturally" by mouth. The aggressive sting receded from the withholding act not simply because the nasogastric tube suddenly appeared inhumane but more fundamentally because the recipient suddenly seemed inhuman—"as good as dead," one might say.

A similar transformation in the conception of the recipient—the transformation of a living "subject" into a lifeless "object"—lay beneath Judge Reinhardt's rejection of the distinction between self-administered

and physician-administered lethal medication. The original purpose of this distinction was also to diminish the aggressive implication of using drugs to kill people, by restricting others' actions to the provision of the drugs and insisting that the dying person must perform the act of self-poisoning. Reinhardt rejected this distinction, however, on the ground that "the patient may be unable to self-administer the drugs and that administration by the physician . . . may be the only way the patient may be able to receive them." He then justified this rejection on the ground that "the critical line [is] between the voluntary and involuntary termination of an individual's life" and the question of "who administers the medication [is] less important" than "who determines whether the terminally ill person's life shall end." That is, according to Reinhardt, so long as the decision to take the lethal dosage is voluntarily made by the recipient, it doesn't matter whether the actual administration is carried out by him or by someone else.

Reinhardt ignores the fact, however, that the originally proclaimed purpose of insisting on self-administered medication was to ensure its voluntary character. He treats the distinction between self and physician as irrelevant to the question of voluntariness, without explaining why it is unnecessary or no longer needed to ensure voluntariness. He would, however, be hard put to provide any such explanation. He could not argue that practical experience had demonstrated that self-administration was not a necessary protection to ensure voluntariness. In 1996, there had been no experience of any form of legalized physician-assisted suicide in the United States; the only empirical guide anywhere in the world was in the Netherlands, where physicians have effectively been authorized to administer and not merely prescribe lethal medications and where, according to Dutch governmental studies, euthanasia has been performed on nonconsenting subjects in some cases.[23]

Reinhardt was not, however, concerned about experience; rather, he was driven by the logic of the self-determination ideal, by the internal imagery or ethos of the ideal. The ideal image is the self-reliant individual who independently controls life's course. For this imagery, the question of who injects a lethal medication is unimportant, even irrelevant. The crucial question, as Reinhardt said, is who decides whether to live or to die. The very idea that an individual could be so disabled that he or she could not self-administer lethal medication itself violates this image of independent self-determination. From the perspective of the ideal image, this kind of disability is a good reason for choosing death, not a basis for withholding the possibility of death.

It did not occur to Reinhardt that helplessness might undermine voluntariness, that an individual's wish for continued life could be clouded by a disability that undermined accustomed self-confidence, even though the diagnostic label of "mental incompetence" might not clearly apply. Reinhardt did not see how the self-administration requirement could provide some measure of protection against the ambivalent inclination of many disabled people to defer to others in devaluing themselves—an ambivalence that would express itself by a passive acceptance of hastened death which they would resist if they were required to act entirely on their own volition. Reinhardt did not comprehend the self-administration requirement as a protective measure; he saw it only as a barrier (even a punishment), not a guarantee to self-determination.

Thus we have two typified individuals, on diametrically opposite sides of the conflict—both incapable of self-administering lethal drugs, but one demanding death because of disability while the other is unable to resist because of disability. Reinhardt did not, however, acknowledge that he was choosing favorites between these two individuals. If he had admitted this, the basis for choice would not have been clear-cut: who is more worthy, more suffering, more vulnerable? Reinhardt broke loose from this conundrum in the same way that Milgram's teacher-subjects decided to follow the experimenter's directive—by ignoring the pained cries of a learner-victim while denying that they were, in fact, making any choice in averting their attention. Just as Milgram's subjects were helped toward this path by their preexisting inclination to prefer scientific authority, so Reinhardt was inclined to prefer strong-willed, self-reliant types for whom death was clearly preferable to prolonged disability. But in both cases the inclination was invested with such force as to make any alternative preference virtually invisible, unthinkable.

In Milgram's experiment this initial disregard for the plausible claims of the learner-victim set the stage for escalating violence and increasingly obvious, though increasingly denied, wrongdoing—not simply wrongdoing from the perspective of an external moral observer but wrongdoing as understood by most teacher-subjects themselves (though they could not hold to this understanding in the embattled enterprise, recurring to it only in shamed retrospect). In Reinhardt's case, it is possible to see this same dynamic unleashed.

The possibility appeared in a footnote at the conclusion of Reinhardt's rejection of the distinction between self-administered and physician-administered lethal drugs. After stating that the critical difference was between voluntary and involuntary death, rather than the identity

of the person administering death, Reinhardt appended the following footnote: "In . . . 'involuntary death,' when the motive is benign or altruistic, we classify the act as 'euthanasia.' . . . We define euthanasia as the act or practice of painlessly putting to death persons suffering from incurable and distressing disease, as an act of mercy, but *not* at the person's request. . . . While we place euthanasia, as we define it, on the opposite side of the constitutional line we draw for purposes of this case, we do not intimate any view as to the constitutional or legal implications of the practice. Finally, we should make it clear that a decision of a duly appointed surrogate decision maker is for all legal purposes the decision of the patient himself."[24] There is a considerable, though unacknowledged, tension in this footnote, between Reinhardt's apparent refusal to address the merits of "involuntary death" and his endorsement of decision making by "a duly appointed surrogate."

The tension initially appeared in the first legal ruling that propelled the "right to die" into general public attention; in the *Quinlan* case, the New Jersey Supreme Court found that Karen Ann Quinlan had a constitutional right to discontinue her respirator, notwithstanding her incommunicative vegetative state, by reasoning that she would have had this right if she had been mentally competent and the fact of her incompetence should not deprive her of the right. The court purported to resolve the apparent anomaly of ascribing volition to Karen Ann by requiring that the court-appointed decision maker must exercise so-called "substituted judgment," reaching the same decision she would have reached if she had been competent to do so, while ignoring the essential indeterminacy of this criterion and obscuring the necessarily "involuntary" character of any decision made on her behalf.

Subsequent efforts to contain decision making for incompetent people within the apparently comforting framework of voluntary self-determination focused on lobbying for legislative enactments that authorized competent individuals to make binding advance directives or to appoint surrogate decision makers, so-called "health care proxies" to regulate any future medical interventions. Although such legislation has by now been enacted in every state, and the Congress endorsed such efforts in 1990 by requiring every hospital to inform patients of their rights under these state laws, in practice relatively few people have taken advantage of these laws.[25] In the pre-*Quinlan* era, physicians would have confidently taken charge of medical decision making for incommunicative people; but this resolution has lost its social approbation. Accordingly, in face of the failure of most people to claim their rights to self-

determination, by 1996 the legislatures in thirty-three states had enacted specific statutes providing for the automatic default appointment of surrogate decision makers for incompetent patients (based on a prescribed scheme, typically with first preference to spouses, then adult children, then other relatives or close friends).[26]

There are practical reasons favoring this legislative approach; and it is not clear that such automatic appointments would lead to abuses of trust. But this is not self-determination. When a default surrogate decision maker exercises this legislatively bestowed authority to discontinue life-prolonging medical treatment, this action would precisely fit the definition that Judge Reinhardt prescribed for "euthanasia"—that is, "an act or practice of painlessly putting to death persons suffering from incurable and distressing disease, as an act of mercy, but *not* at the person's request." Whatever the merits of this result, however merciful it might truly be, this involuntary "putting to death"—this "mercy killing"—is exactly what Reinhardt approved in his endorsement of surrogate decision making, just one sentence after he insisted that he was approving no such thing.

Was this a purposeful elision on his part? Did Reinhardt know about the numerous state statutes already in force that would yield this result? His careful locution, avoiding the customary phrase "mercy killing" in favor of "painlessly putting to death," itself suggests some cosmetic covering-up. But perhaps, as I am inclined to believe, his concealment was as much from himself as from others.

An argument can be made that this kind of involuntary killing should become accepted practice—that the automatic appointment of surrogate decision makers is appropriate because many people fail to anticipate the possibility that they would become incompetent and tethered to life-prolonging medical devices but that this outcome would be abhorrent to them; and, moreover, that a default surrogate should be authorized to consent to physician-assisted suicide as well as withdrawal of life-prolonging treatment because both are logically and morally equivalent ways of intentionally hastening death. This argument is disputable in both logical and moral terms; but it is not implausible. Judge Reinhardt did not, however, make this argument; he made no argument at all in favor of this result and yet slid into it without acknowledgment.

Reinhardt is not unique in his inclination toward this slippery maneuver. This is the way that public deliberation about emotionally charged issues often proceeds—the way that initial, avowedly small steps away from some previously fixed moral position make it easier, almost unno-

ticed, to take larger and then again larger steps, until the old, adamantly held position appears quite empty and completely evaporates. This progression from cautious incremental reform to ultimate wholesale repudiation—from, say, Gorbachev's *glasnost* to Yeltsin's revolution—is not necessarily misleading or malign. But in considering the administration of death, there are special dangers in this kind of progression.

The slippage in Judge Reinhardt's vocabulary illustrates the danger. From insisting that he was doing nothing more than protecting every individual's right to self-determination in controlling death, he moved to endorse one person's control over another person's death. This dying person is literally "out of control"; and so is Reinhardt himself. He is beyond the control of the only governing principle he is prepared to acknowledge, the principle of self-determination; but also, in a deeper way that this principle itself refuses to acknowledge, he is in the grip of death, which is in final analysis the antithesis of self-control. The slippage in his invocation of a self-controlled death ironically, even mockingly, mirrors the ultimate inability of anyone to attain this cherished goal.

The pursuit of this goal, of rational control over one's own life, is a noble endeavor. But pressed beyond sensible limits, this pursuit becomes destructive, as we have seen in the distorted impact—the suffering imposed on dying people—of the noble aspirations of medical science to exert rational control over death. Judge Reinhardt's opinion illustrates how readily the worthy ideal of individual self-determination slides toward unintentional distortions.

.   .   .   .

You Anoint My Head

The deep roots of ambivalence toward chosen death are apparent in the first recorded treatment of assisted suicide in the Western cultural tradition—that is, in the death of King Saul as recounted in the first and second books of Samuel. Two inconsistent versions of Saul's death appear in Samuel. Here is the first version, at the conclusion of the first book:

> [T]he Philistines were battling against Israel, and the men of Israel fled before the Philistines, and they fell slain on Mount Gilboa. And the Philistines followed hard upon Saul and his sons, and the Philistines struck down Jonathan and Abinadav and Malkishua, the sons of Saul. And the battle went heavy against Saul, and the archers, the bowmen, found him, and he quaked with fear of the archers.
>
> And Saul said to his armor bearer, "Draw your sword and run me through

with it, lest these uncircumcised come and run me through and abuse me."
But the armor bearer did not want to do it because he was very frightened,
and Saul took the sword and fell upon it. And the armor bearer saw that Saul
was dead, and he, too, fell upon his sword, and he died with him.

And Saul died, and his three sons and his armor bearer, and all his men
as well, together on that day.[27]

The second book of Samuel shifts the scene to David's encampment,
after his own successful battle against the Amalekites, another enemy of
Israel. Here is the second version of Saul's death, as David learned of it:

> And it happened after the death of Saul, when David had returned from
> striking down Amalek, that David stayed in Ziklag two days. And it hap-
> pened on the third day that, look, a man was coming from the camp, from
> Saul, his clothes torn and earth on his head. And it happened when he came
> to David, that he fell to the ground and did obeisance. And David said to
> him, "From where do you come?" And he said, "From the camp of Israel I
> have gotten away." And David said to him, "What has happened? Pray tell
> me." And he said, "The troops fled from the battle, and also many of the
> troops have fallen and died, and also Saul and Jonathan his son died."
>
> And David said to the lad who was telling him, "How do you know that
> Saul died, and Jonathan his son?" And the lad who was telling him said, "I
> just chanced to be on Mount Gilboa, and, look, Saul was leaning on his
> spear, and, look, chariots and horsemen had overtaken him. And he turned
> around behind him and saw me and called to me, and I said, 'Here I am.'
> And he said to me, 'Who are you?' And I said to him, 'I am an Amalekite.'
> And he said to me, 'Pray, stand over me and finish me off, for the fainting
> spell has seized me, for while life is still within me. . . .' And I stood over him
> and finished him off, for I knew that he could not live after having fallen. And
> I took the diadem that was on his head and the band that was on his arm,
> and I have brought them here to my lord."
>
> And David took hold of his garments and tore them, and all the men who
> were with him did so, too. And they keened and they wept and they fasted
> till evening for Saul and for Jonathan his son and for the Lord's people and
> for the house of Israel because they had fallen by the sword.
>
> And David said to the lad who had told him, "From where are you?" And
> he said, "The son of an Amalekite sojourner am I." And David said to him,
> "How were you not afraid to reach out your hand to do violence to the Lord's
> anointed?" And David called to one of the lads and said, "Come forward,
> stab him." And he struck him down, and he died. And David said to him,
> "Your blood is on your own head, for your mouth bore witness against you,
> saying 'I was the one who finished off the Lord's anointed.'"[28]

One consistency shines through these conflicting accounts—that
Saul asked for assistance in hastening his death and that his motives for

this request appeared reasonable and even praiseworthy. Indeed, the first book of Samuel recounts that when the Philistines found Saul's body, they cut off his head and stripped him of his armor and carried his decapitated body to their city where they impaled it on a temple wall;[29] Saul was clearly correct in anticipating that if the Philistines had found him still alive, they would have tortured him horribly (and thereby put added indignity on Israel by this treatment of its king). There is no criticism to be found in the Biblical account of Saul's wish for a hastened or an assisted death. Even the second version of his death at the hands of an Amalek youth had its own implied justification, since Saul had lost God's favor and his kingship because he had failed to implement God's specific commandment to kill all the Amalekites.

The Biblical criticism is focused instead on those whom Saul asked, or apparently asked, to speed his death. Of Saul's armor bearer, we know only that he was struck with fear by Saul's request, but we are not told the source of that fear. As to the Amelek youth, he may not actually have killed Saul but instead encountered his dead body and stripped it of royal emblems to seek some reward from David, the putative successor. But we clearly do know that the Amelek felt no inhibition in claiming to have acceded to Saul's request; he must indeed have calculated that this account would receive heightened favor in David's eyes.

But David's accusation—"How were you not afraid to reach out your hand to do violence to the Lord's anointed?"—evoked his own troubled relationship with, and fears regarding, Saul. On two prior occasions David could himself have killed Saul and if he had done so, his motives would have appeared entirely justified. After Saul had lost God's favor, he knew that David had been chosen as his successor, and he repeatedly tried to kill him. After numerous murderous assaults against him, David came upon Saul alone and unprotected, relieving himself against the wall of a cave. David did not kill Saul, however, but only cut off a small piece of his cloak; yet even then, we are told, "David was smitten with remorse . . . and he said to his men, 'The Lord forbid me, that I should have done this thing to my master, the Lord's anointed, to reach out my hand against him, for he is the Lord's anointed.'"[30] In a second episode, David and his men came upon Saul asleep in his camp, but David restrained his men, saying "Do no violence to him! For who can reach out his hand against the Lord's anointed and be guiltless?"[31]

These past associations proved fatal to the Amelek youth—not simply in spite of the strong justifications for Saul's death at his hand but because of their very strength, because of the seemingly ineluctable temp-

tation to inflict death without any remorse. As David observed, in the light of his own powerful temptations and equally powerful justifications, who can do such killing and "be guiltless"? When David erupted against the messenger who claimed to have assisted King Saul's suicide, his imprecation—"How were you not afraid to reach out your hand to do violence to the Lord's anointed?"—directly referred to his own fearfulness and self-recrimination when he had inhibited his impulse to kill Saul. In modern guise, this same transaction occurs entirely within one individual's mind in recapturing his or her mature sense of self in imminent confrontation with death, as I discussed in chapter 1. The virtual identity of the psychological processing of one's own death and one's experience of significant other deaths powerfully expresses the confusing shift between first-person and third-person perspectives that Charles Taylor identified as the central conceptual weakness in the modern sense of self. In this confusion are the roots of the psychoanalytic observation that mature individuation necessarily carries some implication of parricide, of guilt-inducing violence directed against the psychologically internalized image of one's parents.[32]

In this melange of feelings induced by the confrontation with one's own death, we can see the vulnerability of modern claims for self-determined death through the lens of King David's punitive, murderous outburst against the embodiment of his own worst fears about himself. As this Biblical transaction is reenacted entirely in one individual's mind, the danger is that this guilt-ridden eruption will be aimed at oneself—that the individual will embrace death as a deserved punishment rather than, in the hopeful spirit of the contemporary reform ethos, as a calmly accepted inevitability. The struggle between these two moods will present an opening for the abuse of dying people reminiscent of discredited past practices. In the confusion of this struggle, terrible suffering can fall on dying people.

CHAPTER SEVEN

THE DEATH PENALTY

Surely Goodness and Mercy Shall Follow

The death penalty is the paradigmatic expression of officially sanctioned involuntary killing. There is, moreover, no pretense of mercy; it is intended as punishment, even though constitutional norms against "cruel and unusual punishment" restrain its administration. We can nonetheless discern important lessons from American efforts during the past thirty years to ensure the "rationality" and "fairness" of capital punishment that provide guidance for thinking about the administration of death more generally. The lessons emerge from the following themes that have been explored in previous chapters: that death conveys an inherent aura of wrongdoing, in persistent counterpoint to claims for its practical or moral worthiness; that suppression of this ambivalent attitude is psychologically possible but nonetheless carries considerable risk that it will erupt into actions which express the underlying sense of wrongdoing, even as it remains unacknowledged; and that rigid commitment to the "goodness" of one's motives and the coherence or "meaningfulness" of one's thinking—that is, the denial of ambivalence or confusion—is a marker for an impetus toward condoning and even escalating actual wrongdoing.

I have thus far developed these themes by focusing mainly on an effort to explain a considerable anomaly—the fact that, during the past century, the well-intentioned efforts of medical science to avert death have carried the unintended consequence of inflicting considerable suffering on many dying people. The common complaint against physicians, which erupted in public discourse around 1970, has been that their protestations of beneficence were virtually transparent masks for

baser motives—for profit seeking or research kudos while using their terminally ill patients as laboratory specimens. From my perspective, this complaint is misguided and, indeed, misses the most important (and troublesome) aspect of this iatrogenic infliction of suffering. The basic problem does not arise from bad motives among physicians; rather, it arises from and is compounded by the consciously intended goodness, the purity, of their motives and their corresponding refusal to acknowledge in their own minds the possibility of any taint of wrongdoing.

Judicial efforts to reform the administration of capital punishment during the past thirty years provide another, sharply etched instance of the more general explanatory hypotheses I have put forward. From an initial acknowledgment in 1972 of the unfairness and irrationality of the death penalty, federal judges (led by the U.S. Supreme Court) have grappled with reform efforts; thirty years later, it is apparent that the courts have done little more than devise new means to shut off public scrutiny of capital punishment, all the while spreading an almost patently false patina of fairness and legitimacy over the enterprise. As with conventional accusations of bad faith against physicians, it is possible to charge these judges with self-conscious hypocrisy. I believe, however, it is more illuminating to understand their conduct as driven by their refusal, their incapacity, to acknowledge that the death-dispensing enterprise carries an inescapable taint of wrongdoing no matter how fervently they want to believe otherwise—indeed, even precisely because of this fervor. Examining the recent rationalizing efforts for the death penalty will bring into sharper focus the paradoxical characteristics and problems of parallel efforts to rationalize the administration of death in the contexts of terminal illness and abortion.

Even more than in these other contexts, the very structure of the administration of capital punishment depends for its moral legitimacy on a well-defined, self-conscious differentiation between "guilt" and "innocence." The rigidity—and the underlying, nagging implausibility—of this differentiation is apparent in the currently resurgent controversy about the possibility that wrongfully convicted people might be executed. Recent advances in DNA testing have led to the exoneration of some death-row prisoners; and intense media attention to these almost-executed innocents has led to some softening of public and official support for capital punishment.[1] Two different reactions are conceivable in response to this possibility that innocent people might be executed. One was offered by George W. Bush during his successful presidential campaign in 2000. Texas leads the country in numbers of executions

and, as governor, Bush signed 135 death warrants—more than any other chief executive in American history.[2] When challenged about this record during his presidential campaign, Bush declared that he was "confident that every person that has been put to death in Texas, under my watch, has been guilty of the crime charged."[3]

The alternative to this staggeringly confident assertion would have been for Bush to assert that, while no guarantee of infallibility was possible, Texas had nonetheless instituted multiple safeguards to ensure that any plausible evidence of innocence would surface and would be seriously evaluated at some stage in the administration of the death penalty—if not at trial, then at some point in post-trial proceedings. For anyone who is passingly familiar with the Texas death penalty regime, this claim would be highly disputable; but it would not be patently fallacious, as was Bush's assertion that he could know with certainty that no future evidence would ever be found to establish the innocence of anyone executed in his state. A realistic defense of the death penalty must rest on the explicit admission that no human institution can ever attain perfect knowledge and that, if American society wants to retain whatever benefits might follow from capital punishment, we must necessarily settle for less than perfection. But then-Governor Bush implicitly understood that this defense would not wash—that he must make a public claim for infallibility, no matter how implausible this claim might be.

This claim for infallibility follows from the eruption of public attention to the administration of the death penalty that the Supreme Court precipitated in its 1972 ruling, in *Furman v. Georgia*,[4] that all extant death penalty statutes violated constitutional norms of rationality. In capital punishment, as in the contexts of terminal illness and abortion, the pre-1970s technique for accommodating the underlying, unacknowledged aura of death's inherent wrongfulness had been to bury the practices away from public view; but by 1970 this appeasing technique no longer had its desired effect. The wrongfulness of the death penalty suddenly appeared palpable, based on the same judicial critique as in the other contexts: the penalty was arbitrary; its decisional processes were wrongly hidden from public view; and it was unjustly inflicted on especially vulnerable people (racial minorities, poor people). The reformist agenda adopted by the judiciary was also the same as in the other contexts: the administration of the death penalty would be brought into public light; rational standards would now be identified and enforced; and this would make it "just," thereby solving the problem of its newly revealed wrongfulness.

After some fifteen years of effort to implement this reformist agenda, the Supreme Court effectively proclaimed in the mid-1980s that the agenda had been successfully achieved and turned away from the enterprise while ignoring clear evidence that the originally identified abuses not only persisted but had been exacerbated. In its public posture thereafter, the Court was as adamant in refusing to admit this reality as George W. Bush was in his more recent claim for infallibility. The Court covered its tracks with legalisms and statistical dust-clouds; but the brittleness of their stance became patent as the 1980s progressed, first, in their refusal to give any credence to overwhelming empirical evidence of jury bias toward guilty verdicts[5] and against racial minority defendants in death cases,[6] and second, in their progressive restriction of the scope of habeas corpus relief in order to close off any windows for seeing the general persistence of arbitrariness.[7]

This judicial shift might seem entirely attributable to changes in national politics, the accession of Ronald Reagan, and his appointment of more conservative judges. But if we retrace this path in some detail from the eruption of the rationalizing reform impulse in the 1970s to its unacknowledged betrayal beginning in the mid-1980s, we will see that this political explanation is too glib, that deeper psychological forces were at work which suggest that the rationalizing enterprise was bound from the beginning to become a mask for renewed wrongdoing, even if there had been no change in judicial personnel.

In the early nineteenth century, the administration of capital punishment was as much a publicly acknowledged and visible feature of American social life as the easy availability of abortions and the deathbed rituals surrounding terminally ill people. The first substantial stirrings of public concern about the death penalty occurred around 1830 — earlier than for these other contexts. Carnival-like public executions, attended by thousands of people, were then common throughout the country; but a newly organized group of death-penalty abolitionists began to denounce its degrading social impact by pointing to "fearful spectacles of a tense and ribald crowd, hooting and cheering a criminal at the gallows."[8] In 1834, Pennsylvania became the first state to end public executions, followed the next year by New York. It seemed at the time that ending public executions would be a first step toward abolition. By 1853, three states had eliminated capital punishment, and until 1860 there was significant public agitation and legislative activity toward this end in several other states.

The Civil War had a transformative impact on this movement, as it

had on other aspects of American life; the "widespread enthusiasm and evangelical fervor" for abolishing the death penalty virtually vanished immediately after the war.[9] In its place, a new public policy took hold which had direct parallels with the treatment of death in its newly medicalized dispensation for abortions and for terminally ill people—that is, capital punishment persisted but was now hidden from public view, with exclusive custody of the enterprise turned over to specialized administrators acting in secret. By the end of the nineteenth century, most state legislatures had shifted from public to private executions behind prison walls, with only a handful of designated official witnesses.[10] In the late 1880s, several states even banned newspaper accounts of executions, notwithstanding constitutional objections based on freedom of the press. These so-called gag laws also required that there be no prior public announcement of scheduled executions and that they take place at midnight or early dawn, when most people were, of course, asleep.[11]

The same impulse toward secret administration also took hold in the decision-making processes for imposing the death penalty. In 1800 the typical state criminal code contained an extensive, specific listing of crimes for which conviction automatically carried the death penalty; in 1794, Pennsylvania became the first state to substantially reduce the number of capital offenses and provide a scheme of graduated severity regarding murders that essentially gave juries open-ended discretion whether or not to impose a death sentence. During the next half-century, many other states followed Pennsylvania's example as an alternative to outright abolition.[12] At this same time, however, the growth of the penitentiary movement and the resulting possibility of long-term imprisonment as an alternative to the death penalty markedly changed the context of criminal sentencing. While juries had, in effect, played the principal social role in deciding both guilt and punishment under the old regime, the new arrangement gave most sentencing decisions exclusively to judges. Most notably, however, the death penalty remained within the jury's province—but now as a discretionary dispensation rather than an automatic consequence of a guilty verdict. During the course of the nineteenth century, this fundamental distinction became a deeply ingrained feature of state criminal codes; judges dominated all sentencing matters except for discretionary decisions to inflict death, which remained firmly in the hands of juries.[13]

Nineteenth-century state legislatures could, of course, have shifted sentencing responsibility to judges in all criminal matters, capital as well as noncapital cases. By treating capital offenses differently, legislators

gave the power to inflict death to anonymous decision makers who deliberated in secret and were never expected (or provided formal opportunity) to give any public explanations for their decisions. At the same time that the specific application of the death penalty retreated behind the closed doors of the jury room, public attention to the policy question regarding the existence of capital punishment also faded away. Though there were occasional flurries of abolitionist activity in state legislatures between 1870 and 1917, only Wisconsin, Maine, and North Dakota remained abolitionist states thereafter, although Michigan effectively abolished the death penalty by restricting it to cases of treason.[14] Nonetheless, after 1930 the actual infliction of the death penalty markedly declined (from an annual average of 178 during the five-year period 1935–39 to an average of 61 in 1955–59 and 36 in 1960–64); moreover, about half of all executions between 1930 and 1969 were concentrated in the Southern states.[15] We seemed embarked on a path of unacknowledged abolition—one might say, a publicly invisible path.

Here too there is an intriguing parallel with the evolution of abortion policy and practice. By 1969, a trend toward unacknowledged abolition of abortion restrictions had apparently taken hold in state legislatures. Without much general public attention to the issues, medical professional groups had successfully sponsored liberalizing legislation in some sixteen states which was so broadly permissive as to effectively end restrictions but without acknowledgment as such.[16] In 1970, moreover, legislatures in four states entirely repealed any restrictions for first-trimester abortions, thus explicitly endorsing "abortion on demand"—and one of these states, New York, had no residence requirement for women who wanted an abortion. With abortion effectively available to any woman who could travel to New York (or to California, whose exceedingly liberalized new statute similarly had no residence requirement), the nationwide restrictive regime appeared effectively—if only implicitly—undermined.

The invisibility of this trend toward the abolition of both the death penalty and abortion restrictions was dramatically shattered by the Supreme Court in the early 1970s. Ironically enough, however, the judicial rulings that proclaimed the abolition of both the death penalty (*Furman v. Georgia,* in 1972) and abortion restrictions (*Roe v. Wade,* in 1973) led to an outpouring of public resistance and legislative enactments across the country to reinstate capital punishment and impose new restrictions on the availability of abortions. It is tempting to blame the Court itself for this unruly popular arousal and legislative backlash;

but something more is at work here than populist outrage at judicial authoritarianism. A comparison might be made to the court's extraordinary intervention against race segregation in *Brown v. Board of Education*,[17] where the initial resistance to that 1954 decision had turned to ultimate legislative and public endorsement by 1968. By contrast, fifteen years after the Court's decisions in *Furman* and *Roe*, there was no equivalent national consensus for abolishing the death penalty or eliminating abortion restrictions, and the Court itself had substantially retreated from its initial positions on the two issues. Unlike *Brown*, moreover, the justices had not anticipated much public resistance for their death penalty and abortion rulings; indeed, they initially seemed beguiled by the public invisibility of these issues into believing that their own rulings would (after a brief flurry of media commentary) essentially slip by unnoticed.

When the justices decided *Brown*, they clearly anticipated the intense controversy that followed. In both *Furman* and *Roe*, however, the justices did not see the explosive underlying force of the questions that they were drawn into—the unsettled and suddenly fragile quality of the social arrangements about the administration of death that had seemed so solidly, so invisibly, resolved over the course of the preceding hundred years. In their apparent eagerness to put a public seal of moral legitimacy on the implicit but unacknowledged trends regarding the death penalty and abortion, the justices themselves offered some testimony to the contemporary force of these issues—as if they could not restrain themselves and simply allow the silent social processes to work toward their own apparent goals, as if they were drawn like proverbial moths into this consuming flame.

In *Furman*, the Court ruled by a narrow 5-to-4 majority that all existing state and federal death penalty statutes were unconstitutional because they were arbitrary, without any guiding rational standards, in their administration.[18] In the confusing melange of separate opinions among the majority justices, it appeared that this ruling left no room for legislative efforts to devise rational standards. The majority justices' opinions read as if they meant to endorse the de facto abolition of capital punishment that had already occurred; in the same way that the Court majority in *Roe* originally saw itself as endorsing the existing de facto discretionary authority of physicians in performing abortions, the *Furman* majority appeared to believe that it was ratifying rather than dramatically unsettling conventional attitudes.

In both abortion and capital punishment, however, a Court major-

ity quickly sensed a new direction to public opinion and jumped in front of the parade. By 1975, two years after it had decided *Roe,* the Court had recast its decision as an affirmation of a woman's unencumbered right to choose abortion for herself, though without admitting that it was doing anything more than reaffirming *Roe.*[19] In 1976, the Court was more open in acknowledging its changed direction regarding the death penalty; but it strove nonetheless to claim consistency with its prior rulings, on the ground that *Furman* had been concerned with arbitrariness in the administration of the death penalty and new state statutes promised to remedy this concern.[20]

Within two years of the *Furman* decision, the legislatures in thirty-five states had reenacted their death penalty statutes, with varying alterations designed to meet the apparent objections raised by the *Furman* majority. In *Gregg v. Georgia,* a Court majority found that the new state statutes, which provided specific lists of "aggravating" and "mitigating" circumstances and bifurcated trial procedures to separate the jury's deliberations on guilt and on punishment, did on their face, at least, adequately promise to "guide and regularize" death sentencing. At the same time, the Court rejected newly enacted statutes that purported to remove all discretion by mandating a death sentence whenever the jury found a defendant guilty of certain specific crimes. Four justices were prepared to constitutionally validate these mandatory statutes as well as the "guided discretion" versions in other states (Burger, Rehnquist, and Blackmun—all of whom had dissented in *Furman*—and White, who had joined the abolitionist majority in that case). Justice Stewart concluded, however, that the mandatory statutes in practical effect "simply papered over the problem of unguided and unchecked jury discretion" because jurors would adjust their votes for or against guilt based on their willingness to impose death; they would, that is, disguise their exercise of discretion which, Stewart asserted, would "exacerbate the problem identified in *Furman* by resting the penalty determination on the particular jury's willingness to act lawlessly."[21] Stewart was joined in this conclusion by Justices Powell (a *Furman* dissenter) and Stevens (new to the Court, replacing Justice Douglas); since Justices Brennan and Marshall voted to invalidate all death penalty statutes, a Court majority was stitched together to overturn the mandatory statutes while a differently constituted majority approved the new "guided discretion" statutes.

This patchwork assemblage of majorities, composed of different groups of justices unable to agree among themselves on a consistent set of ruling principles, did not speak well for the possibility of devising ra-

tional standards to "guide and regularize" the administration of the death penalty. Nonetheless these unstable voting majorities held together within the Court for some seven years; between 1976 and 1982 fifteen capital cases were fully argued and decided on the merits by the Court and all but one of these rulings reversed or vacated the death sentence as imposed.[22] The Court's rulings during this time narrowed the application of the penalty to murders, explicitly excluding rapists,[23] and to those who intended to kill, excluding co-felons vicariously liable for murder.[24] The Court also struck down any limitations on the kinds of mitigating evidence a defendant might present in sentencing proceedings[25] and overturned restrictions on the defendant's access to all information provided to the sentencer.[26]

On their face, these results suggested that the Court was engaged in a sustained, searching inquiry about the rationality and fairness of the application of state death penalty statutes. In fact, two justices (Brennan and Marshall) had announced at the outset that no such statute could be rationally or fairly administered; and three others so regularly voted to sustain these statutes (Burger, Rehnquist, and White) that it seemed they were not at all committed to a scrutinizing enterprise. This apparent rationalizing task was, then, embraced only by three justices (Stewart, Powell, and Stevens), occasionally joined by a fourth (Blackmun). In 1983, however, this plurality itself unraveled, and a newly constituted Supreme Court majority effectively (though not admittedly) abandoned the rationalizing enterprise.

Justice Stewart had retired from the Court in 1981 and was replaced by Sandra Day O'Connor who, throughout her tenure, almost always voted to uphold the imposition of the death penalty. But this one vote was not enough to alter the Court's direction; in 1983 Justice Powell visibly shifted his disposition, joining the invariable supporters of capital punishment. With three others then on the Court (Burger, Rehnquist, and White), a stable group of five justices was thus constituted to turn aside objections to both the general structure and the particular applications of death penalty statutes; notwithstanding changes in Court's membership during the next fifteen years, this result has remained essentially constant.

Thus, little more than a decade after *Furman* apparently abolished capital punishment by overturning every extant death penalty statute, a fixed majority on the Court effectively (though without explicit acknowledgment) turned away from probing supervision of the administration of capital punishment. Was it inevitable that the death penalty could not be successfully subjected to rationalized control? Was there

no real middle ground between judicial deference to unexamined jury discretion and judicial abolition of the death penalty? An answer to these questions can be pursued by close attention to the stresses encountered and the strategies adopted by lower courts in attempting to carry out the Supreme Court's rationalizing mandate. We can see with particular clarity the intrinsic obstacles to rational ordering of the death penalty and the forces that lead to added disorder in the actions that occurred around the first execution of an unwilling prisoner since 1967, five years before *Furman* had been decided.

The state of Florida killed John Spenkelink on May 25, 1979.[27] In 1973 Spenkelink had been convicted of murdering a traveling companion who, he had alleged, had previously stolen money from him and forced him to engage in homosexual acts. Spenkelink claimed that the two were struggling together when he shot in self-defense, but the state contended that the other man was sleeping when he had been killed.[28] Spenkelink's conviction was affirmed on direct appeal two years later;[29] by May 1979 his subsequent petitions had been denied twice by the Florida Supreme Court[30] and twice by the Fifth Circuit, with review denied by the Supreme Court.[31] Notwithstanding these prior defeats, attorneys on his behalf predictably filed new motions in both state and federal courts as his scheduled execution loomed. Less predictably, perhaps—in light of their repeated prior reviews—these courts showed considerable strain in rejecting Spenkelink's final appeals.

This strain, and the obstacles it revealed toward devising an orderly, regularized regime for administering the death penalty, appear with particular vividness in an account of the case provided by Arthur England, Chief Justice of the Florida Supreme Court in 1979. England had twice previously concurred in his court's denial of relief to Spenkelink.[32] He told about his final concurrence at a Yale Law School seminar in 1985:

> I got a call at two o'clock in the morning from some attorneys who wanted to make an argument that [Spenkelink's] . . . execution should be stayed. I did not deny them that right. I was foggy, it was late at night, but I said, "Fine, be at my house at seven o'clock." I hung up and I realized I'd said, "be at my house." What am I doing holding court in my house? But I had said it.
>
> I called the other members of the court. I called my research aide, and I said, "Mike, do what's necessary to have coffee and pencils. We're having court at seven a.m." And at seven a.m. that morning—he was scheduled to be executed, I believe, at ten o'clock—my front yard was filled with cars, the Attorney General of the state, assistants, . . . some lawyers who were arguing . . . [for Spenkelink]. One of the first questions that came to my mind was, "Who are these lawyers? By what authority do they represent him?

There've been lawyers in this case for years." But we didn't want to waste time with that. We just wanted to hear what they had to say.

In my living room we heard arguments from both sides. We had no place to adjourn in my house. We don't have a back room. So we adjourned there. They went out in the yard. And we sat and deliberated on what points they had raised. We concluded they were not a basis for a stay and called them back in and told them that was that.

The phone rang. The Governor had been advised, of course, by the Attorney General that there was this hearing and needed to know to tell the warden what to do at Raiford State Prison or not. We only had one telephone line in the house—three extensions but only one line. My daughters had their phone in their room. The Governor wanted to be sure our line was open. And the Attorney General reported to him what had happened.

We immediately got another call from some people in New Orleans who wanted to argue another ground for a stay of execution. I didn't want to deny them the right to do it. I was scared to death to deny them the right to do it. I didn't know what they wanted to say. Maybe it would be the basis upon which we would stay the execution.

How do you do that—seven Justices in the living room and three phones? Well, you put three of them on the line and listen to the argument. The Attorney General can't hear what they're saying and we had to come back and translate what the motions were and get their reactions to the telephone motions and the grounds that were being considered. We adjourned them again to the front yard.

. . . [Then] we went out to get them. . . . The Governor was frantic trying to get through to us while we were on this call. Everything was chaotic. Finally we made our last decision, I think, thirty, thirty-five minutes before the scheduled execution. The Attorney General called the Governor and confirmed that was the result.

This was to be on television. There was a television set in our living room. I don't think anybody wanted to watch it. But we didn't know what to do. Nobody wanted to leave: the attorneys for Spenkelink, the Attorney General and all his assistants. Everybody was immobilized by this process.

So we watched what happened on television. We couldn't see the execution. What we saw was the outside of the prison and that sort of stuff. After it occurred, there must have been silence—just—I don't know what it was. It was an immobile silence for five or ten minutes. Nobody wanted to go anywhere, to do anything. Nobody had any idea what they were to do next. Nobody on the court wanted to go in the office and decide cases.

Fifteen, twenty minutes later we got a call from the Attorney General's office, that his wife and children had been threatened, that they were being protected, that they had been spirited away, and that it was not advisable for him to come to the office. The same with some of his assistants.

We didn't get such threats. But it was emotionally devastating to be a part of this process. And I can't even capture it in words. I can't even give you a sense of what it was like. We walked around like zombies for a day—I'm sure

all of us did. We were pinned down—even people who were advocating capital punishment repeatedly in the courts and had been doing so for five, ten years, and who believe it's in the public interest. The toll-taking is very, very heavy.

It occurs to me that I may be wrong on some of these steps. It's just dawned on me. I may have them out of sequence or I may not have them accurately—because I was living them at the time and my recollection may be off. It would be interesting . . . to see if [others] remember two hearings. I'm sure it was in the house. After that I really don't know. It would be interesting to find out.[33]

Around this same time there were also federal court proceedings in Spenkelink's case, pursued by attorneys acting separately from those appearing in the state supreme court. This extraordinary infusion of lawyers came, of course, because of Spenkelink's notoriety as the case that might end the twelve-year moratorium. The hectic, last-minute character of the infusion came specifically because it had not been clear until little more than a week before his scheduled execution that Spenkelink, rather than some other prisoner in Florida (or in some other state), would be first in line to break the moratorium. Numerous attorneys not previously involved in his case were suddenly drawn into it.

One of these new attorneys was Ramsey Clark, a former attorney general of the United States. Clark had flown to Florida on May 22, not to represent Spenkelink, but to participate in a protest vigil—as he put it, "to bear witness"[34]—at Spenkelink's anticipated execution. When Clark arrived in Jacksonville, however, he received an emergency call from an American Civil Liberties Union attorney in Atlanta who had pored through Spenkelink's records for the first time and had found possible grounds for appeal in previously unnoticed aspects of the original murder trial. Clark subsequently wrote this magazine account of what happened:

> She began a litany of allegations familiar to all who have followed capital trials in the United States these last years. John Spenkelink's trial attorneys were court-appointed. They lacked sufficient resources to prepare and conduct the defense. . . . [Clark then listed a lengthy series of strategic errors that experienced counsel would never have committed: failure to challenge the composition of grand and petit juries, failure to request severance from trial with a co-defendant later acquitted, errors in arguments to the jury and the like.] . . .
>
> Then came what was for me the clincher. Spenkelink's father was a paratrooper in World War II. . . . The war weighed heavily on him. Life wasn't easy thereafter. To his son he was a hero.
>
> One day, when John was 11, his father went into the garage, attached a

hose to the car exhaust, started the motor, put the hose in his mouth and asphyxiated himself. John found his father dead on the garage floor with the hose in his mouth. The troubled youngster began a career of minor crime. Prison psychiatrists examining him over the years wrote that his criminal behavior was in large part due to the suicide of his father and that he was amenable to treatment. Incredibly, when the sentencing phase of the case was tried, these facts were not presented to mitigate the punishment. A jury would not give a death penalty in the face of such evidence. John Spenkelink was a second-generation casualty of World War II.[35]

On this basis, Clark concluded that Spenkelink had been denied his constitutional right to effective assistance of counsel. He agreed to fly immediately to Atlanta to present a new petition with this allegation to a federal judge there. Federal and also state judges were even closer at hand in Florida. But Clark, as the phrase goes, went shopping for the most favorably inclined forum; his choice was Elbert Tuttle, a federal court of appeals judge who not only sat in Georgia but had long since retired from active service. Clark knew and admired Tuttle from the old civil rights battles of the 1950s and 1960s.

At 11 P.M. on May 22, Clark presented himself at Tuttle's home with a petition to stay Spenkelink's execution:

> Mrs. Tuttle answered the door, and graciously led us to her living room. As we settled down with Judge Tuttle, she retired. I had not seen him in a decade. Now in his early 80's, Judge Tuttle was as erect, dignified, alert and interested as ever. He knew of course why we were there. He stated at the outset that he was pleased to meet with us, that he would read our petition and hear our plea. But he cautioned us that he had not granted a writ of *habeas corpus* since assuming senior status a dozen years earlier and did not see how he could do so now. Then he asked why we had come from Florida to bring a Florida case to him. . . .
>
> I gave him a hard, straight answer. This case had been in the courts for six years. The Federal district judges in Florida had reviewed it at length time and time again. It had been rejected on other grounds just the day before by the District Court in Florida. The Legal Defense Fund had made prodigious efforts at the District, Appellate and Supreme Court levels.
>
> Now we were eight hours away from an execution and a new and difficult question, never raised in the case, and one courts and lawyers alike abhor, was raised. Did Spenkelink's court-appointed Florida lawyers represent him effectively? There was little chance that judges with six years' involvement behind them would consider this new issue. We needed a very courageous, very independent, open-minded and fair judge. That is why we chose Judge Tuttle. That is what I told him.[36]

Clark's answer satisfied Tuttle. He then heard the substantive allegations on which Clark based his claim and immediately stated that he would grant the stay to permit an evidentiary hearing on the allegations. The statute on which Tuttle grounded his jurisdiction provided that an independent appellate judge could either assign this hearing to an appropriate district judge or conduct it himself.[37]

Immediately the next morning, the Florida attorney general flew to Washington to present a petition to the Supreme Court to vacate Tuttle's order. The Court declined the following day, May 24, with Justice Rehnquist noting his dissent. In a subsequently filed opinion, Rehnquist was harsh to the point of caricature in his criticism of any attorney who would seek this last-minute stay:

> It strains credulity to suppose that six years and countless courthouses after his trial, respondent suddenly determined that his trial attorney had been ineffective. Either he does not believe the claim himself or he had held the claim in reserve, an insurance policy of sorts, to spring on the federal judge of his choice if all else fails. This Court has disapproved of such tactics before . . . [as] "needless piecemeal litigation . . . whose only purpose is to vex, harass, or delay."[38]

Rehnquist did not specify which of these malicious intentions, to vex, harass, or delay, he would ascribe to Ramsey Clark—perhaps all three. For Judge Tuttle, Rehnquist's criticism was more restrained but equally pointed:

> [B]ecause the imposition of the death penalty is irreversible, I respectfully suggest that there may be a tendency on the part of individual judges or courts . . . to create or assume [constitutional] . . . doubts where in fact there are none.
>
>   . . . [T]here are several hundred federal judges in the United States who have authority to issue stays. . . . As the new execution date approaches, new claims are conceived and, at the last minute, new stay applications are filed. Understandably, because no mortal can be totally satisfied that within the extremely short period of time allowed by such a late filing, he has fully grasped the contentions of the parties and correctly resolved them, judges are inclined to grant such 11th-hour stay applications. Then, again, new execution dates must be set and the process begins anew. This now familiar pattern could in fact result in a situation where States are powerless to carry out a [constitutionally valid] death sentence.[39]

Rehnquist characterized the systemic implications of both Clark's conduct as an attorney and Tuttle's as a judge to be "at odds with a government of law."[40]

Rehnquist filed his opinion on May 25, the day after the Court had acted and the very day that Spenkelink was executed. The execution occurred because Judge Tuttle's stay was vacated by the swift action of a three-judge panel of the Fifth Circuit, an action which itself strained the boundaries of governance under law. As if in response to Tuttle's (and Clark's) disregard for the ordinary conventions against forum-shopping and their implicit disrespect toward the federal judges sitting in Florida, the panel itself was inattentive to the ordinary conventions governing judicial conduct.

On May 23, the same day it asked the Supreme Court to vacate Judge Tuttle's stay, the State of Florida also sought the same result from the Fifth Circuit Court of Appeals. The state's motion was routinely assigned to a panel consisting of Judges James Coleman (based in Mississippi), Peter Fay (in Florida), and Alvin Rubin (in Louisiana). Late that afternoon, the state's written motion with supporting papers was delivered to the court clerk in New Orleans. A deputy clerk read the material by telephone to Judge Coleman that afternoon and to Judge Fay the next morning; a copy of the material was forwarded to Judge Rubin that same morning. The judges conferred among themselves by phone. Though the court rules did not require any oral argument regarding such motions, Coleman and Rubin agreed on May 24 to convene a telephone conference call with the parties. Judge Fay indicated that he could not be available for the call but asked the other judges to tell him what occurred. The conference call was accordingly convened at 7 P.M. on May 24.

This is Ramsey Clark's account of it:

The telephone conference was a nightmare. We were told at the beginning not to record what was said. The court did not have our papers. We had not seen the State's papers. Some factual statements in the State's papers were in error, but we could not know this until we saw them some days later. We were asked whether we had gone to Spenkelink and urged him to attack his trial lawyers, to which we replied, if so, discipline us, do not kill him without determining his rights. There was loose, unstudied, uninformed discussion about whether Judge Tuttle had jurisdiction, whether he entered a final order, whether the Court of Appeals had power to review his order.

It soon became clear that the bizarre late-night argument over long-distance phone among lawyers and judges who had not seen the papers in the case nor been briefed on the issues was worse than meaningless; it was dangerous. I complained and Judge Coleman replied that he was not legally required to give us the opportunity to discuss the matter over the telephone. We asked for time to file affidavits and a response to the State's motion. The merits of our petition for a writ of *habeas corpus* had been barely discussed.

A representative of the Attorney General's office, . . . [the other ACLU attorneys,] and I made some emotional conclusory statements and the call was
over shortly after 8 p.m.[41]

Three hours later the panel entered an order vacating Judge Tuttle's
stay, indicating that its "reasons will hereafter be stated in a formal opinion" and noting that Judge Rubin "reserves the right to dissent for reasons to be assigned."[42] No such opinions ever were issued. The panel
postponed the effectiveness of its order until 9:30 the next morning,
May 25. Clark drove during the night from New York to Washington
where, at 7 A.M., he presented a petition to the Supreme Court to overturn the panel's decision and reinstate Judge Tuttle's stay. At 10 A.M.,
Clark was notified that the Court had denied his petition, with Justices
Brennan and Marshall noting their dissents.[43] Within the hour, Spenkelink was dead.

In the hectic last moments leading to John Spenkelink's execution,
two details particularly illuminate the intrinsic obstacles to rational ordering of the death penalty. The first, from Chief Justice England's nar-
rative, is the oddity that the proceedings before his court occurred in
his home. England explained this misstep as a result of his "fogginess"
at 2 A.M. when Spenkelink's attorneys called him. There are many possible answers to the question England immediately asked himself, "What
am I doing holding court in my house?" Some of these answers would
be unique to England himself—perhaps some greater comfort he felt in
his home that prompted him to move the proceedings there or some
wish that he could remain at home rather than confronting the difficult
decision that attendance at his office implied or who knows what. But
there is one general explanation for England's confusion, one that is not
unique to him—that the special stress of this pending execution pressed
against his capacity to separate his personal and his official identities.
For reasons unique to him, Chief Justice England may have had more
difficulty in sustaining this separation than others involved in the proceeding; and he may accordingly have overstated the personal impact on
others—that it was "emotionally devastating to be part of this process
. . . we walked around like zombies for a day," that even for those who
had been long-time advocates for the death penalty, "the toll-taking is
very, very heavy." But for anyone—except perhaps a true "zombie"—
some added emotional energy is required to maintain the distinction
between personal and official in the highly charged atmosphere of a
pending execution.

The social importance of preserving this distinction is, moreover, not

restricted to judges or to others with obvious official roles in the enterprise, such as defense or prosecuting attorneys or the prison wardens
who carry out the death sentences. Crime victims also, for example, have
designated social roles that require them to differentiate between their
personal impulses (perhaps to strike out in retaliatory rage or to run
away in terror for their own safety) and their official responsibility (to
testify in court proceedings, to sit quietly in the courtroom a few feet
away from the perpetrator). These role imperatives are not themselves
unique to capital punishment cases. The need to differentiate between
personal and official is a pervasive feature of social life, as is the similarly
structured distinction between public and private realms. Chief Justice
England's collapse of the public and the private in choosing a location
for the final hearing in Spenkelink's case testifies to a common difficulty
of maintaining the clarity of this ordinary differentiation in the face of
extraordinary emotional stress.

The second detail from the events just before Spenkelink's execution
speaks more directly to the tenuousness of the public/private distinction, but in a different and darker register. The detail is the fact that Spenkelink's father had killed himself and that his son had discovered the body
in the family garage. The ways in which John Spenkelink, the eleven-year-
old son, might have subsequently been impelled to give public expression to his internal psychological turmoil arising from this event—public expression, perhaps as Ramsey Clark speculated, through a life of
escalating criminal activities—is one aspect of this detail. A second aspect is the ways in which other people involved in Spenkelink's life dealt
with the implications of this past event in his present circumstances. By
Clark's account, some people knew about this event but chose to ignore
it—this is clearly so for the federal judges in his final appeal. And some
people, according to Clark, did not know but should have known—the
sentencing jurors and perhaps his initial defense attorneys, assuming
that they had failed to investigate Spenkelink's background rather than
purposefully deciding to withhold this information from the jury. My
own speculation is that this biographical detail is emotionally distressing for almost everyone—except perhaps the proverbial "zombie"—
and that addressing it (whether to give it some evaluative weight or to
dismiss it as utterly irrelevant) requires some added emotional energy
beyond the imperatives of other elements in Spenkelink's life history.

We can understand the implications of this biographical detail by first
spending some time exploring the difficulty identified by Arthur England, the difficulty in separating his home from his office. In observing
the dynamics of this difficulty more closely, we can come to some gen-

eralizations about the inherent obstacles to rational ordering in the administration of the death penalty.

By his account, Chief Justice England succumbed to this difficulty in a specific moment of extraordinary stress—during a late-night call from lawyers representing a man scheduled for imminent death, which, if it actually occurred, would be the first execution during England's own tenure as a judge. It is possible for us to trace the evolution of this same difficulty for another judge over a much longer time—for Justice Harry Blackmun during twenty-two years, almost his entire tenure, on the Supreme Court. Blackmun's first writing about the death penalty as a justice came in *Furman v. Georgia,* where he dissented from the majority's ruling; in refusing to follow their abolitionist course, Blackmun spoke explicitly about a conflict between his personal inclinations and his judicial role obligations.

Describing his brief dissenting opinion as "somewhat personal comments," Blackmun recited an enumerated catechism of his experience and attitudes regarding the death penalty:

1. Cases such as these provide for me an excruciating agony of the spirit. I yield to no one in the depth of my distaste, antipathy, and, indeed, abhorrence, for the death penalty, with all its aspects of physical distress and fear and of moral judgment exercised by finite minds. That distaste is buttressed by a belief that capital punishment serves no useful purpose that can be demonstrated. For me, it violates childhood's training and life's experiences, and is not compatible with the philosophical convictions I have been able to develop. It is antagonistic to any sense of "reverence for life." Were I a legislator, I would vote against the death penalty. . . .

2. Having lived for many years in a State that does not have the death penalty . . . capital punishment had never been a part of life for me. In my State, it just did not exist. . . .

3. I, perhaps alone among the present members of the Court, am on judicial record as to this. As a member of the United States Court of Appeals, I first struggled silently with the issue [in 1962]. . . . I struggled again with the issue, and once more refrained from comment, in my writing for an en banc court [in 1967]. . . .

4. . . . [U]ntil today capital punishment was accepted and assumed as not unconstitutional per se under the Eighth Amendment or the Fourteenth Amendment. . . . Suddenly, however, the course of decision is now the opposite way. . . . My problem, however, . . . is the suddenness of the Court's perception . . . since decisions of only a short while ago.

5. To reverse the judgments in these cases is, of course, the easy choice. It is easier to strike the balance in favor of life and against death. . . . This, for me, is a good argument, and it makes some sense. But it is a good argument

and makes sense only in a legislative and executive way and not as a judicial expedient. . . . We should not allow our personal preferences as to the wisdom of legislative and congressional action, or our distaste for such action, to guide our judicial decision in cases such as these. The temptations to cross that policy line are very great. In fact, as today's decision reveals, they are almost irresistible.[44]

In 1994, twenty-two years later, Blackmun concluded that the death penalty was inconsistent with the commands of the Constitution. Once again he spoke in personalized terms: "From this day forward, I no longer shall tinker with the machinery of death. For more than 20 years I have endeavored—indeed, I have struggled—along with a majority of this Court, to develop procedural and substantive rules that would lend more than the mere appearance of fairness to the death penalty endeavor. Rather than continue to coddle the Court's delusion that the desired level of fairness has been achieved and the need for regulation eviscerated, I feel morally and intellectually obligated simply to concede that the death penalty experiment has failed."[45] Blackmun did not assert in this opinion that after decades of struggle, he had decided to succumb to his initial temptation to read his personal morality into the language of the Constitution. By his own testimony in 1994, he had come to believe that his judicial role obligation and his personal inclinations were now in harmony.

Blackmun did not, however, provide a clear map to explain the progression of his views, this transmutation from the personal morality of the private Harry Blackmun into the official morality of the public Justice Blackmun. Moreover, in some parts of his 1994 opinion, he seemed to maintain that capital punishment was not intrinsically outside rational ordering but only that a Court majority since 1983 had betrayed this possibility.[46] Nonetheless, his predominant conclusion was, as he said, "It seems that the decision whether a human being should live or die is so inherently subjective—rife with all of life's understandings, experiences, prejudices, and passions—that it inevitably defies the rationality and consistency required by the Constitution."[47] The reasons Blackmun set out to explain this conclusion strongly support it—with even greater force than he himself acknowledged.

The essential reason that the death penalty was outside rational ordering, according to Blackmun, could be found in the self-contradictory commands that the Court itself had imposed since *Furman*. On the one hand, he observed, the Court had demanded a regime of controlled discretion—"procedural rules and objective standards to minimize the risk

of arbitrary and capricious sentences of death."[48] At the same time, the Court had insisted that juries must make individualized determinations regarding a defendant's "character and record . . . or the circumstances of the particular offense" in order to keep open "the possibility of compassionate or mitigating factors stemming from the diverse frailties of humankind"; this was rationale that the Court had put forward in 1976 when it struck down so-called mandatory death penalty statutes while upholding the new "guided discretion" statutes.[49] In 1978 the Court had elaborated this proposition that the jury must have access to, and remain clearly open to consideration of, any "mitigating factor . . . that the defendant proffers as a basis for a sentence less than death."[50] The consequence of these two directives was, as Blackmun put it, "that strict restraints on sentencer discretion are necessary to achieve the consistency and rationality promised in Furman but . . . that, in the end, the sentencer must retain unbridled discretion to afford mercy."[51]

This is the same contradiction that Justice John Marshall Harlan had originally seen in his 1971 opinion for the Court in *McGautha v. California,*[52] refusing to require rationalized standards for capital punishment, just one year before a transformed Court majority came together in *Furman* to invalidate all such statutes. In 1971 Harlan saw an inherent conflict between the commands of Justice and of Mercy derived from the difference in their internal logical structures;[53] and he (joined by a Court majority) was prepared to resolve the contradiction by simply opting for one of these dichotomous poles, to favor Mercy by approving unstructured jury discretion. This resolution fell apart within a year's time because it was no longer plausible to assert that compassionate regard by traditional caretakers and caretaking institutions was a reliable feature of our social life. It was no longer plausible, that is, to believe that officials would act mercifully.

Harlan's resolution of this contradiction was not, however, the only logical possibility. There are two others. One was embraced by Justice Antonin Scalia—to opt for Justice rather than Mercy, to overrule the Court's prior ruling against mandatory death penalty statutes and implement a general regime of rigid restrictions on the permissible criteria for imposing or withholding a death sentence. Scalia had first taken this position in 1990 and reiterated it as a specific rejoinder to Blackmun's conclusion in 1994;[54] Justice Clarence Thomas had taken this same position in 1993.[55] But beyond these two justices, this angle for slicing the Gordian knot did not appeal to other members of the Court. A second possibility is not so rigorously logical but it is nonetheless well within

the usual practice of social institutions—to "muddle through" with contradictory policies, tacking this way or that as the prevailing winds shift.

In his 1994 opinion Blackmun rejected both these possibilities. To
follow the Scalia/Thomas logic would cure the conundrum but at an
unacceptable cost, "offensive to our sense of fundamental fairness and
the respect for the uniqueness of the individual." [56] As to persisting in
the "muddling-through," Blackmun had two responses: that the Court
majority had not been truly engaged in this meliorative enterprise and
that, in any event, he no longer had the stomach for it—he was done
"tinker[ing] with the machinery of death." [57] These are strong and ultimately convincing arguments, but Blackmun did not adequately spell
out the case for them.

To see this case, we should begin with an assumption that for the
same historical reasons it is no longer plausible to believe in the compassion of traditional caretakers—to believe in official administrations
of Mercy—it is also implausible to believe that death can be justly inflicted. I have maintained that this belief in the inherent wrongfulness
of death is a persistent strain in Western culture; and though never the
univalent view, this aura of wrongfulness has sometimes readily, and
sometimes less successfully, been suppressed from most people's conscious awareness. In chapter 3, I invoked Freud's perception of the de-
moralizing impact of the First World War in Europe—that it "created a
disturbance in the attitude which we have hitherto adopted towards
death" [58]—and I suggested that events in this country, culminating in
the late 1960s and clustering around attitudes toward the Vietnam War,
had similarly swept away our comforting conventions for the treatment
of death. The public eruption of doubts about the "just-ness" of administrations of death in various contexts has still not been appeased, as
contemporary disputes about physician-assisted suicide and abortion
especially attest. We remain as Freud portrayed Europe in 1915: "unable
to maintain our former attitude towards death, and . . . not yet [having]
found a new one." [59]

The Supreme Court's prolonged encounter with the administration
of the death penalty can best be understood in these terms—and Harry
Blackmun's personal pilgrimage offers an especially revealing account of
these underlying tensions, however differently expressed, that have affected all of the justices. In 1972, when a bare Court majority seized the
day in *Furman* to embrace a new attitude toward death—to abolish capital punishment in a lightning strike—Blackmun constrained himself,
falling back on conventional conceptions of judicial authority to criticize

the majority for the "suddenness" of their conversion to abolitionism. In 1973, Blackmun broke loose from this restraint in *Roe v. Wade,* leading a Court majority suddenly and unexpectedly to strike down abortion restrictions. As I have noted, however, the justices' underlying goal in *Roe* was to rehabilitate traditional ideals of medical caretaking. In the context of the death penalty, Blackmun pursued the same effort to keep faithful to old attitudes in the face of new pressures by the simple expedience of silence. Until 1983, Blackmun said almost nothing in any of the Court's death penalty cases. This was akin to Learned Hand's approach to the moral status of euthanasia in the *Repouille* case, his insistence that "not much is gained by discussion." Hand, however, was able to rest comfortably on unquestioned assumptions about the solidity of social caretaking arrangements; in the 1970s Blackmun could not maintain his silence on the basis of this unspoken reassurance. Unlike Hand, Blackmun could not confidently hold to the distinction between his personal views and his official responsibilities, because the distinction itself had lost its social salience, because the "responsibility of officials" no longer had a confident, self-evidently beneficent social content.

Blackmun was thus led back—or perhaps it is more apt to say fell back—into his personal revulsion against accepting responsibility for killing another human being, into the "distaste, antipathy, and, indeed, abhorrence, for the death penalty" to which he had testified in his original *Furman* dissent. He could not rely on extrinsic social supports to shield him from the pull of the empathic identification at the core of abolitionism, "the shuddering recognition of a kinship: here but for the grace of God, drop I." [60] From this perspective, the opening paragraph of Blackmun's valedictory opinion in 1994, refusing any longer to "tinker with the machinery of death," was much more than a rhetorical flourish:

> On February 23, 1994, at approximately 1:00 a.m., Bruce Edwin Callins will be executed by the State of Texas. Intravenous tubes attached to his arms will carry the instrument of death, a toxic fluid designed specifically for the purpose of killing human beings. The witnesses, standing a few feet away, will behold Callins, no longer a defendant, an appellant, or a petitioner, but a man, strapped to a gurney, and seconds away from execution. [61]

Whatever the direct witnesses to Bruce Edwin Callins's execution might have perceived, Harry Blackmun saw a man strapped to a gurney; and the conventional social supports, the structure of social meanings, that had surrounded the very idea of death in earlier times, were no longer

available to help Blackmun see this man only as "a defendant, an appellant, or a petitioner"—only, that is, in the context of their official relationship. Blackmun's stripped vision of this dead man conveys the same sense as the stark listing of names without affiliations on Maya Lin's Vietnam War Memorial.

The same collapsed distinction between personal and official led Chief Justice Arthur England to hold court in his living room; but England nonetheless concurred in John Spenkelink's execution. Even so, England spoke of the emotional devastation that he experienced; and this itself is testimony to the absence of conventional social supports to sustain participants in this death-dispensing enterprise. But if Freud's diagnosis truly applies to this contemporary undertaking, emotional tension must somehow affect all the participants, not only those who abandon it, like Blackmun, or acknowledge devastation, like England.

If we look for this more pervasive expression of tension, it can be seen in the further events surrounding John Spenkelink's execution—and these events exemplify the currently prevalent judicial response to capital punishment. Blackmun's abolitionism is only one way, and not the currently typical way, to turn away from the death penalty. The other way is more figuratively to turn away—to look away, that is, by an act of self-blinding. This kind of willful inattention is not indifference, and it cannot be casually sustained. It requires active effort, and escalating effort, to suppress unwanted knowledge; and in this sense, it betrays an underlying, nagging tension.

Two kinds of self-blinding have been characteristic of the post-1983 death penalty jurisprudence in the Supreme Court. The first is purposeful disregard for evidence presented about the persistence of active bias in the practical administration of the death penalty. In 1986, a Court majority refused to credit empirical findings that capital juries excluding members invariably opposed to the death penalty were "conviction-prone"—that is, more likely to find guilt regarding the substantive offense than juries that included death penalty opponents. After raising a flurry of questionable objections to the statistical reliability of this finding, Chief Justice Rehnquist assumed for purposes of argument the existence of jury bias toward guilt and then inexplicably insisted that this bias had no constitutional significance.[62] In addition, the data in the case showed that capital juries were also less likely to include women or minority group members, but the Court dismissed the significance of this finding as well. Justice Marshall in dissent accused the Court of displaying "a glib nonchalance ill-suited to the gravity of the issue presented

and the power of [the empirical] claims";[63] but beneath the apparently casual dismissiveness of Rehnquist's prose was a grim determination to suppress all doubts about the fairness of the capital punishment system.

This determination was even more adamantly expressed in a 1987 ruling that disregarded evidence of persistent racial bias in the administration of the death penalty. In *McCleskey v. Kemp,* the Court was confronted with an intensive, statistically sophisticated (and generously funded) empirical study which found race discrimination in the disproportionate rate of death sentences imposed for murders where blacks killed whites as compared to same-race murderers or where whites killed blacks.[64] In an opinion by Justice Powell, the Court followed the same strategy as Rehnquist had deployed in the conviction-prone jury case: that is, a dust-cloud of objections were tossed up about the statistical findings, which were then assumed correct "for purposes of this opinion" but inexplicably disregarded.[65] For this latter purpose, Powell asserted that the statistical evidence could not prove the existence of racial bias in any particular case but only as a general systemic characteristic, and that the Court would only credit evidence of bias intentionally directed against specific defendants (presumably provable only by direct testimony from jurors admitting to racially biased motivations). The Court thus claimed the high ground of moral opposition to racial discrimination while imposing an impossible burden for obtaining evidence to prove the existence of such discrimination.[66]

The Court's second strategy for self-induced blindness was even more effectively conceived. In these two bias cases described above, the Court acknowledged the existence of the evidentiary claims even though it immediately trashed them. In a more extensive series of post-1983 rulings, however, the Court constructed a labyrinth of procedural obstacles that made it almost impossible for anyone to offer evidence of injustice. The Court essentially eviscerated the availability of the traditionally generous habeas corpus review of state convictions at the same time that it dismantled the procedural obligations it had previously imposed on state tribunals to monitor the internal operation of their capital punishment systems.[67]

In his 1979 dissent in the *Spenkelink* case, Justice Rehnquist had set out the background premises for this second strategy—"a tendency" that he had detected "on the part of individual judges or courts" in death penalty cases "to create or assume . . . doubts where in fact there are none." In 1981 Rehnquist offered a procedural solution to combat this judicial proclivity; he proposed that the Supreme Court should

grant certiorari and thus provide full substantive review in every capital case coming from any state court in order instantaneously to dispose of "all issues of fact or law" regarding any federal constitutional claim. In this way, Rehnquist observed, "the jurisdiction of the federal courts . . . would be at an end, and . . . petitioner's sentence . . . would presumably be carried out."[68] Since 1976, when *Furman* had been displaced with a promise of judicial supervision to cure the inequities in the capital punishment system, the Court had granted certiorari in an average of two capital cases each term; if Rehnquist's proposal had been followed, this number would have jumped from less than 2 percent to more than half of the Court's fully argued cases.[69] Rehnquist was apparently willing to inundate the Court's docket with death cases because he saw a deep threat to the ideal of the rule of law in what he called "the natural reluctance of state and federal habeas judges to rule against an inmate on death row"; this "stalemate in the administration of federal constitutional law," he said, constituted a "mockery of our criminal justice system," undermining government's capacity to "provide security to our people in the streets or in their homes [so that] we are rapidly approaching the state of savagery."[70]

There was an apparent factual predicate for Rehnquist's hyperbolic concern. From 1976 to 1981, between 60 and 75 percent of death-sentenced defendants had obtained reversals at some point in their appeals, either in state or federal tribunals. This proportion was roughly ten times the reversal rate in federal noncapital criminal appeals and almost one hundred times the reversal rate for general felony convictions in typical states such as California.[71] These extraordinarily high rates of judicial reversals in capital cases clearly testified to some disturbance in the operation of our criminal justice system—some collapse of usual assumptions about the integrity of its functioning.

It was an open question whether these disturbing results reflected (a) systemic injustices that did not typically occur in noncapital cases, (b) injustices that occurred with equal frequency but were typically unnoticed in noncapital cases, or (c) false findings promoted by unscrupulous abolitionist attorneys and endorsed by gullible or actively complicit judges. After 1983 a majority of Supreme Court justices clearly opted for alternative (c). This conclusion was emphatically expressed in a direct rebuke administered in 1992 to the judges of the United States Court of Appeals for the Ninth Circuit. On April 19, 1992, the State of California was poised to execute Robert Alton Harris—the first imposition of the death penalty in that state since the national moratorium had been im-

posed in 1967. The imminence of Harris's execution, like Spenkelink's thirteen years earlier, produced a blizzard of last-minute legal appeals before various federal judges. Between April 19 and 21, four different stays of execution were entered by different judges on the Ninth Circuit; the state immediately appealed each of these stays to the Supreme Court, which, in turn, immediately overturned each one. At the fourth iteration, the Supreme Court issued an unprecedented order; not only did the majority reverse this specific stay but it stated, "no further stays of Robert Alton Harris' execution shall be entered by the federal courts except upon order of this Court."[72] This preemptive strike against the possibility of any future interventions by lower-court federal judges was an extraordinary and virtually unprecedented action by the Supreme Court.[73]

In 1981 Justice Rehnquist had complained that "judicial decisions" impeding the administration of the death penalty "had focused so much on controlling the government that we have lost sight of the equally important objective of enabling the government to control the governed." This was the predicate for his conclusion that American society was "rapidly approaching the state of savagery." In the extraordinary expedient deployed in the 1992 *Harris* case, a Supreme Court majority clearly viewed the judges of the Ninth Circuit as themselves spinning out of control—perhaps not "savages," but lawless nonetheless.[74] At the same time, the justices' unprecedented improvisation pushed lower court judges to surmise that the Court itself was acting lawlessly.[75]

This intense public struggle between the Supreme Court justices and the judges of the Ninth Circuit reiterated the difficulty that Justice Blackmun and Chief Justice England had experienced—the difficulty in separating official and personal attitudes toward the administration of the death penalty. The *Harris* case presented this difficulty in a different register—not so much as a struggle between official role and personal empathy for the condemned man, but more as a conflict between obedience to the impersonal commands of law (respect for the judicial hierarchy from the lower-court judges, respect for past precedent from the members of the Supreme Court) and the obligation to do justice according to the individual conscience of each judge. It seems virtually certain that each of the judicial antagonists in the *Harris* case believed he or she was acting according to norms of justice; and it seems equally clear that neither the Ninth Circuit judges nor the Supreme Court justices were prepared to credit this motive in their adversary. Each, that is, appeared to ascribe their differences to personal willfulness rather than an honestly held disagreement in interpreting their official responsibility.

This kind of personalized argument is not unique to disagreements about capital punishment; it has become almost commonplace in contemporary polarized disputes both within the judiciary and in our political institutions generally. The *Harris* case nonetheless revealed a special intensity in the ways these accusations, these mutual recriminations, of lawlessness have emerged among judges in their consideration of the death penalty.

The presence of a pervasive sense of injustice in these judicial deliberations appeared in a different guise in the opinions of two justices who were more at the center of the Court's death penalty work than either Rehnquist (who has been an adamant supporter of capital punishment throughout)[76] or Blackmun (who moved into dissent after 1983). Justices Byron White and Lewis Powell changed their views at crucial moments in the progression of the Supreme Court's treatment of the death penalty. White's conversion occurred in 1976; he had been the fifth vote in *Furman* to overturn all extant death penalty statutes, and just three years later he completely reversed direction, voting to uphold all of the newly enacted statutes, though a Court majority was prepared to accept only those new laws that promised to confine jury discretion. In the course of explaining his revised position, White stated, "Petitioner's argument that there is an unconstitutional amount of discretion in the system . . . seems to be in final analysis an indictment of our entire system of criminal justice. Petitioner has argued, in effect, that no matter how effective the death penalty may be as a punishment, government, created and run as it must be by humans, is inevitably incompetent to administer it. This cannot be accepted as a proposition of constitutional law."[77]

The defining shift for Powell came ten years later, in 1987. Unlike White, he had dissented in *Furman;* and unlike White, he had subsequently engaged in detailed scrutiny of newly enacted statutes, voting to overturn some but uphold others, based on his differential evaluation of their fairness and effectiveness in confining jury discretion. Powell's abandonment of this scrutinizing enterprise, which began in 1983, was the critical move in creating a new Court majority; but the full extent of Powell's disaffection from his prior position was not clear until the 1987 ruling in *McCleskey v. Kemp,* the racial bias case, for which he wrote the Court's opinion. In the course of explaining his position (and the Court's), Powell stated, "McCleskey's claim, taken to its logical conclusion, throws into serious question the principles that underlie our entire criminal justice system. . . . [I]f we accepted [his] claim that racial bias

has impermissibly tainted the capital sentencing decision, we could soon be faced with similar claims as to other types of penalty. . . . [T]here is no limiting principle to the type of challenge brought by McCleskey."[78]

The position of both White and Powell comes close to asserting that, regardless of the intrinsic merits of the specific challenges to the death penalty (for excessive jury discretion or for racial bias), acceptance of these challenges would amount to an indictment of the entire criminal justice system—and that, as Justice White stated, "cannot be accepted as a proposition of constitutional law." Justice Brennan, dissenting in *McCleskey,* characterized Powell's similar position as "a fear of too much justice."[79] I would reverse this characterization: Powell and White were afraid of too little justice—too little justice, that is, in any of our social arrangements, a generalized indictment that would be revealed by close attention to the administration of the death penalty.

This is, as Justice Brennan put it, a "dismaying" and "apocalyptic" vision;[80] no wonder that a Supreme Court majority would turn away from it. To believe not simply that the death penalty is in itself unjust but that its insufficiencies reveal the injustice of our entire system of criminal justice is to stumble into a lawless and uncivilized world. This is essentially the same vision, though approached from a different angle, that the Supreme Court majority thought it encountered in the resistance of the Ninth Circuit to Robert Alton Harris's execution—a vision, that is, of lawlessness among federal judges sworn to uphold the law. This is the nightmare, though also seen from a different angle, that Justice Rehnquist invoked—that because of judicial fault-finding in the administration of capital punishment "we are rapidly approaching the state of savagery."

In all of these "dismaying" and "apocalyptic" visions regarding the death penalty, we can see the same difficulties that afflicted the subject-teachers in the Milgram experiments—the looming threat of disorder for ordinary ways of understanding social relationships and the consequent impulse to deny incomprehensibility by shutting off any awareness of injustice in one's actions. We have seen in previous chapters how this threat of incomprehensibility is especially provoked by the imminence of death, how it casts an aura of wrongfulness surrounding death, and how it expresses itself in injurious, wrongful actions toward dying people by physicians and by dying people toward themselves. This is the truth underlying La Rochefoucauld's maxim that "death, like the sun, should not be stared at"—that death is inherently disorienting, that there is something inescapably incomprehensible about it, and that close

involvement in it undermines the sense of justice, of moral order, in the world.

These are the reasons why intense engagement with the death penalty provoked images of lawlessness among its supporters as well as its opponents. The opponents combat these images by the apparently simple expedient of abolishing the death penalty. The supporters have taken two different approaches. The first was to rationalize the enterprise, to craft substantive standards and procedural safeguards to eliminate or at least appease the apparent lawlessness. This approach has now clearly been abandoned in favor of the second—to suppress all doubts by ignoring evidence of injustice and, even more rigorously, to eliminate opportunities for the presentation of such evidence. The apocalyptic imaginings and heated rhetoric that led supporters to this repressive effort are in themselves indications of the reasons why the first approach—the rationalizing effort—was actually unavailable, was a false and misleading alternative at the outset. From the first moments in the early 1970s when the conventional cultural understandings about death and its discomforts suddenly broke loose from their stabilized moorings, there was no way that the indictment of death's inherent wrongfulness could be directly and convincingly refuted. The old arrangements had served as a more or less successful appeasement, an apparent refutation, of this indictment. The disintegration of those understandings meant that the indictment, always persistent even though muted, had suddenly and insistently reemerged.

The slow but seemingly inexorable decline in public support for and interest in the death penalty during the preceding half-century had occurred in the comforting context of the stable cultural understandings about death generally. The collapse of this background context in America—but not in Europe, which has followed a different time sequence on death-related issues during this century—explains why our public treatment of the death penalty suddenly and so radically diverged from their calmly continuous downward trajectory toward abolition.[81] The American effort to remain calm in the face of our sudden storm took the form of falling back on efforts at rational self-control, the cool voice of reason. The task was, however, beyond rationalizing capacities, for it was no less than to refute the insistent belief in the injustice, the wrongfulness, of death. But this belief is in fact irrefutable. It can be appeased, disguised, attenuated in its forcefulness in our personal and social arrangements. All of these mollifying goals were achieved by the previously stable cultural understandings; but these arrangements did not,

and could not, exculpate the indicted enterprise. Death might be assuaged, its inflictions might be disguised or denied; but it could not be freed from the indictment of guilt as charged.

The urgency of this underlying indictment arises from the deep-rooted cultural assumption about the inherent evil of death as such; and the force of this assumption provides the most plausible explanation for the great surge in public support for the death penalty immediately following the Supreme Court's apparent abolitionist strike in its 1972 *Furman* decision. The Court's ruling brought the death penalty into heightened public visibility at virtually the same moment that other death-dispensing social arrangements also came into unaccustomed public attention. As I have noted in earlier chapters regarding terminal illness and abortion, the existing social modality for appeasing underlying assumptions about the inherent wrongfulness of death had been to bury all the transactions away from public view—"don't ask, don't tell." When this modality broke down generally in the late 1960s, one candidate alone appeared to offer a convincing new possibility for appeasing this stubborn, suddenly visible sense of guilt surrounding death. That candidate was the death penalty. Unlike terminal illness or abortion, a clear-cut case could be made that the dying person—the convicted criminal—deserved to die.

Before 1972, American public opinion had apparently turned away from this moralistic judgment; during the preceding forty years, there had been a steady decline in public support for capital punishment and in actual numbers of executions.[82] The increased public support and legislative endorsement for the death penalty immediately following *Furman* cannot be adequately explained as a resentful backlash against an activist Court. As with *Roe v. Wade* for abortion, the Court's action brought into high public visibility the weakness of existing social arrangements for dispensing death. The emergence of the national "right to life" movement directly provoked by *Roe* was one response to the breakdown of prior social arrangements for addressing the wrongfulness of death; since, that is, abortion practice could no longer be hidden from public view, abortions must be unambiguously defined as "murder" and entirely prohibited. The pro-choice rejoinder took a different tack toward the same goal of appeasing the inherent wrongfulness of death, by insisting that the aborted fetus is not killed because it is not a human being capable of dying. The diametric conflict between these two modes of address did very little to appease the aura of guilt surrounding death. If anything, the openly waged conflict only intensified this nag-

ging sense of wrongdoing in the escalation of mutual recriminations among the partisans themselves and, in a different vein, by provoking a belief among the middling general public that partisans on both sides were wrong and that abortions should not be forbidden but should be "rare."

For the death penalty, however, a much more promising route initially appeared for appeasing, for escaping, this same sense of death's wrongfulness—that killing a killer was not wrong, that the convicted criminal had done wrong and the social retaliatory response was therefore a guiltless act. If American culture in 1972 had not been so desperately in need of finding new ways to placate the suddenly resurgent aura of guilt surrounding death generally, we would have followed our prior path toward abolitionism—the path that our Western European allies took at this same time and that the Supreme Court had definitively marked out in *Furman*. But we needed a new way of appeasing guilt and paradoxically, of course, at the same time finding new ways to acknowledge guilt by enmeshing ourselves more deeply in patently wrongful conduct. This was the alternative course that American legislatures initially chose in direct response to *Furman* and that the Supreme Court obligingly facilitated in its subsequent charade of imposing rational control over the death penalty.

This prolonged deceit could not and has not erased an underlying guilt-ridden discomfort with the infliction of death. This unease has recently found heightened public expression in highly visible concerns about possible executions of wrongly convicted people; these concerns are fueled by unrealistic demands for perfect accuracy in determining guilt yet in fact reflect the persistently nagging sense of wrongdoing that insistently demands appeasement in any death-dispensing enterprise. Pressed by this new concern for the "killing of innocents," contemporary public opinion may be edging back toward abolitionist sentiments.[83] Abolition of capital punishment is, of course, no more capable of erasing death's taint than attempting to rationalize it or suppressing inquiry into its administration. But if we dig deeper into the psychological premises that I have already set out, we can see how abolition is likely to be the safer course for social action—more likely, that is, to allay and contain the impulse toward escalated wrongdoing than continued social engagement in inflictions of the death penalty. From these premises, we can understand why the current American regime for administering the death penalty is inclined toward escalating wrongdoing and specifically why the course traveled by the contemporary Supreme

Court—the failed attempt at rationalization followed by the suppression of inquiry—has led to even greater injustice than the troublesome practices of the prior regime.

The measure of this greater injustice is not in the increased numbers of people sentenced to death and actually executed since *Furman*, though this escalation in itself does testify to some spiraling impetus arising from the insistently proclaimed justifications for the death penalty that have also followed *Furman*. Nor is its full measure in the Court's rigid refusal to enforce even minimal standards of competency for attorneys in capital cases, notwithstanding repeated demonstrations of the inadequate funding for state-appointed counsel and the disproportionate numbers of impoverished defendants under death sentences. Nor is the escalating injustice fully gauged by the Court's imposition of increasingly stringent obstacles to post-trial consideration of newly discovered evidence of innocence, notwithstanding that even minimally competent (or even minimally paid) counsel would have found this evidence before trial. Nor is the injustice fully encompassed by the repeated experience that, in the majority of states with elected judiciaries, numerous state trial or appellate judges who dared to rule in favor of death-sentenced defendants have been pilloried by political opponents and subsequently ejected from office—surely a "chilling effect" on the possibility of independent state judicial oversight to ensure justice in the administration of the death penalty.[84] All of these characteristics of the current capital punishment regime obviously impeach its fairness, while the Court refuses to acknowledge this patent evidence of pervasive injustice.[85]

But even beyond these indicia, the true full measure of the escalated injustice is the charges of bias whose truth the Court was impelled to admit in 1986 and 1987, at the same time that it refused to accept these charges: the bias toward finding guilt among jurors who supported the death penalty (in *Lockhart v. McCree*) and racial bias in the infliction of the death penalty (in *McCleskey v. Kemp*). By assuming the truth of these charges—even though only "for purposes of argument"—the Court has insisted that there is no injustice in a criminal enforcement regime where juries primarily composed of white men (since minorities and women are disproportionately excluded in "death-qualified" juries) impose the death sentence disproportionately on blacks who murder whites. The Court has thus effectively endorsed a regime of law enforcement where the most serious and publicly visible cases are entrusted to groups of white men who value white lives more than black—who visibly appear, indeed, most concerned with the containment of black violence against

whites. This is a clear reiteration of American social arrangements before the abolition of slavery—a regime that, by contemporary values, is the prototypical representation of injustice.

It may be that the current Court majority has refused to acknowledge any of this evidence of the pervasive injustices in the regime of capital punishment because it is so firmly convinced of the intrinsic social value of the death penalty, whatever its imperfections. This rationale would only apply, however, to intrinsic imperfections; it would not justify turning away from the effort to distinguish between correctable and inherently uncorrectable flaws in the system. The current Court majority has, however, turned its face against this entire enterprise. This kind of self-blinding suggests a different explanation—that the justices are willing to appear passive in the face of obvious wrongdoing in the administration of the death penalty. They are willing, in other words, to appear complicit in the wrongdoing.

The manifold injustices in the current death penalty regime are so patent, the Supreme Court justices are so obviously refusing to acknowledge the plain evidence before their eyes, various justices are so vehemently proclaiming that a state of "savagery" will erupt, that the entire criminal justice system would be impeached if these wrongs are admitted. There is, in short, such a pervasive sense of lawlessness and fear of anarchy that we might find the best explanation for the justices' current treatment of the death penalty in Freud's account of the paradoxically inverted relationship between guilt and wrongdoing. As with the physicians who paralyze their patients before removing them from respirators, as with Milgram's experimental subjects who inflict possibly lethal shocks on an innocent learner, so too the justices are embracing wrongdoing in their administration of the death penalty without being able to admit their self-condemnatory motivation. They too may be understood in Freud's terms, as "criminals from a sense of guilt."

Their guilt would come from the same discomfort that Justice Blackmun and Chief Justice England had experienced in their confrontations with the death penalty—from an inability to maintain sharp distinctions between their personal and official involvement without the exertion of considerable emotional effort. Blackmun and England may be "softer" than other judges in their willingness to acknowledge the effort demanded of them. But the source of their discomfort is not unique to them; it arises from the deepest roots of the Western cultural account of death and its intrinsic wrongfulness. This culturally embedded conviction does not univocally lead to revulsion toward capital punishment; to

the contrary, the revulsion can be a strong impetus for imposition of the death penalty as a response to killing. In this response, however, there is an inherent problem for social order and for personal repose—that the infliction of death, whatever the provocation, carries an inevitable taint of wrongdoing and this taint must somehow be appeased or contained in order to arrest the impulse toward escalating (self-accusatory) wrongdoing.

Abolishing the death penalty would not eradicate this sense of guilt; failure to meet murder with murder can itself feed irrational belief that the passive witness has been an active accomplice in the crime. If, however, social arrangements are generally weak for appeasing a pervasive belief in the inherent wrongfulness of death, the safest course is to avoid direct engagement in death's infliction in order to forestall self-punitive, escalated wrongdoings. As Justice Blackmun finally understood, continuous "tinkering with the machinery of death" breeds no good for the officials directly involved or for the community at large.

CHAPTER EIGHT

ALL THE DAYS OF MY LIFE

Our publicly proclaimed motives are impeccable: the death penalty must be administered without arbitrariness, without discrimination against racial minorities or poor people, and only with the most intense scrutiny by impartial judges to assure that the entire enterprise is beyond reproach. This was the explicit commitment that the United States Supreme Court first made in 1972. The reality is, however, far distant from this ideal—and the Court itself, beginning in the early 1980s, adopted one measure after another to ensure that this ugly reality would remain hidden from public view. The dynamic could not be clearer: a public commitment to moral purity coupled with actions that undermine that commitment but without any acknowledgment of the contradiction.

Our commitment to moral purity is, paradoxically, the core problem with the death penalty. We are unwilling to settle, honestly and openly, for systemic imperfections and injustice because the death penalty is an intentional, unambiguous infliction of death on a human being; in embracing it openly, there is no psychological space for self-protective ambivalence. The pre-1970s social ethos of invisibility was never more than a marginally effective instrument for expressing ambivalence about capital punishment specifically or the presence of death generally. But once this ethos had lost its grip, we had no choice regarding capital punishment but directly to acknowledge its clear volitional character. At that point, we had only one next choice: either abolish the death penalty or lie to ourselves and others about the attainability of perfect justice, of an absence of wrongfulness, in its administration. Because the administration of the death penalty requires strictly dichotomous allocation of

moral guilt and innocence and because there is no possibility that this dichotomy can be sustained, the death penalty cannot be reformed. It cannot be cleansed. It must either be accompanied by persistent wrong-doing or abolished; there is no middle ground. We have chosen, however, to pursue this illusory middle ground—led and deluded by the Supreme Court since 1976—and we thereby set ourselves on a path of escalating falsehoods, coupled with a virtually irresistible impulse to betray our guilty consciences by engaging in increasingly obvious injustice which, of course, we are impelled to deny with increasing intensity. And so down, down the slippery slope.

Two general guidelines can be extrapolated from this conclusion and applied in contexts beyond capital punishment. The first is that inten-tional, unambiguous infliction of death in any context should be rigor-ously avoided and socially disapproved. The second is that, where death cannot be avoided, ambivalence about its moral status is also unavoid-able and should, accordingly, be self-consciously and visibly honored through the design of practical techniques for highlighting and even amplifying its inevitable presence.

These are the premises that implicitly guided Judge Learned Hand in his rejection, in the *Repouille* case, of Judge Jerome Frank's dissenting claim that "ethical leaders" might properly bestow definitive moral ap-proval on a purposeful infliction of death and in Hand's preference in-stead for openly avowed ambivalence. We can now explicitly draw out three interlocking dimensions of Hand's disposition: its psychological virtues, in both individual and social terms; its value in democratic the-ory; and its significations in the rituals for approaching death.

Psychological Virtues

Applying Hand's guidelines to social arrangements regarding abortion might seem to lead to the same conclusion that I have reached for the death penalty. Abortion could conceivably be prohibited, just as the death penalty could be abolished. Some people argue, of course, that there is no direct parallel because capital punishment involves the death of a human being while abortion does not. But even if we assume that abortion involves human death, there is one salient difference from capi-tal punishment. Abolishing abortion in order to protect fetal life involves the direct imposition of coercion and suffering on another person—on the pregnant woman who is forced to carry the fetus to term. If permit-

ting abortion necessarily involves denying the humanity of the fetus (treating it as nothing but disposable biological protoplasm), prohibiting abortion necessarily involves denying the humanity of the unwilling pregnant woman (treating her as nothing but a biological container).

It is true that abolishing the death penalty would inflict suffering on the family of murder victims who might have a powerful need to remove the murderer from among the living. This infliction would not, however, be so clear or extensive an assault on their status as human beings as the imposition on an individual of an enforced pregnancy. Abolishing the death penalty does not imply a complete turning away from the suffering of the victim's family; it is still possible, and indeed all the more imperative, to respond to their suffering by long-term or even permanent imprisonment of the murderer. Prohibiting abortion, by contrast, involves a much more complete disregard for the suffering of the woman during and after her term of enforced pregnancy. Abolishing the death penalty is not inconsistent with finding a rough middle ground between protecting the humanity of the murderer and honoring the suffering of the victims and their families. This is not "perfect justice," but it is visibly structured ambivalence—a middle ground steered between two guilt-inducing alternatives. This kind of ambivalence is not simply an adequate arrangement; it is a much preferable and safer social arrangement than the self-deceptive and ultimately self-betraying pursuit of "perfect justice," of moral purity.

In final analysis, I believe this is the central failing—the well-motivated but ultimately self-deceptive and socially harmful failing—of pro-life advocates for abolishing abortion. Their commitment to the innocence and purity of the fetus is so single-minded that they close their minds entirely to the suffering that the presence of the fetus inflicts on the unwilling pregnant woman. The dichotomy between innocent fetus and guilty woman is too rigid; it provides no psychological or moral space for ambivalence, for intimations of blameworthiness on both sides of the relationship (the unwanted fetus inflicts harm on the pregnant woman, while her abortion harms the fetus). By contrast, social arrangements that permit abortion but restrict it to early stages of pregnancy provide a visible structure of ambivalence. Though it is possible in this regime to maintain one's innocence while committing abortion, by insisting that the fetus is not a human being and nothing has been killed, this proposition is difficult to hold on to. It is difficult even for most people who favor legalized abortion to ignore the violence inherent in the act; and yet, at the same time, the restriction of abortion to the earliest stages of

pregnancy provides some tenuous comfort in the plausible proposition that it is potential life more than actual life that is being destroyed. Legalized early abortion does not demand suppressing any intimation of violence; it permits and can even promote conscious acknowledgment of ambivalence, and this acknowledgment exerts a protective psychological force against escalating abuse.

My proposed guidelines—requiring social disapproval for intentional, unambiguous infliction of death and visibly structured ambivalence where death cannot be avoided—also provide a framework for evaluating the rules enacted by Congress in 1984 requiring medical treatment of seriously ill newborns. This issue arose in the 1970s as an ironic consequence of the new public visibility of, and apparent commitment to remedy, the prior abuses inflicted on retarded people. In 1976, just three months after the New Jersey Supreme Court authorized discontinuance of mechanical respiration for Karen Ann Quinlan, the Massachusetts Supreme Judicial Court ruled that potentially life-prolonging chemotherapy for leukemia should be withheld from a severely retarded resident of a state institution because of its painful side effects, even though the court acknowledged that virtually all mentally normal people would have accepted the pain for the possibility of longer life. The court held that hastened death would be a kinder result for this man, Joseph Saikewicz, in light of his retardation and consequent incomprehension of the reasons for painful treatment—in effect, a mercy killing, though the court did not use this term.[1] Saikewicz's illness would have remained undiagnosed but for the public light on institutional conditions brought by class action litigation; his illness was only discovered as a result of a court-ordered health screening to remedy long-standing general medical neglect of residents in the state institution. For Saikewicz, at least, the new ethos of visibility for retarded people meant that hastened death as a result of unacknowledged withholding of medical treatment was supplanted by publicly avowed hastened death.

Around the same time, this same ironic twist to the new ethos of visibility was also applied to mentally and physically disabled infants. In 1973 an article explicitly endorsing mercy killing of disabled infants appeared in the *New England Journal of Medicine,* the preeminent publication in the medical profession. Two physicians in charge of the newborn intensive care nursery at Yale–New Haven Hospital, Raymond Duff and A. G. M. Campbell, publicly announced that of the 299 deaths in their nursery from January 1970 through June 1972, 43 (or some 14 percent) of the infants had been intentionally allowed to die, although their lives

could have been prolonged by available technology. After identifying the various circumstances of these deaths (including a newborn with Down's syndrome whose parents refused relatively simple life-saving surgery to correct its inability to ingest food), Duff and Campbell stated that they were acting "as physicians have done for generations" and that there had been "public and professional silence on [this] major social taboo," which they had now "broken." They concluded, "That seems appropriate, for out of the ensuing dialogue perhaps better choices for patients and families can be made. If working out these dilemmas in ways such as those we suggest is in violation of the law, we believe the law should be changed."[2]

In 1982 the Indiana Supreme Court propounded the law as Duff and Campbell had proposed. In rejecting a petition by a local prosecuting attorney seeking an order to compel corrective surgery for a newborn with Down's syndrome, the court ruled that parents had the right to refuse treatment; the infant, known only as Baby Doe, died as the prosecutor was pursuing an emergency appeal to the United States Supreme Court.[3] This 1982 ruling embraced a new guise for imposing invisibility on retarded people—in place of the old mode of extruding them into the custody of physician-led institutions, this new mode gave explicit moral approval to parental custody, to the "right" of parents to decide for or against the death of their retarded child without any external societal supervision. The Indiana ruling carried forward the logical possibility offered by the U.S. Supreme Court's abortion ruling, awarding a constitutional right to pregnant women for externally unsupervised decisional authority regarding the continuance of their pregnancy—a logic extended in the *Quinlan* case to endorse a parent's authority to decide for his adult child's death, as if he were speaking for that child rather than on his own behalf.

This new guise for hidden decision making for the death of retarded people did not, however, take hold in 1982. The Indiana Baby Doe case attracted considerable public attention. President Ronald Reagan seized on it as a dramatic example of the consequences following from the judicially imposed policy of freely available abortions; as an extension of his pro-life opposition to abortion, he saw this as proof that court-sanctioned maternal choice to abort fetuses slides into court-sanctioned parental choice to kill unwanted newborns. Pro-choice abortion proponents were eager to refute this proposition, and the Baby Doe case quickly crystallized a political consensus that such parental choices should be forbidden. Congress enacted, by a virtually unanimous vote,

the Child Abuse Amendments of 1984 requiring that states, as a condition for receiving certain federal funding, must compel the provision of medical care to all infants unless, in effect, treatment would be futile.

The practical impact of this law is not clear. Some pro-life advocates have alleged that the practice of purposefully withholding medical treatment from seriously disabled infants was simply driven back away from public visibility or acknowledgment.[4] Others have maintained that typical clinical decisions to withhold medical treatment are more incremental and thus less amenable to legal regulation than the rigid categorization of "treat / don't treat" in the federal statutory formulation.[5] In actual practice, moreover, the respective roles of physicians and parents in making these incremental treatment decisions are uncertain; whatever formal legal authority parents might plausibly claim to decide the "futility" of treatment,[6] physicians can easily dominate decision making by shaping the information they provide to or withhold from parents. Current arrangements are thus "messy." Unlike the definitive resolution requested by Drs. Duff and Campbell and provided by the Indiana Supreme Court in the Baby Doe case, there are no clear lines of authority or clearly designated moments for explicit decisions to end a gravely ill infant's life. The 1984 federal law effectively forbids such highly visible decisions, permitting the termination of treatment only when death appears inevitable in any event. Decisions in favor of death can still occur, but only in a context of ambiguity about the existence of or responsibility for such decisions.

This is one way to provide what I would call visibly structured ambivalence, as a preferred alternative to authorizing the intentional, unambiguous infliction of death. As with abortion and capital punishment, any legal arrangement providing such clear-cut authority must necessarily insist on the moral purity, the blamelessness of the actors authorized to administer death. (In this context, the parents' or physicians' motives must be composed of nothing but beneficent concern for the "best interests" of the seriously ill child.) The current arrangement, by contrast, permits only halting and indirect decisions by parents or doctors in favor of death, if formulated as a determination that treatment would be futile. It thereby in effect accepts and even promotes conscious acknowledgment of mixed motivations, of guilt as well as innocence, of self-interest as well as altruism, of wrongdoing as well as purity.

This same analysis applies to the contemporary campaign for legalizing physician-assisted suicide. Legalization of this practice also ostentatiously depends on the moral purity of all authorized actors: the dying person must be entirely free from tainted motives, from anything in-

terfering with uncoerced choice; and those around the dying person (whether family or physician) must be equally pure and single-minded, without any self-interested wish to hasten that person's death. This is the breeding ground for unacknowledged abuse—for self-abuse by the dying person or abuse by others. By contrast, the context of decisions to forgo life-prolonging treatment provides an equally clear illustration of what I would call structured ambivalence. It is plausible to believe that no one's action in refusing or withdrawing treatment is the actual cause of death; it is plausible to assert that the illness, and not any human agency, is the cause. At the same time it is clear that human beings are doing something by refusing or withdrawing treatment and that something is clearly implicated in the onset of death. It is also clear that insistence on continued treatment—by physicians, family, or the patient—also can bring terrible, pointless, and therefore wrongful suffering. It is thus very difficult—not impossible, but very difficult—for anyone involved in this decision making to avoid some conscious acknowledgment of ambivalence, of a sense of wrongdoing as at least a muted counterpoint to the impulse to believe in high-minded innocence.

The contrast I am drawing between forgoing life-prolonging treatment and physician-assisted suicide is only a matter of degree, of relative intensities. I do not believe that the arrangements around refusing or withdrawing treatment are free from the impulses toward abuse which I have described. The practice of paralyzing patients in the course of withdrawing ventilator support, documented in the *New England Journal of Medicine* article I discussed in the first chapter, is contemporary evidence of this abuse; and I believe we have been too uncritical over the last ten years in accepting the new willingness to forgo treatment. But I do not believe these practices are inherently abusive, because of the way that ambivalence is likely to be understood not only as inevitable but also as consciously acceptable among all the participants. This acknowledged ambivalence can contain the impulses for abusive acting-out in ways that are not likely to apply to physician-assisted suicide.

Advocates for physician-assisted suicide or direct euthanasia commonly argue today that there is no adequate logical distinction between these practices and the already approved practices of refusing or withdrawing life-support, and that justice therefore requires this next, logically consistent step.[7] From my perspective, however, it is precisely the tenuousness of the logical distinction that recommends its preservation, as a way of giving expression to the inherently limited force of rationality in regulating the administration of death.

The underlying resistance to acknowledging ambivalence about death

is apparent not only in the existence of any regime legalizing euthanasia or physician-assisted suicide. We can see it in administrative details of such regimes. Take, for example, three details of the new Oregon statute legalizing physician-assisted suicide. The statute provides that the evaluating physician may, but is not required to, refer the requesting patient to a mental health professional before issuing a lethal prescription; the statute specifies an exceedingly narrow definition of mental competency to constrain any mental health evaluations that might be performed by the initial physician or referral professionals; and the statute provides that family members should be informed of the patient's request for a lethal prescription only if the patient agrees.[8] There are sensible principled and practical reasons behind each of these statutory provisions—concerns about endless diagnostic evaluations that could obstruct and even ultimately defeat the patient's claim of the statutorily granted right or about intrusions by mental health professionals or family members on matters that the requesting patient would prefer to keep private. These reasons support the statute's "streamlined" procedures—minimizing the numbers of people involved in the death-dispensing decision; denying the legitimacy of mental health professionals to quarrel with the patient's determination to end his life by narrowly constricting the definition of mental competency the professional is authorized to explore; denying the legitimacy of family members quarreling about the decision by giving the patient unilateral authority to keep them uninformed about his determination. But this compressed format also serves to abet the denial of ambivalence, both by the requesting patient and by any evaluating physicians or mental health professionals.

This impulse to deny ambivalence is, of course, not restricted to arrangements for physician-assisted suicide. We can see the same impulse in other statutory provisions for end-of-life decisions. Consider this detail from the model statute proposed by the U.S. Commissioners on Uniform State Laws and the American Bar Association. If an incompetent patient has not formally designated any proxy decision maker, section 5 of the act provides for automatic appointment of family members in a descending order: first, the patient's spouse (if reasonably available and not "legally separated"); second, an adult child; third, a parent; and fourth, an adult brother or sister. The act further provides that if, for example, there is no spouse but the patient has several adult children who are unable to agree on a decision, then the "supervising health-care provider shall comply with the decision of a majority of the members of that class"; and if the class is "evenly divided," then decision-making au-

thority descends to the next statutory class (the parent, for example) until an unambivalent decision and decision maker can be found.[9]

This statutory provision may seem to express nothing but the most obvious common sense: a health-care decision must be made (to turn off the respirator or not, to provide nutrition and hydration or not) and so a decision maker must be found who is able to choose between inconsistent binary alternatives. There is, however, an alternative possibility: if there is more than one member of a designated class and unanimous agreement is not reached among these members, then a default rule could follow that would, as far as possible, preserve the incompetent patient's status quo until and unless the class members were able to unanimously agree on a different course. This is, of course, a much messier solution than the model law proposes; and it would in practical effect favor those family members who would not endorse termination of life-prolonging treatments, since theirs would be the default decision. It is true that the prolongation of treatment might impose suffering on the patient without any commensurate likelihood of benefit; but categories of "suffering" and "benefit" are rarely self-defining, and family members may well disagree among themselves in making this calculus. Ultimately, then, it is not clear as a general proposition that treatment rather than non-treatment in deference to majority preference is the more accurate or more "just" result.

More fundamentally, however, insistence on family unanimity as a precondition for terminating care has two distinct advantages from the perspective I have set out: First, this decisional rule blurs individual responsibility for the purposeful infliction of death. (It gives vivid expression to the moral of Agatha Christie's tale *Murder on the Orient Express*, that if every suspect is guilty of the crime, then all are somehow innocent—or at least, that the collective guilt attenuates the guilt of each individual.) Second, a unanimity rule gives heightened visibility and conscious force to ambivalence about the infliction of death, to ensure against the impetus toward suppression and subsequent uncontrollable eruptions of the negative valences that inevitably accompany any death-dispensing decisions. In this seemingly small, practical detail about voting rules for designated health-care proxies, we can see a model for choosing between social arrangements likely to suppress ambivalence and those likely to bring it into awareness in the administration of death.

The same choice is present in considering resolution of the dispute between those who claim that intractable pain suffered by terminally ill people can only be remedied by legalized physician-assisted suicide and

those who assert that the medical practice of so-called terminal sedation is an adequate and preferable arrangement. For the minority of patients whose physical or psychological suffering cannot otherwise be alleviated, it is technologically possible to administer sufficient narcotics to render them unconscious and to maintain this state until they die—in effect to permanently anesthetize them or, in the medical vernacular, to terminally sedate them. From an ideological perspective, this possibility does not satisfy the claim for self-determination of those patients who want a hastened death rather than a prolonged stupor before death; and ideologically minded proponents for assisted suicide reject it on this ground. From a more practical perspective, these proponents assert that narcotics dosage sufficient for terminal sedation often, perhaps even always, hastens death by suppressing respiration and that there is no logically supportable difference between "quickly hastened" and "slowly hastened" death—between "euthanasia" and "slow euthanasia." [10]

The ideological and practical components of these objections cannot easily be disentangled. It is, first of all, not clear that the administration of terminal sedation necessarily or even typically involves any hastening of death; this question, at the least, has not been subjected to rigorous empirical investigation. [11] But even if there are some cases where terminal sedation does have this "slowly hastening" effect, there are important practical differences between "slow" and "fast" assisted suicide. The standard differentiation focuses on the intent of the administering physician: if the intent behind the administration of narcotics was to alleviate suffering rather than to hasten death, then the "unintended" though clearly foreseeable consequence is irrelevant in assessing the physician's conduct. This is the so-called double effect argument by which "foreseeably but unintentionally" hastening someone's death is not viewed as murder or assisted suicide. [12]

The psychological foundation for this distinction is even more tenuous than the claimed difference between "action" and "passivity" when physicians withhold life-prolonging treatment. If I know that my action will bring an undesired result and yet I take this action, it is hard (though not wholly implausible) for me to say that I did not intend this result—and if the result is the death of an inevitably dying and terribly suffering person, it is even harder (and close to implausible) for me to claim that I did not "want" this result at the same time I "intended" it. My motives may be clearly mixed, but weighing the specific gravity of one motive against the other is very difficult as a matter of personal introspection, and almost impossible from an external observer's inde-

pendent inspection.[13] Proponents of assisted suicide can convincingly argue that the physicians' motives in "quickly hastened" deaths are equivalent—to alleviate suffering and only unintentionally, regretfully, to cause death.

I take a different approach to this question. I begin by conceding that it is impossible to disentangle these "beneficent" and "murderous" motives in any individual case; and I then ask how the format for decision making can be structured so that this ambivalence, this tension, can be most effectively and visibly preserved. On this score, terminal sedation has clear advantages over physician-assisted suicide.

Regardless of the administering physician's "true intent," the technical demands of terminal sedation require close and persistent monitoring, not only by a single attending physician, but by an entire corps of medical personnel who maintain an around-the-clock vigil—the very opposite of a death watch—to ensure that the narcotics dosage remains precisely titrated so that the patient does not reawake but at the same time is not pressed toward a quicker death. This titration point is very difficult to maintain, perhaps even is illusory in many cases. But the technical definition of the practice requires that this elusive middle ground—the self-conscious maintenance of this difficult distinction between alleviating suffering and hastening death—be persistently (even if unattainably) pursued.

By contrast, the technical requirements of physician-assisted suicide have no such ambivalence-preserving constraints. The required medication dosage is intentionally lethal (notwithstanding that the "true motive" of both physician and patient is only "unintentionally" lethal); and the administration is a quick and readily private transaction requiring no prolonged vigil, no direct participation or even observation by anyone except the individual physician and patient. The very structure of the statutory regulations for physician-assisted suicide demands strict binary determinations—demands resolution, that is, of any possible ambiguity and ambivalence—regarding the "true beneficence" of the intended killing, both from the patient's perspective (whether he has "competently and rationally" determined that death is in his best interest) and from the physician's (whether he is sure that the patient is truly dying and truly competent).

When the Supreme Court unanimously overturned the circuit courts' rulings in the 1997 assisted-suicide case, three of the justices specifically concurred on the ground that the legalized availability of terminal sedation effectively accomplished all that the plaintiffs demanded. Justice

Sandra Day O'Connor stated, "a patient who is suffering from a terminal illness and who is experiencing great pain has no legal barriers [under New York and Washington laws] to obtaining medication, from qualified physicians, to alleviate that suffering, even to the point of causing unconsciousness and hastening death. . . . [T]here is [accordingly] no need to address the question whether suffering patients have a constitutionally cognizable interest in obtaining relief from the suffering that they may experience in the last days of their lives." [14]

O'Connor was mistaken on two counts here. First, state narcotics laws have often been rigidly applied in ways that obstruct physicians' ability to provide effective pain palliation (although immediately following the Supreme Court's rulings, many states—including New York—specifically liberalized their narcotics laws for this purpose, thus converting O'Connor's erroneous observation into a self-fulfilling prophecy).[15] Second, the constitutional claim for self-determination in hastening death is not fully satisfied by the legal availability of terminal sedation. The heart of that claim, as the Ninth Circuit described it, was for the "right [of] . . . controlling the time and manner of one's death" on the same basis that the Supreme Court had previously grounded the right to self-determination in abortion, that "the most intimate and personal choices a person may make in a lifetime, choices central to personal dignity and autonomy, are central to the liberty protected by the Fourteenth Amendment." [16] However effective terminal sedation might be in eradicating any awareness of suffering, this option for prolonged dying would not satisfy everyone's conception of a "dignified" or "autonomous" death.

Justice O'Connor's reasoning may not have fit the conventional model of judicial rationalism; but in its almost palpable self-contradiction, she intuitively grasped the psychological and social protective function of visible ambivalence in these matters. O'Connor understood that the availability of the mediating alternative of terminal sedation— even though it does not fully satisfy some claimants' demands for autonomous control in approaching death—was a dispositive consideration against the legalization of assisted suicide.

This positive valuation of ambivalence and purposeful design of social arrangements to heighten its visibility has implications beyond the structuring of specific practices. This criterion provides a general evaluative guide for competing allocations of decision-making authority between physicians and patients. In the now-discredited past, decision-making authority was unilaterally vested in the medical profession, to

the exclusion of all other conceivable participants; and within the profession exclusive authority rested in the sole person of the attending physician. The currently dominant reform agenda ostentatiously rejects this medical authoritarianism; driven by the catchphrase "whose life is it, anyway," the new agenda offers sole controlling authority to the self-determining patient. In actual practice, most patients have been much less willing to exercise this social authority than attending physicians, their specifically authorized predecessors, had been. Many explanations have been offered for this contemporary reticence—most notably, the unwillingness of physicians to give more than lip service to the new regime and the feelings of distress and dependency induced by serious illness among patients that lead them to cede their authority to others.[17] If these explanations are correct—and they are certainly plausible—this is an undesirable state of affairs from my perspective, insofar as the new regime has failed to dislodge the old ethos of unilateral authority vested in physicians.

But even the lip service, the ritual bow toward patient autonomy, now required of physicians is itself a significant break with past practice and contains at least the seeds of an important corrective. The ideal of "shared decision-making authority" between physician and patient approximates the goal that I would prescribe.[18] In the way this ideal is typically described in contemporary reformist literature, however, it still reflects assumptions about the desirability and practical necessity for univalent loci of authority. Physicians, that is, are typically understood as technical authorities, and patients are viewed as "value-choosing" authorities; physicians set out the data on which cost-benefit calculations can be made, and, using this data, patients do the calculus. These tidy divisions have little correspondence to actual practice in physician-patient relations. But insofar as the prescriptive ideals do have some impact on practice, these jurisdictional boundaries within the ethos of shared decision making should be abandoned. Conceptual tidiness, with its handmaiden of administrative efficiency, is precisely the wrong guide for action here. Explicitly overlapping and competitive grants of decision-making authority offer the best way to promote the acknowledgment and expression of ambivalence as death approaches. This may be administratively messy, even a bureaucratic nightmare, for physicians and hospital administrators who have limited time and limited tolerance for debate or challenges to their authority. This may be offensive in principle to advocates for patient self-control who object to any derogation of patient autonomy—to any legitimated role for physicians or family

members to argue with patients about the value for them, for example, of discontinuing or persisting in life-prolonging treatment. But clean lines of decision-making authority are not next to godliness in these matters.

At the same time, however, explicit grants of overlapping authority can readily be transformed in practice to univalent authority vested in a single dissenter. The trick for prescriptive techniques to highlight ambivalence is to keep all participants enough off balance in their decisions about the approach of death that psychological space remains open for conflicting purposes to become visible for all participants, without utterly disabling the participants from ultimately choosing some path among these conflicting directions. As we have seen through illustrative examples in this chapter regarding unanimity rules for family proxies or the practice of terminal sedation, it is indeed "tricks"—that is, cleverly designed stratagems embedded in the detailed processes of decision making—that must be relied upon for this purpose.

This criterion provides a guide for thinking about decision making to withdraw or withhold life-prolonging medical treatments through the new vocabulary of patient choice. The format of this choice making is not as clearly troublesome as the movement for assisted suicide because in these settings no one directly inflicts death on a human being—no one, that is, directly engages in what we must understand as an inherently guilty act. Nonetheless, however important this distinction is, it can often seem gossamer thin, and the prospects for hidden abuse cannot be casually dismissed. In our current self-congratulatory embrace of the right to forgo life-prolonging medical treatment, however, we have too quickly and too casually dismissed the possibility of an abusive undertow. Where is the intensive empirical research into the actual implementation of these newly proclaimed rights, to make sure that elderly people or poor people or psychologically vulnerable people are not being pressured by this new ethos into premature self-abandonment? Where is the skepticism that should temper our enthusiastic embrace of this new guise for the rational mastery of death? [19]

Our enthusiasm for advance directives should similarly be subjected to this wash of "skeptical acid." For this purpose, I would distinguish between two different goals of advance directives. One goal—in my view, a foolish and possibly dangerous goal—is to specify in advance exactly what treatments an individual does and does not want as death comes closer. This is almost a caricature of the pursuit of rational mastery. For this reason alone, it is not surprising that in actual practice, nei-

ther physicians nor patients themselves appear to take these advance directives very seriously.

There is another goal for advance directives, however—and this goal seems to me both worthwhile and a possibly important corrective to the abusive potentials that I have identified. The goal is not in the specifics of the directives or in the apparent effort to exert rational control over one's ultimate death. The goal is to have open, serious, and intensive conversation between seriously ill people and their families, friends, and physicians about the prospects of death and the way that everyone expects to behave as death comes closer. The underlying protection here is not in the specifics of what is said, but in the fact that people are talking—and thereby assuring one another that, as death comes closer, no one will flee in terror from the dying person, including the dying person him- or herself.

This is not so much an advance directive as it is talk-in-advance to offer reassurance against the inevitable impulses toward the abandonment and isolation of the dying person. The breeding ground for abuse of dying people—for guilt and blame and degradation, for self-abuse and others' inflictions of abuse—is in the silences engendered by this social isolation. Effective counteracting of this social isolation does not depend on rational mastery of death. It depends on enlarging everyone's tolerance for their inability to achieve this mastery; it depends on reassuring everyone that their fears, their guilt, their desperation, are shared experiences that can be tolerated, or at least are less terrifying, because they are shared rather than isolated ordeals.

These considerations point to another practical prescription for averting the powerful impulses toward abuse of dying people. I have already noted the nonpublic character, the secrecy of the old regime of medical decision making about death and the ways in which the new regime of patient self-determination reiterates this nonpublic, this secret characteristic—especially in the reliance on the ideal of privacy and the absence of any structured guidance, of any social accompaniment, for the "private, uniquely personal" decisions about when and how death should come for each individual. This private, this secret and therefore socially isolated, format is the problem, not the solution, in confronting death. This isolated format for rational decision making—whether by physicians or by individual patients—in practical effect is the give-away for, the implicit acknowledgment of, the persistent force of unreasoned convictions about the inherent evil of death and our ultimate inability to exert rational control over it. We make a public show of our confi-

dence in our capacity for rational control, but we then retreat into a private place to make these decisions, where we can hide from others and from ourselves the underlying reality that this kind of control is a vain and empty ambition—a private place where we can punish ourselves and others for our failure to achieve this much-wished-for, socially acclaimed goal of rational mastery.

The corrective for this impulse is—to borrow a phrase from diplomatic history—"open decisions, openly arrived at and openly implemented." This prescription indicates, from yet another direction, the inappropriateness and abusive potential in physician-assisted suicide. The decision making is cloaked in the confidential relationship between physician and patient. (Recall, for example, the provision of the Oregon statute that the examining physician is not permitted to notify the patient's family that he or she is requesting suicide unless the patient agrees beforehand.) And once the decision is made, it can be carried out in an entirely private setting—in the suicidal person's own home, even without the physical presence of the physician, who has done nothing more than prescribe the lethal dose of medication.

Again, one of the great strengths of terminal sedation as an alternative to assisted suicide is that this response to a dying, intensely suffering person cannot be carried out in private, in a socially isolated setting. By its nature terminal sedation is an intensely public transaction—by the very fact that it is a complex medical regime requiring the participation of many people and around-the-clock monitoring. This public character thus serves as a potential corrective to the impulse toward irrational infliction of abuse on dying people—an impulse that encounters no resistance in the privacy of the transactions involved in physician-assisted suicide.

Democratic Values

Thus far we have been discussing decision making in a microcosmic context—that is, individual clinical decisions about or by specific patients. If we shift consideration to the macrocosmic context—that is, in communal deliberations about the generality of cases, conducted in large-scale institutional settings such as legislatures, courts, and executive agencies—we can apply the same criteria regarding the preferred role of visibly structured ambivalence in the administration of death. These criteria in particular provide a way for thinking about the role of

the Supreme Court in adjudicating the constitutional status of laws prohibiting abortion and physician-assisted suicide. We can see in particular how the conventional conception of the judiciary as the definitive moral arbiters of American social arrangements—the role Judge Frank extolled in his dissenting opinion in *Repouille*—is inconsistent with democratic values of participatory decision making and how honoring these values, as Judge Hand did, serves the socially protective function of visibly structuring ambivalence in social arrangements regarding death.

Proponents of a constitutional right to assisted suicide built their case on an analogy with the abortion right; and on its face there is a close fit with the constitutional rule that the state cannot obstruct a mentally competent pregnant woman's choice for an abortion, that the woman has a protected "privacy right" or a "liberty interest" to control the integrity of her own body. Indeed, if there is a constitutional right based on "privacy" or "liberty" to control one's bodily integrity, it would apply with greater force and coherence to assisted suicide than to abortion. A choice to hasten one's own death is more clearly a "private" act involving one's own "liberty of action" without imposing on others than is aborting a fetus, even if the fetus is understood only as a "potential life."

This argument can, however, be turned upside down. If a constitutional right to choose an abortion cannot coherently rest on a self-determination claim because of the plausibility (but not the certainty) that the fetus is a separate "self," then the claimed right for self-determination in choosing death should equally falter on the plausible (even though not certain) proposition that the "self" becomes conceptually incoherent in attempting to choose its nonexistence. Put another way, in both instances—in the constitutional claims for assisted suicide and for abortion—the focus on self-determination is too abstract, too removed from the psychological and social meanings of the act, to serve as an intelligible framework for understanding the choice itself.[20] The self-determination framework requires suppressing awareness of uncomfortable contradictions about the "self's" independent integrity or coherence in the very act of choosing either death or abortion. In abortion there are too many selves at stake and in assisted suicide there are too few for self-determination to be a reliable guide to action.

The restrictive abortion regime of the late nineteenth century was incompatible with the socially protective goal I advocate of keeping these contradictions in high social visibility, because it sought to sup-

press awareness of the pregnant woman's personal stake in the abortion decision. Her "self" was obliterated in the service of protecting the perfect integrity, the "independent" existence, of the fetus's "self." The restrictive abortion laws were, moreover, part of a larger legal and social imposition of subordinated status on women. *Roe v. Wade* should properly be understood as an effort by the judiciary to correct this imbalance, to end the social invisibility of women in the abortion context where that invisibility and consequent powerlessness had been most starkly imposed.[21]

As noted in chapter 4, this was not the Supreme Court's initial understanding of its enterprise in *Roe;* the Court's enshrinement of the individual physician's discretion in the abortion decision was itself at odds with this understanding. The Court's subsequent reinterpretation of *Roe* as based on the woman's right to self-determination was more to the point—useful as a corrective to the past suppression and invisibility of the woman's stake but awkward and imprecise nonetheless. The proper goal was to supplant the false, destructive univalence of physician dominance in abortion decision making without substituting a different single-mindedness in self-determination.

If the Court had understood and pursued this goal, there were many possible paths toward it. The Court could have invalidated all abortion restrictions on the ground that the statutes were constitutionally required to give more focused attention to the pregnant woman's wishes, without necessarily dictating that those wishes were the only relevant criterion. The Court could have ruled that states were obliged to provide specific reasons—and opportunities for women to challenge those reasons—for overriding their choice rather than permitting abortion only to save the woman's life, as in the most of the then-extant statutes, or to safeguard her vaguely defined "physical health" (and sometimes also "mental health") as in the more recently liberalized statutes enacted by 1973 in about one third of the states. This kind of judicial intervention would have required that every state legislature redraft its abortion restrictions, whereas in *Roe* itself the Supreme Court devised its own nationally uniform trimester-based abortion statute. The benefit of judicial insistence on revision by the legislatures themselves, guided only by an injunction to give specific, and even preferential, attention to the woman's wishes, is not that the statutes would thereby be more "rational" or more "virtuous" than the Court's own version. It is, rather, that the unilateral perspective on abortion in existing statutes, in which women's specific voices were utterly silenced, would be supplanted by a

new regime where multiple voices would be more clearly and avowedly heard—both in the legislative processes of redrafting, where newly active women's rights advocates would be given some greater political advantage as a result of the Court's intervention, and in the ultimate statutes themselves.

The possibility that differing state statutes might emerge from this required redrafting would be a further benefit from this process. Variation among states would be wrong only if there is a single morally or constitutionally correct perspective on the abortion decision; my own view is that there is a single correct perspective but only in the limited sense that this correct perspective requires explicit acknowledgment of multiple voices—some kind of visibly structured ambivalence—in the decision making. The possibility that some states might give greater weight than others to fetal or to maternal interests is in itself one way of providing a visible structure to the requisite multiplicity of perspectives on abortion. Indeed, before the Court ruled in *Roe,* there was already strong indication that a new national regime of multiple perspectives was emerging—not only from the sudden explicit enactment in 1971 of freely available first-trimester abortions in four states but also from the implicit freedom clearly provided by the administration of the 1968 statutory reforms in California and, even more importantly, by the absence of prior residence requirements in both the California and New York statutes, which meant that women anywhere in the country could freely obtain abortions in either place.[22] A more modest judicial intervention than the Court chose in *Roe* could have fostered this evolution toward a practical accommodation of all the competing interests—so that pregnant women intent on abortions could obtain them by traveling to the closest "free-choice" state while other states could maintain their separate, more restrictive regimes giving greater weight to fetal than maternal interests for specific reasons found.

This is, roughly speaking, the national regime we have ultimately come to as the Court itself has backed away from the initial strictures of *Roe* to abandon the trimester system as such and to validate the imposition of "reasonable" restrictions on women's free choice.[23] But this retreat from *Roe* has not been visibly guided by any principled commitment to the superior virtues of multiplicity and ambivalence in abortion decision making. It has been apparently without any principled direction, responsive only to the inflamed political pressures engendered by *Roe* and the vagaries of the appointment processes for new justices coming to the Court. This politicized reevaluation, moreover, has had the

utterly unprincipled effect of imposing new and almost insurmountable burdens specifically on the most vulnerable women, those too poor to afford abortions or to travel in search of the increasingly few physicians or facilities willing and brave enough to provide them.[24] The ostensibly new regime of constitutionally protected self-determination for women has turned out to have some close family resemblances to the old regime, where only women with financial resources and social connections could find abortions. The restrictive appearance of the old regime was belied in practice for these socially favored women; the hypocrisy of the new regime is that its universally proclaimed right of self-determination is much more readily available in practice for the same group of socially favored women.

Hypocrisy can be understood as another word, though more pejorative, for ambivalence. This hypocritical outcome of the Supreme Court's effort to suppress ambivalence about the death-dispensing implications of abortion can itself be viewed from the social psychological perspective I have been pursuing here. The notable resurgence of an injustice that *Roe v. Wade* set out to correct—the arbitrary availability of abortion with discriminatory impact on poor women—can be understood as the consequence of the inevitably unsuccessful attempt to suppress some sense of wrongdoing implicated in the practice of abortion.

This sense of wrongdoing was, of course, directly expressed in the old regime on the face of the restrictive statutes. But it found a further expression in the old regime that has been carried over into the new regime of individual choice. I suggested in chapter 4 that the old restrictive statutes set the pattern for general medical custody of death during the past century by proclaiming that all fetuses were fully human from the moment of conception but nonetheless giving physicians secret authority to abort fetuses as they alone saw fit, and that the hidden character of this medical control betrayed the underlying belief that physicians were committing a shameful act, a murder, when they aborted these human beings.[25] The new pro-choice regime takes an apparently different path—but it leads to the same end.

The old regime of medical control relied on a format of privacy, of abortion decisions carried out away from public view; and this kind of privacy was an unacknowledged contradiction to the pro-life public face of the statutes. By contrast, the new regime of individual self-control relies on the idea of privacy as its central public justification. But the privacy ideal has a peculiar character in its application to the abortion issue. The central moral question in the public debate about abortion remains

the same today as in the nineteenth century when the restrictive statutes were originally enacted: this question is whether the fetus is a fully recognizable human being from the moment of conception. The privacy ideal does not, however, directly address that question; it avoids it, quite ostentatiously, by proclaiming that the personhood of the fetus is an issue that cannot be publicly resolved but can only be answered in private, by each individual woman deciding on the basis of her own personal values. This invocation of the privacy ideal to sidestep the question of the personhood of the fetus in effect leaves the question open, unresolved—and by avoiding this central moral issue, implicitly betrays an underlying source of uneasiness about the true moral status of this private (and in this sense "secret") decision to commit an abortion.

Even in the regulatory regime directly proclaimed by the Supreme Court in *Roe,* ambivalence is apparent in the Court's grasping hold of the odd proposition that fetal viability—that is, the biological capacity of a fetus to survive outside its mother's womb—somehow was a sufficient justification for forcing the mother to retain the viable fetus in her womb. Ambivalence about the moral status of abortion was virtually enshrined by the Court in this fragile, and technologically shifting, line between the fetus as a "human being" worthy of social protection and a being of another sort, subordinate to its mother's dispositional choice. This virtually visible ambivalence does have some measure of the psychologically and socially protective function that I would prescribe. From my perspective, nonetheless, it would have been preferable if this ambivalence had arisen, not as an unintended consequence of moral confusion, but as a self-consciously calculated social choice; and if this had been self-consciously understood as the proper social goal, the virtues of greater deference to majoritarian institutions, though insistently prodded by judicial interventions, would have been more apparent.

In the 1997 assisted-suicide decisions, all of the justices had apparently absorbed some lesson from the Supreme Court's past engagement with the abortion issue. But their greater caution in approaching assisted suicide may have come primarily from a political calculation—from the polarized battles between pro-life and pro-choice forces that were precipitated by *Roe*—rather than from a deeper understanding of the unruly forces inevitably propelled by any socially visible dispensation of death. The justices' caution in the assisted suicide cases was, however, justified by much more than a reflexive aversion to politicized conflict. Their deference to legislative initiative was justified by the underlying virtue in democratic practice of enhancing the possibility, through pub-

lic legislative debate and electoral contests, of empathic understanding among people with divergent, and even contradictory, perspectives. The moral basis for democratic practice takes root in this social function of promoting empathic connection through the deliberative structure of formal institutional arrangements.

We can appreciate the working of this moral imperative in the Supreme Court's response to the dispute about physician-assisted suicide. At its core, the dispute engages two diametrically opposed antagonists whose conflicting interests appear to demand utter victory for one side and utter defeat of the other. The first type are ideological combatants— people with no immediate practical and personal stake, though nonetheless passionately committed to the ideal of self-control or of the untouchable sanctity of life. These antagonists—in effect, the pro-choice and pro-life camps—know one another well from the abortion wars. Each side claims moral superiority to the other; but in the secular realm of democratic politics, neither side has higher moral standing. Assuming, as the Supreme Court unanimously ruled, that there is no individual constitutional right to assisted suicide, there is no moral barrier to resolving this dispute by majority vote. To the contrary, the moral imperative of equality among citizens requires majority resolution.

The second type of antagonists on this issue are people with quite immediate practical and personal stakes—on the one side, terminally ill, mentally competent people who want assistance in hastening their deaths; on the other, terminally ill people who do not want hastened death but, because of social and personal vulnerabilities, would find it difficult or impossible to resist if this option were legally and routinely available. Proponents of assisted suicide claim that there is no conflict here, because screening mechanisms to ensure mental competence and voluntariness would be sufficiently sensitive to protect these vulnerable people. This is, however, a disputed proposition.[26] For the reasons I have already set out, I believe that these screening mechanisms will not achieve their proclaimed protective goals in the routinized practice of assisted suicide and that a perversely escalating guilty dynamic will make failure both psychologically desirable and socially invisible. I cannot definitively prove that this will occur; but if this outcome appears at least plausible, then there is a clear moral imperative that should guide the resolution of the assisted suicide controversy.

The imperative most clearly appears in the biblical parable of the good Samaritan; but the moral force of this imperative is not dependent on any theological grounding or on this sectarian basis. The Christian

parable is a version of the so-called Golden Rule of doing what you would want from others, of an empathic identification with others' neediness and a consequent willingness to accept some lesser personal sacrifice in the service of meeting another person's greater need. In the assisted-suicide dispute, there is neediness on both sides of the argument—in the person who desperately and adamantly wants hastened death and in the person desperately unable to resist the offered possibility. The moral obligation of empathic identification rests equally on each claimant, and the question is the same: given that both needs cannot be met because they diametrically conflict, how much self-sacrifice would be required—how much could tolerably be accepted—to satisfy the other's desperate, legitimate need? The available option of terminal sedation is crucial to this calculus on both sides. Because, as a practical matter, this option can only operate at the very end stages of terminal illness, is relatively onerous to administer, and requires coordinated effort by large numbers of people, it is less threatening than legalized assisted suicide to people unable to resist the possibility of hastened death. On the other side, this option does not provide hastened death for those who clearly want it; but terminal sedation does reliably promise that as death approaches on its own, any accompanying physical or psychological suffering can be ended.

The final tally on this calculation cannot vary for individual transactions; it must be made on a collective basis because the controversy itself is addressed to the collective arrangement—the general legality or not of assisted suicide—that provides the framework for all individual transactions. In this collective deliberation, there is a constant danger that the spirit of self-sacrifice in the service of mutual support will be swamped by narrowly conceived self-interest and that the majority will simply ignore the minority's needs and wishes, however desperate and minimally disruptive to majority interests. There is a proper role here for judicial intervention, to serve as a kind of balance wheel by providing various protections and advantages to the minority in pressing the moral worth of its claims on the majority. This is the core function of the judicial role in protecting "discrete and insular minorities" who are so socially isolated or disrespected that their interests are reflexively disregarded by others.[27]

"The dying" are not such a group, although they do have some resemblances to scorned social groups that have warranted special judicial protection. The paradigmatically protected group is African Americans, and dying people have been spatially segregated in hospitals and widely

feared by others in ways similar to the indignities historically imposed on African Americans. (Indeed, the very status of slavery has been powerfully illuminated by the sociologist Orlando Patterson as a form of "social death.")[28] Nonetheless, dying people cannot be kept confined as persistently or rigidly as racial minorities; and there are more obvious bases for cultivating empathic connections between those still living and those obviously embarked on dying, even though these connections have been often denied. On this ground, the Supreme Court was right to withhold any special judicial protection from terminally ill people claiming a self-determination right to assisted suicide and to remand them to majoritarian institutions to pursue those claims.

Ritual Significations

In the campaign to legalize assisted suicide, there has been little attention to the question of why physicians should be the chosen instrument for the task. Proponents of legalization treat the issue as self-evident; opponents claim that assisted suicide would undermine the physician's traditional role as healer, but they don't use this argument as a springboard for preferring some other professional or paraprofessional in the enterprise. In fact, assisted suicide is not a high-tech procedure. Insofar as the proposed statutes require a diagnosis of terminal illness and a limited survival prognosis as preconditions for eligibility, physicians do have special expertise, and their involvement does seem appropriate, even necessary. But prescriptive choice of lethal drugs by physicians as such and some direct role in their administration or oversight of their self-administration does not necessarily follow. A statutory scheme could readily be crafted with physicians limited to a preliminary eligibility determination but insulating them from further participation as prescribers or supervisors. In light of the intense opposition to legalization from the American Medical Association and other representatives of organized medicine, it is striking that proponents of legalization have not sought to bypass the medical profession. Proponents might, for example, have argued that the hostility of the medical profession was an adequate reason for the legislative approval of a new cadre of specialized assisted-suicide practitioners, just as the narrow-minded hostility of obstetric professionals to home births had prompted legislatures to authorize nurse-midwives trained to provide this service.

It is possible, of course—perhaps even likely—that the medical pro-

fession would be legislatively bypassed if assisted suicide became widely accepted and medical professionals generally remained hostile to its implementation. But the current, virtually unquestioned assumption that physicians have an irreplaceable role in any assisted suicide schemes illuminates an underlying cultural norm regarding the ritual function of physicians in approaching death. The current assumption about physicians' role in assisted suicide demonstrates that we remain in the grip of the norm that first took firm hold in the mid-nineteenth century, when physicians displaced clergy as the principal and even exclusive custodians of death and dying.

As I discussed in chapter 5, this new role for physicians brought them for the first time into direct contact with the aura of wrongdoing surrounding death—a taint that the profession had previously avoided by formally withdrawing from attendance after diagnosing a patient as terminally ill. In displacing clergy as custodians of death, the medical profession also gained social permission to breach other taboos surrounding death. Physicians had long sought access to cadavers but were pilloried for their efforts and relegated to midnight grave-digging expeditions. After the mid-nineteenth century, the general social taboo against handling corpses did not disappear, but physicians as such were exempted from it. State legislatures gave physicians legitimated access to cadavers for medical training and experimentation as well as through autopsies for public health or criminal law enforcement purposes. The ethos of science dictated that physicians' contact with corpses was a "clean" enterprise—benevolently justified as an instrument for enhancing social welfare through rational inquiry. Scientific handling of corpses is thus isomorphic with the "clean" conception of death—as a morally neutral biological process, a natural inevitability, and a rationally controllable event—at the core of contemporary efforts at generalized demystification. There is, however, a different way to understand the special social dispensations for physicians—but not others—to handle corpses and assume custody of death and dying. The scientific dispensation can be understood not as a generally applicable social cleansing of death but instead as a specialized set of practices which permit its initiates (and only its initiates) to cross the contamination boundaries that remain intact against the lay public. We can understand the special role of physicians, that is, as a ritual practice that reinforces the boundary between health and death for the laity by giving permission to physicians (and only physicians) to violate that boundary—in effect, to patrol it through regular border crossings.

This ritual function for initiates is illuminated by Mary Douglas's classic anthropological account of the "concepts of pollution and taboo." Douglas portrays general social practices regarding pollution beliefs as setting social boundaries between "purity" and "danger"—as ways, that is, to map a safe course through a threatening world. Some version of socially constructed categorical differentiations between "purity" and "danger" are, by her account, universal features of human social organizations. Moreover, she observes, "the focus of all pollution symbolism is the body" and therefore "the final problem to which the perspective of pollution leads is bodily disintegration. Death presents a challenge to any metaphysical system."[29] Douglas also identified a special role for priestly castes in many societies as enforcers and, at the same time, as approved transgressors of those categorical boundaries.

Of all the purity practices Douglas discussed, she found the greatest fascination and profundity in the pangolin cult of the Lele tribe of the Congo. I want to set out her account at some length in order to suggest some parallels between this cult and the ritual role of physicians as custodians of death in our culture:

> [The Lele] are a people who are very pollution-conscious in secular and ritual affairs. Their habitual separating and classifying comes out nowhere so clearly as in their approach to animal food. Most of their cosmology and much of their social order is reflected in their animal categories. Certain animals and parts of animals are appropriate for men to eat, others for women, others for children, others for pregnant women. Others are regarded as totally inedible. One way or another the animals which they reject as unsuitable for human or female consumption turn out to be ambiguous according to their scheme of classifications. Their animal taxonomy separates night from day animals; animals of the above (bird, squirrels and monkeys) from animals of the below: water animals and land animals. Those whose behaviour is ambiguous are struck off someone's diet sheet. . . .
> [Lele formal rituals] lead through a series of cults which allow their initiates to eat what is normally dangerous and forbidden, carnivorous animals, chest of game and young animals. In an inner cult a hybrid monster, which in secular life one would expect them to abhor, is reverently eaten by initiates and taken to be the most powerful source of fertility. . . . [T]he benign monster to which Lele pay formal cult [is] the pangolin or scaly ant-eater. Its being contradicts all the most obvious animal categories. It is scaly like a fish, but it climbs trees. It is more like an egg-laying lizard than a mammal, yet it suckles its young. And most significant of all, unlike other small mammals its young are born singly. . . . Instead of being abhorred and utterly anomalous, the pangolin is eaten in solemn ceremony by its initiates who are thereby enabled to minister fertility to their kind. . . .

[In this] inner cult of all their ritual life, . . . the initiates of the pangolin, immune to dangers that would kill uninitiated men, approach, hold, kill and eat the animal which in its own existence combines all the elements which Lele culture keeps apart.[30]

As the specialized custodians of death in our culture, modern physicians serve equivalent functions to the Lele initiates who are authorized to devour the pangolin. Our physicians, like the Lele initiates, bring together in an uneasy yet celebratory tension, elements of life and death which our ordinary culture "keeps apart." Physicians' handling of corpses and their authorization to invade the live bodies of their patients—to commit fearsome mayhem without any overt imputation of wrongdoing—are the most dramatic expressions of this specialized role. In these transgressions of the ordinary categories demarking "purity" from "danger," the specialized work of physicians also cuts across ordinary distinctions between "self" and "non-self" (e.g., their role in combating the invasion of alien disease in our seemingly intact, even impregnable, bodies), between "active choice making" and "passive choicelessness" (e.g., controlling disease through active intervention versus powerlessness in contesting the inevitability of death).

In addressing these categorical distinctions, physicians might try to accentuate one polarity to the virtual exclusion—the psychological suppression—of its opposite. There is no universal cultural command or invariable psychologic imperative for giving even implicit representation to these polarities as such. Our culture is free to disregard the ritual opportunities seized by the Lele initiates in their pangolin cult. But if we do take this restrictive course, we will be turning away—as Douglas observes—from a "common urge to make a unity of all [human] experience and to overcome distinction and separation in acts of atonement." In this refusal, this rigid insistence on the purity and power of our conventional conceptions of rational self-control and rational control over natural forces, we will miss what the Lele have grasped. As Douglas saw,

The dramatic combination of opposites is a psychologically satisfying theme full of scope for interpretation at varying levels. . . . [A]ny ritual which expresses the happy union of opposites is also an apt vehicle for essentially religious themes. The Lele pangolin cult is only one example, of which many more could be cited, of cults which invite their initiates to turn round and confront the categories on which their whole surrounding culture has been built up and to recognise them for the fictive, man-made, arbitrary creations that they are. . . . By the mystery of [the pangolin] rite they recognise some-

thing of the fortuitous and conventional nature of the categories in whose mould they have their experience. If they consistently shunned ambiguity they would commit themselves to division between ideal and reality. But they confront ambiguity in an extreme and concentrated form. They dare to grasp the pangolin and put it to ritual use, proclaiming that this has more power than any other rites. So the pangolin cult is capable of inspiring a profound meditation on the nature of purity and impurity and on the limitation on human contemplation of existence.[31]

For us, the lesson of the pangolin cult is to turn away from the fantasy that we can control our attitudes toward death—that we can suppress a sense of ambivalence and contaminating mystery—by a self-willed act of rational intellectual mastery. Our Book of Genesis tells us that it was eating "of the tree of knowledge of good and evil" that brought death to humanity; knowledge, that is, was contaminating, death-inducing, not an antidote to our mortality.[32] If we dare to grasp the opportunity, our cultural resources can sustain what John Keats called "negative capability . . . that is, when a man is capable of being in uncertainties, mysteries, doubts, without any irritable reaching after fact and reason."[33] Learned Hand displayed this capability in his conception of "liberty [as] the spirit which is not too sure that it is right" and his understanding that, in addressing the status of death, this spirit demanded the rejection of any moral certainty, that "the outcome must needs be tentative."[34]

We should accept the persistence of irrational fears and aversions about death rather than trying to conquer, to eliminate, these fears—a vain pursuit which can only succeed in burying them more deeply away from conscious awareness and thereby entangling ourselves further in them. Admitting the existence and power of these irrational forces does not mean that we should return to the past practices of hidden deaths. Those practices were simply another version of social efforts to control death—efforts as much doomed to failure as the current campaign to exert rationalized control, efforts whose inevitable failure produced terrible suffering and patent wrongdoing which are likely to be reiterated in the new formats of rationalized control. Death should be visible. Social arrangements should be structured so as to promote the visibility of death—but in formats where the essential truths about the inherent unruliness of death and the persistence of individual and social ambivalence about death are given full expression.

We cannot abandon the ambition for rational mastery over death. It is too deeply ingrained in our culture and in our selves—and it is not intrinsically bad. But we must somehow learn to temper this ambition

in order to avoid its impulses toward abuse of self and others. Unfortunately, the only tool available to us for learning this lesson is our capacity for rational mastery and self-control. Here is our problem. Here is the paradox that we must somehow learn to live with in regulating death— that we must teach ourselves, through our rational intellectual capacities, that our rational intellect cannot adequately comprehend, much less adequately control, death. We are no more compassionate, honorable, or intelligent than our predecessors who embraced the pursuit of rational mastery over death and were led, without acknowledgment, into unreasoned evil. We would do better to admit, as W. H. Auden acknowledged, that "Death is not understood by Death; nor You, nor I."[35]

NOTES

1. Good Death

1. See Philippe Aries, *Western Attitudes toward Death: From the Middle Ages to the Present* 94–103 (Baltimore: Johns Hopkins Univ. Press, 1974).

2. Jay Katz has invoked Dostoevsky's Grand Inquisitor—who exercises dictatorial authority in order to protect mankind from the vulnerabilities and terrors of freedom—as an analogue of the physician's culturally approved role in protecting patients against the terrifying realities of sickness and death. *The Silent World of Doctor and Patient* 127, 164 (New York: Free Press, 1984).

3. *Roe v. Wade,* 410 U.S. 113 (1973); this case is discussed generally in chapter 4, infra.

4. *Furman v. Georgia,* 408 U.S. 238 (1972).

5. Ronald Dworkin, *Life's Dominion: An Argument about Abortion, Euthanasia, and Individual Freedom* 237 (New York: Knopf, 1993).

6. See Sheila Rothman, *Living in the Shadow of Death: Tuberculosis and the Social Experience of Illness in American History* (New York: Basic Books, 1994).

7. B. J. McNeil et al., *On the Elicitation of Preferences for Alternative Therapies,* 306 (21) New Eng. J. Med. 1259–62 (1982).

8. Leo Tolstoy, *The Death of Ivan Ilych and Other Stories* 129 (Signet Classic ed.; New York: New American Library, 1960).

9. Sigmund Freud, *Thoughts for the Times on War and Death* (1915), in 14 Standard Edition of the Complete Psychological Works of Sigmund Freud 285 (James Strachey, ed.) (London: Hogarth Press, 1964).

10. Id. at 299.

11. See Valentin F. Bulgakov, *The Last Year of Leo Tolstoy* (Ann Dunnigan, trans.) (New York: Dial Press, 1971).

12. See Hans W. Loewald, *Psychoanalysis and the History of the Individual* 16 (New Haven: Yale Univ. Press, 1978).

13. Freud first posited the existence of a "death instinct" in his 1920 book

Beyond the Pleasure Principle, chapter 6. In his earlier thinking he had explained human aggression as one face of an instinct for self-preservation; by 1920, he had come to see aggression in a different light, as an independent and self-destructive psychological imperative. See James Strachey, Introduction, in Sigmund Freud, *Civilization and Its Discontents* 8–9 (New York: W. W. Norton, 1962 ed.).

14. Id. at 104.

15. Compare Jonathan Lear's incisive critique of Freud's conception of the death instinct, that "there is a more austere hypothesis that better fits the evidence: that the mind has a tendency to disrupt itself, that these disruptions are not *for* anything—they are devoid of purpose. Indeed, insofar as mind is teleologically organized, these disruptions disrupt teleology . . . because the mental efforts to lend meaning to a meaningless disruption—an external trauma or internal self-disruption—abort." *Happiness, Death, and the Remainder of Life* 77 (Cambridge, Mass.: Harvard Univ. Press, 2000). I would say that the imminent prospect of death, for oneself or for significant others, commonly provokes the kind of disruption that Lear portrays.

16. Taylor observes, "Here we see the origin of one of the great paradoxes of modern philosophy. The philosophy of disengagement and objectification has helped to create a picture of the human being, at its most extreme in certain forms of materialism, from which the last vestiges of subjectivity seem to have been expelled. It is a picture of the human being from a completely third-person perspective. The paradox is that this severe outlook is connected with, indeed, based on, according a central place to the first-person stance. Radical objectivity is only intelligible and accessible through radical subjectivity." *Sources of the Self: The Making of the Modern Identity* 176 (Cambridge, Mass.: Harvard Univ. Press, 1989).

17. Id. at 315.

18. See Robert A. Paul, *Moses and Civilization: The Meaning Behind Freud's Myth* 1–4 (New Haven: Yale Univ. Press, 1996).

19. Thus Hans Loewald, one of the most influential post-Freudian psychoanalytic theoreticians, has observed, "the assumption of responsibility for one's own life and its conduct is in psychic reality tantamount to the murder of the parents, to the crime of parricide, and involves dealing with the guilt incurred thereby. Not only is parental authority destroyed by wresting authority from the parents and taking it over, but the parents, if the process were thoroughly carried out, are being destroyed as libidinal objects as well." *The Waning of the Oedipus Complex,* in Papers on Psychoanalysis 389 (New Haven: Yale Univ. Press, 1980).

20. As Loewald states, "Reconciling parricide with love for [one's] father, and . . . the quest for emancipation and self-responsibility with . . . desire for identification and becoming one with [one's] father [requires] a confluence and integration of conflicting needs. . . . To master all of these currents permanently and without the aid of degrees and waves of repression appears to be beyond human capacity." Id. at 391–92.

21. For a neurological account of the intimate linkage between "body

sense" and "sense of self," see Robert Pollack, *The Missing Moment: How the Unconscious Shapes Modern Science* (Boston: Houghton Mifflin, 1999).

22. Compare Nietzsche's connection between these seemingly distinct categories of error: "I am afraid we are not rid of God because we still have faith in grammar." Friedrich Nietzsche, *Twilight of the Idols*, in The Portable Nietzsche 483 (Walter Kaufmann, ed. & trans.) (New York: Viking Press, 1968). I am grateful to Kenji Yoshino for this citation.

23. Genesis 3:15, 22.

24. Revelation 21:4. See Eberhard Jungel, *Death: The Riddle and the Mystery* 74 (Philadelphia: Westminster Press, 1974) ("That death is the wages of sin is something which is asserted only in the New Testament. . . . Nevertheless, through the entire Old Testament, death is specifically related to man's guilt which he must bear throughout his life and which he cannot explain.") In the Jewish tradition, contact with death—such as touching corpses or even being in the same enclosure with dead bodies—violates purity laws. Among Talmudic scholars, there is dispute about whether "the human corpse is by far the greatest source of impurity" or, more generally, whether "every source of impurity functions as a form of death." Hyam Maccoby, *Ritual and Morality: The Ritual Purity System and Its Place in Judaism* 1 (Cambridge: Cambridge Univ. Press, 1999). Maccoby maintains that there is a clear distinction between ritual impurity and moral wrongdoing; but this seems too rationalistic to capture the underlying psychological connection between the two categories. As Mary Douglas observes in her general anthropological account, although "it is true that pollution rules do not correspond closely to moral rules," nonetheless "pollution has indeed much to do with morals." *Purity and Danger: An Analysis of the Concepts of Pollution and Taboo* 130 (London: Routledge & Kegan Paul, 1966).

25. D. Hilfiker, *Healing the Wounds: A Physician Looks at His Work* 61 (Omaha, Neb.: Creighton Univ. Press, 1998). This same set of attitudes has been observed among psychiatrists whose patients have committed suicide. According to research interviews reported by Dr. Herbert Hendin, medical director of the American Foundation for Suicide Prevention, "for most of the therapists, having a patient commit suicide was 'the most traumatic event' of their professional lives. It is troublesome how long the difficulty stays with people. . . . They don't seem to get the kind of working through you would think people would get in a professional situation." A co-investigator, Dr. John T. Maltsberger, observed, "Doctors are ashamed of this. . . . There is a feeling in the [psychiatric] profession that if you lose a patient to suicide, you probably did something wrong." Erica Goode, *Patient Suicide Brings Therapists Lasting Pain*, N.Y. Times, Jan. 16, 2001, F6.

26. Mildred Z. Solomon et al., *Decisions Near the End of Life: Professional Views on Life-Sustaining Treatments*, 83 Am. J. Pub. Health 14, 17 (1993).

27. Id. at 18.

28. See also Howard Brody et al., *Withdrawing Intensive Life-Sustaining Treatment—Recommendations for Compassionate Clinical Management*, 336 (9) New Eng. J. Med. 652–67 (1997) ("It has been relatively difficult to con-

vince health care professionals that it is appropriate to withdraw artificial nutrition and hydration, despite ethical guidelines and court decisions that support the practice . . . [and notwithstanding] that death after the withdrawal of artificial nutrition and hydration will usually be comfortable and . . . continued treatment may cause considerable discomfort from fluid overload or when restraints are required." Id. at 655).

29. Solomon et al., supra note 26, at 19–20.

30. *In re Quinlan,* 355 A.2d 647 (N.J. 1976).

31. See Joanne Lynn, *Unexpected Returns: Insights from SUPPORT,* in To Improve Health and Health Care (S. Isaacs & J. Knickman, eds.) (San Francisco: Jossey-Bass, 1997); this article is discussed generally in chapter 6, infra.

32. Compare this observation regarding the new self-determination regime from Daniel Callahan, *The Troubled Dream of Life: In Search of a Peaceful Death* 35 (New York: Simon & Schuster, 1993):

> Consider . . . what we have come to. You ask: "What does death mean?" The answer: "That is for you to choose." You ask again, not entirely satisfied: "But what should I think about?" The answer: "That is your right to decide." You ask once more, by now becoming restless: "What kind of person should I be to ask such questions and have such rights?" The answer: "Who knows?" The more publicly sanctioned our right to choose death, so it seems, the more buried, the more hidden, the meaning of that death in our lives, and the more excluded from any common, public discourse. The more public becomes the espousal of choice, the more private the content and substance of that choice.

33. Cited in Dave Grossman, *On Killing: The Psychological Cost of Learning to Kill in War and Society* 3–4 (Boston: Little Brown, 1995).

34. Id. at 16.

35. Id. at 29.

36. Id. at 35, 251.

37. T. J. Pendergast & J. Luce, *Increasing Incidence of Withholding and Withdrawal of Life Support from the Critically Ill,* 155 Amer. J. Respiratory & Critical Care Medicine 15 (1997).

38. R. D. Truog et al., *Pharmacologic Paralysis and Withdrawal of Mechanical Ventilation at the End of Life,* 342 (7) New Eng. J. Med. 508–11 (2000). See also N. L. Cantor & G. C. Thomas, *The Legal Bounds of Physician Conduct Hastening Death,* 48(1) Buffalo L. Rev. 83–173 (2000), at 142–43.

39. Sigmund Freud, *Criminals from a Sense of Guilt,* in 14 Standard Edition of the Complete Psychological Works of Sigmund Freud 332 (James Strachey, ed.) (London: Hogarth Press, 1964).

40. Peter Brooks, *Troubling Confessions: Speaking Guilt in Law and Literature* 115 (Chicago: Univ. Chicago Press, 2000).

41. H. Taylor, *Doctor-Assisted Suicide: Support for Dr. Kevorkian Remains Strong and 2-to-1 Majority Approves Oregon-Style Assisted Suicide Bill* (New York: Louis Harris, 1995). See also D. Meier et al., *A National Survey of Physician-Assisted Suicide and Euthanasia in the United States,* 338 New Eng. J. Med. 1193 (1998).

42. Or. Rev. Stat. Sec. 127.800(6) (1998).

43. See Jack D. McCue & Lewis M. Cohen, *Freud's Physician-Assisted Death,* 159 Archives Internal Medicine 1521 (1999); the authors continue:

> Just as Freud chose to live as long as life was personally meaningful, and die the death he chose at the hands of his trusted physician, Max Schur, we believe that it is inevitable that more terminally ill patients will demand physician assistance in a quick, controlled, and reconciled death when life's potential has been exhausted and death is imminent. . . . We conclude that Freud's choice of physician-assisted suicide was not merely an interesting historical event, but one of paramount rationality, and one that is relevant to our contentious contemporary debates concerning euthanasia and physician-assisted suicide. . . . [F]or individuals like Freud who insist on writing their own life's script, a controlled and reconciled death is of grave importance. (1521, 1525)

See also Adam Phillips, *Darwin's Worms* 105–6 (New York: Basic Books, 2000) ("Freud's death was another triumph for medicine. . . . If acceptance of the reality principle means anything it must mean acceptance of death. Freud was, his biographers intimate, at one with his ideas; he embodied his beliefs. He had unified himself.")

44. Ernest Jones, 3 *The Life and Work of Sigmund Freud* 245–46 (New York: Basic Books, 1957).

45. Max Schur, *Freud: Living and Dying* 529 (New York: Int'l Universities Press, 1972). In describing his contribution to Jones's biography regarding this "last chapter," Schur stated that "a great deal was left unsaid." Id. at 7.

46. The letter from Schur to Anna Freud of March 19, 1954, was cited by Peter Gay in his biography *Freud: A Life for Our Time* 740 (New York: W. W. Norton, 1988).

47. Personal communication by Kathleen Foley, M.D., chief of pain and palliative care, Memorial Sloane-Kettering Cancer Center, New York, N.Y., July 15, 2000. See Susan Anderson Fohr, *The Double Effect of Pain Medication: Separating Myth from Reality,* 1 J. Palliative Medicine 315, 320 (1998).

48. Gay, supra note 46, at 650–51 and note at 739.

49. Id. at 740.

50. Id. at 651.

51. As Adam Phillips observed regarding these misleading biographical accounts of Freud's death, "it was part of the Freudian revolution . . . to undermine this particular genre of the heroic ideal; consistency, coherence, integrity in Freud's redescription of them begin to look complicit with everything that undoes them. . . . Freud's candidates for the making of a life—unconscious desire, the life and death instincts, infantile sexuality, the unconscious, language, primal helplessness, family relationships, chance—do not lend themselves to straightforward intelligibility." Supra note 43, at 106.

52. Sigmund Freud, *Civilization and Its Discontents* 104 (New York: W. W. Norton, 1962 ed.)

2. Hidden Death

1. See Robert A. Burt, *Pennhurst: A Parable* in In the Interests of Children: Advocacy, Law Reform, and Public Policy 265 (R. Mnookin, ed.) (New York: W. H. Freeman, 1985).

2. *Despairing Father Kills Imbecile Boy: Elevator Operator Tells the Police His Son, 13, "Just Like Dead All the Time,"* N.Y. Times, Oct. 13, 1939, 25, col. 7.

3. *Guilty in Mercy Killing: Father Convicted for Chloroforming Imbecile Son, 13,* N.Y. Times, Dec. 10, 1941, 27, col. 7.

4. *Father Goes Free in Mercy Slaying: Gets Suspended Sentence for Chloroforming Boy, 13, Who Was a Blind Imbecile: But He Is Disappointed: Says Jury Should Not Have Convicted Him—Appeals for Job to Support Family,* N.Y. Times, Dec. 25, 1941, 44, col. 7.

5. *Says He Slew Son At God's Command: Greenfield Testifies "Voices" Ordered Him to Stop Young Imbecile's Suffering: Tells of Love for Youth; Killing Violated Man's Law but Not God's, He Declares—Both Sides Rest at Trial,* N.Y. Times, May 11, 1939, 10, col. 2.

6. *Father Acquitted in Mercy Killing: Jury Frees Greenfield, Slayer of Imbecile Son, After Four Hours of Deliberation,* N.Y. Times, May 12, 1939, 1, col. 6; 22, cols. 3-4.

7. *$5,000 Bail Is Set in "Mercy Killing": Elevator Operator Detained for Hearing on Homicide Charge in Son's Death,* N.Y. Times, Oct. 14, 1939, 21, col. 2. The jury in Repouille's case heard evidence that Repouille had discussed this prior case before killing his son. *Tells of Killing Son: Father Pressed Cloth of Chloroform on Ill Boy's Face,* N.Y. Times, Dec. 6, 1941, 34, col. 2.

8. *Stepfather Slays Boy, 5, by Drowning: Surrenders to Patrolman, Saying He Feared the Child Was Going Crazy: Read of Mercy Killings: Admits He Had Been Drinking—Neighbors Assert Victim Was Normal Youngster,* N.Y. Times, Oct. 16, 1939, 3, col. 2.

9. *Gets Bail in Mercy Death: Repouille, Who Killed Imbecile Son, Freed on $5,000,* N.Y. Times, Oct, 16, 1939, 3, col. 2.

10. N.Y. Times, supra, note 4.

11. On the general systemic function of the jury in giving protective invisibility to agonizing issues of public morality, see Guido Calabresi & Phillip Bobbitt, *Tragic Choices* 57–62 (New York: W. W. Norton, 1978).

12. The government's brief relied on *In re Ross,* 188 Fed. 685, 686 (M.D. Pa. 1911), where citizenship had been denied to a man who had pled guilty to second degree murder fourteen years earlier and had completed a prison term of nine years. The *Ross* court gave no details about the crime itself and observed that both "before the commission of the offense, and since, the conduct of the petitioner reveals no cause for censure"; nonetheless, the court held, "Citizenship is not to be debauched by conferring on the criminal class its sacred privileges. The crime of which the petitioner admitted his guilt, is so abhorrent to human nature and society that this court will not bestow on him the rights of an American citizen." The government ended its brief in *Repouille* with this peroration.

13. Memorandum from Augustus N. Hand in *Repouille v. United States,* Nov. 19, 1947, in the papers of Jerome Frank, Yale University Library.

14. Memorandum from Jerome Frank in *Repouille v. United States,* Nov. 21, 1947, in the papers of Jerome Frank, Yale University Library.

15. *United States v. Francioso,* 164 F.2d 163, 163–64 (2d Cir. 1947).

16. Learned Hand memorandum, Oct. 17, 1947, quoted in Gerald Gunther, *Learned Hand: The Man and the Judge* 635 (New York: Knopf, 1994).

17. *United States ex rel. Iorio v. Day,* 34 F.2d 920–921 (2d Cir. 1929).

18. Gunther, supra note 16, at 629.

19. *United States ex rel. Guarino v. Uhl, Director of Immigration,* 107 F.2d 399 (2d Cir. 1939); see Gunther, supra note 16, at 635–36.

20. *Schmidt v. United States,* 177 F.2d 450 (2d Cir. 1949).

21. *Posusta v. United States,* 285 F.2d 533 (2d Cir. 1961).

22. *Yin-Shing Woo v. United States,* 288 F.2d 434 (2d Cir. 1961).

23. Memorandum from Learned Hand in *Repouille v. United States,* Nov. 21, 1947, in the papers of Jerome Frank, Yale University Library.

24. Gunther, supra note 16, at 632.

25. *Repouille v. United States,* 165 F.2d 152 (2d Cir. 1947).

26. Id. at 152–53.

27. Id. at 153.

28. Id. at 153–54.

29. This was the clear holding of *In re Ross* (supra note 12), cited for this proposition by the government in its Repouille brief, at p. 9. In 1952 Congress enacted a new provision to the naturalization statute explicitly providing that in judging moral character, "the court shall not be limited to the petitioner's conduct during the five years preceding the filing of the petition, but may take into consideration . . . the petitioner's conduct and acts at any time prior to that period" (codified as 8 U.S.C. sec. 1427(e)). This provision was part of a comprehensive revision of the Immigration and Nationality Act; the committee report accompanying the statute gave no reason for the enactment of this specific provision (see H.R. Rep. 1365, 82d Cong. 2d Sess. [1952], at 189), but it seems likely that this amendment was enacted in specific response to the Second Circuit's decision in *Repouille* just five years earlier.

30. *In re Taran,* 52 F. Supp. 535, 539 (D.Minn. 1943), cited in a law clerk's memorandum (signed RHP) regarding Repouille's case in the Jerome Frank papers, Yale University Library.

31. 165 F.2d at 154.

32. Learned Hand letter to Felix Frankfurter, Dec. 9, 1947, quoted in Gunther, supra note 16, at 631–32.

33. This address was delivered in Central Park before 150,000 newly naturalized citizens, accompanied by more than a million others—the largest gathering ever assembled in New York; the address received extensive subsequent media coverage and became Hand's best-known public presentation. See Gunther, supra note 16, at 548–49.

34. *Buck v. Bell,* 274 U.S. 200, 207 (1927).

35. See Robert N. Proctor, *Racial Hygiene: Medicine under the Nazis* 97–

101 (Cambridge, Mass.: Harvard Univ. Press, 1988).

36. Id. at 285–97. See also Stefan Kuhl, *The Nazi Connection: Eugenics, American Racism, and German National Socialism* (New York: Oxford Univ. Press, 1994).

37. See Gunther, supra note 16, at 444, 490–91.

38. Memorandum from Augustus N. Hand, supra note 13.

3. Death at War

1. *Buck v. Bell,* 274 U.S. 200, 207 (1927).

2. See Joel Williamson, *A Rage for Order: Black-White Relations in the American South Since Emancipation* 117–51 (New York: Oxford Univ. Press, 1986).

3. By the 1930s, the NAACP Legal Defense Fund had initiated a sustained effort to present Black claims of wrongful oppression to courts. See Mark Tushnet, *The NAACP's Legal Strategy against Segregated Education* (Chapel Hill: Univ. N. Carolina Press, 1987). The signal act of recognition was the Supreme Court's decision in *Brown v. Board of Education,* 387 U.S. 483 (1954).

4. The founding of the National Association for Retarded Children in 1950 marked the emergence of parents from shamed silence and social segregation and the beginning of their public claims for support of their mentally disabled children. The signal acts of judicial recognition came in the 1970s in a series of lawsuits protesting abusive conditions in state residential institutions; congressional recognition came in the 1976 enactment of the Education for All Handicapped Children Act, overturning prior state policies of excluding mentally disabled children from public schools. See Robert A. Burt, *Pennhurst: A Parable,* in In the Interests of Children: Advocacy, Law Reform, and Public Policy 265–363, (R. Mnookin, ed.) (New York: W. H. Freeman, 1985).

5. Sigmund Freud, *Thoughts for the Times on War and Death,* in 14 Standard Edition of the Complete Psychological Works of Sigmund Freud 289 (James Strachey, ed.) (London: Hogarth Press, 1964).

6. Id. at 281.

7. Id. at 289.

8. Id.

9. Id. at 291.

10. See Robert A. Burt, *The Constitution in Conflict* 211 (Cambridge, Mass.: Harvard Univ. Press, 1992) and the sources cited there.

11. On the pervasiveness of the imagery of birth, death, and rebirth in Lincoln's Gettysburg address, see Garry Wills, *Lincoln at Gettysburg: The Words That Remade America* 62 (New York: Simon & Schuster, 1992).

12. "Actual war coming, blood grows hot, and blood is spilled. Thought is forced from old channels into confusion. Deception breeds and thrives. Confidence dies, and universal suspicion reigns. Each man feels an impulse to kill his neighbor, lest he first be killed by him. Revenge and retaliation follow. . . . Every foul bird comes abroad, and every dirty reptile rises up. These add

crime to confusion." Abraham Lincoln, 2 *Speeches and Writings* 523 (Don E. Fehrenbacher, ed.) (New York: Library of America, 1989). See Wills, supra note 11, at 180–81.

13. See Gary Laderman, *The Sacred Remains: American Attitudes toward Death, 1799–1833* 83–85, 144–48 (New Haven: Yale Univ. Press, 1996).

14. Id. at 153.

15. Martin Pernick, *Back from the Grave: Recurring Controversies over Defining and Diagnosing Death in History*, in Death: Beyond Whole-Brain Criteria 21 (Richard M. Zaner, ed.) (Boston: Kluwer Academic Publishers, 1988).

16. Id. at 20. "[W]hen classical and medieval physicians spoke of . . . the 'signs of death,' they did not mention heartbeats, pulse, or breath, but repeated the portrait of impending death painted in Hippocrates' *Prognostikon*. Then as now, the 'signs of death' indicated when the doctor's job was finished, but for classical physicians these 'signs' did not mean the patient was actually dead. For most of Western history, the actual diagnosis of death was primarily a non-medical function." Id.

17. Id. at 43, 47.

18. Paul Starr, *The Social Transformation of American Medicine* 7–8 (New York: Basic Books, 1982).

19. Id. at 80.

20. "[B]y the late 1890s, medicine was making a difference in health, primarily through its contributions to public hygiene. The role of physicians, however, should not be disparaged. In recent years it has become the fashion to argue that the great drop in mortality in the late nineteenth and early twentieth centuries was due to changes in the standard of living or to general public health efforts. . . . But this is to draw an exaggerated distinction between medicine and public health during this period and to assume that the effectiveness of medicine depended solely on the possession of 'magic bullets.' By providing more accurate diagnosis, identifying the sources of infection and their modes of transmission, and diffusing knowledge of personal hygiene, medicine entered directly into the improved effectiveness of public health. In two diseases, diphtheria and tetanus, the introduction of antitoxins was followed by a rapid decline in mortality. . . . The value of diphtheria antitoxin depended on early and accurate diagnosis; medical expertise in a case might mean the difference between life and death. For understanding the growth of medical authority, it may be irrelevant that doctors could not cure most sore throats. Informed parents would still want a physician to take a look at a child's sore throat even if the probability of diphtheria was only small. Moreover, it is not difficult to understand how this dependence could become generalized into areas in which physicians claimed expertise on less justifiable grounds." Id. at 138–39.

21. In the late eighteenth century, according to Starr (id. at 30–31), American physicians tried to emulate their English counterparts by organizing medical schools and exercising licensing powers, but

they failed . . . to establish themselves as an exclusive and privileged profession. The licensing authority doctors secured had little more than honorific value, and

during the Jacksonian period in the 1830s and 1840s, their claims to privileged competence evoked a sharp backlash that crippled their ambitions for the next half century. State legislatures voted to do away with medical licensure entirely. No profession was being allowed. . . . Lay practitioners, using native herbs and folk remedies, flourished in the countryside and towns, scorning the therapies and arcane learning of regular physicians and claiming the right to practice medicine as an inalienable liberty, comparable to religious freedom.

22. See James C. Mohr, *Abortion in America: The Origins and Evolution of National Policy, 1800–1900* 147–48 (New York: Oxford Univ. Press, 1978).

23. Id. at 200.

24. Id. at 157, 187. Mohr's historical account has gotten caught up in the contemporary polemics of the abortion debate. His depiction of the primary motivation of the AMA physicians in their anti-abortion campaign—that they were most concerned with shutting off a lucrative source of practice for their "non-scientific" competitors—readily lends itself to the contemporary pro-choice charge that organized medicine deployed its high social status to fool a gullible public into passing restrictive abortion laws after the Civil War. Marvin Olasky has convincingly refuted this caricatured history; see his *Abortion Rites: A Social History of Abortion in America* (Washington, D.C.: Regnery Publ. Co., 1992). It is more plausible to take the AMA campaigners at their word, that they were morally and scientifically convinced that life begins at conception. They might well have had an accompanying, even equally strong, conviction that public acceptance of this view would enhance their own social and economic status; but in embracing this happy coincidence of high moral altruism and narrow self-interest, the AMA physicians would have followed a time-honored role among public policy advocates of "doing well by doing good." Olasky is also correct that the AMA advocates succeeded because they found a readily receptive public for their anti-abortion campaign, not because the public was predisposed to defer to their judgment. The physicians' success in this campaign was in fact a step toward enhancing their social status, not a consequence of it. Olasky is not, however, convincing in his account of legal restrictions on abortion before the Civil War; the extensive case law and prosecutorial practice discussed by Mohr do not give dispositive force to the moment of conception, unlike the post–Civil War statutes. In any event, it is indisputable that some forty state and territorial legislatures adopted explicit restrictive statutes between 1860 and 1880; even if Olasky is correct that the legislators only intended to reemphasize a prior common law rule, the new statutes clearly reflected a general judgment that some legal change was needed in order to effectively prohibit abortion from the moment of conception.

25. Phillippe Aries, *The Hour of Our Death* 570–71 (New York: Oxford Univ. Press, 1981). Regarding American practice specifically, "in 1949, national statistics revealed that 49.5 percent of deaths occurred in institutions (39.5 percent in general hospitals and the rest in psychiatric and other kinds of hospitals and nursing homes); by 1958, the comparable figure had risen to 60.9 per-

cent (46.7 percent for general hospitals). Final mortality statistics for 1980 indicated that 74 percent of deaths occurred in institutions (60.5 percent in hospitals and 13.5 percent in other institutions)." Committee on Care at the End of Life, Institute of Medicine, *Approaching Death: Improving Care at the End of Life* 39 (C. Cassel & M. Field, eds.) (Washington, D.C.: National Academy Press, 1997).

26. Starr, supra note 18, at 169–70. See also G. H. Brieger, *Introduction: Hospitals* in Medical America in the Nineteenth Century 233–34 (G. H. Brieger, ed.) (Baltimore: Johns Hopkins Univ. Press, 1972): ("The average nineteenth-century physician, practicing before about 1885, probably did not have much direct contact with hospitals or their problems. . . . In 1873 one survey revealed only 178 hospitals in the United States. . . . The greatest rise in the number of hospitals occurred in the twentieth century and was related to increasing urbanization and to those technical advances in surgery, radiology, and laboratory diagnosis, that make the hospitals the essential centers of medical practice.")

27. Starr, supra n. 18, at 74–76.

28. On the Civil War, see James M. McPherson, *Battle Cry of Freedom: The Civil War Era* 760–73 (New York: Oxford Univ. Press, 1988); for the Vietnam War, see Michael S. Sherry, *In the Shadow of War: The United States since the 1930s* 284–336 (New Haven: Yale Univ. Press, 1995).

29. It was in this latter sense that the Civil War quickly came to be seen as a defeat for all American forces, as the white North withdrew its military occupation and reclaimed brotherhood with the white South by permitting and even actively conniving at the virtual reenslavement of black Southerners. Thus even the recently freed blacks were forced to see the Civil War as meaningless, though in a different way from the dominant conviction of the whites. For a representative expression of this attitude among Northern whites at the time, see Henry Adams's observation of the attractions of Darwinian "Natural Selection" in 1866: "Such a working system for the universe suited a young man who had just helped to waste five or ten thousand million dollars and a million lives, more or less, to enforce unity and uniformity on people who objected to it." *The Education of Henry Adams* 225–26 (New York: Modern Library, 1931 ed.). For the tenacity until the 1960s of this historical evaluation of the worth of the Civil War, see Eric Foner, *Reconstruction: America's Unfinished Revolution, 1863–1877* xix-xxv (New York: Harper & Row, 1988).

30. Starr, supra note 18, at 142.

31. Robert H. Wiebe, *The Search for Order, 1877–1920* (New York: Hill & Wang, 1967).

32. Starr, supra note 18, at 140.

33. See Robert N. Proctor, *Racial Hygiene: Medicine under the Nazis* 97–101 (Cambridge, Mass.: Harvard Univ. Press, 1988).

34. See Gunnar Myrdal, *An American Dilemma: The Negro Problem and Modern Democracy* 1015–18 (New York: Harper & Row, 1944).

35. Thus, for example, in the nationally televised address on June 11, 1963, anticipating his submission to Congress of the legislation ultimately enacted as the Civil Rights Act of 1964, President John Kennedy stated, "We preach freedom around the world, and we mean it, and we cherish our freedom here at home, but are we to say to the world, and much more importantly, to each other that this is a land of the free except for the Negroes; that we have no second-class citizens except Negroes; that we have no class or caste system, no ghettoes, no master race except with respect to Negroes?" John F. Kennedy, *The Peaceful Revolution,* in "'Let the Word Go Forth': The Speeches, Statements, and Writings of John F. Kennedy 194 (Theodore Sorensen, ed.) (New York: Delacorte Press, 1988).

36. See Lawrence Douglas, *The Memory of Judgment: Making Law and History in the Trials of the Holocaust* 38–94 (New Haven: Yale Univ. Press, 2001).

37. Thus Gunnar Myrdal, the Swedish sociologist recruited during World War II by the Carnegie Corporation to study American racial policy, observed in his massive and influential 1944 report, "in fighting fascism and nazism, America had to stand before the whole world in favor of racial tolerance and cooperation and of racial equality. It had to denounce German racialism as a reversion to barbarism. It had to proclaim universal brotherhood and the inalienable human freedoms." Supra, note 34, at 1004.

38. Gar Alperovitz, *Atomic Diplomacy: Hiroshima and Potsdam* (New York: Simon & Schuster, 1965); for discussion of the popular visibility and influence of this book, see Barton Bernstein, *The Atomic Bomb: The Critical Issues* xvii (Boston: Little, Brown, 1976). Alperovitz's critique was subsequently extended to include American saturation bombing of civilian targets in Europe during World War II; see Eric Markusen & David Kopf, *The Holocaust and Strategic Bombing: Genocide and Total War in the 20th Century* (Boulder, Co.: Westview Press, 1995).

39. Henry Beecher, *Ethics and Clinical Research,* 74 New Eng. J. Med. 1354 (1966).

40. See Evelyn Shuster, *Fifty Years Later: The Significance of the Nuremberg Code,* 337 New Eng. J. Med. 1436, 1438 (1997).

41. "Any undergraduate who was at Yale when I started there in 1977–78 saw one or two men always etching out the names of the alumni from Yale or of the Yale students who had been killed in Vietnam. As you walked through [Woolsey Hall] to and from classes, you'd register that there were these two men etching in the names. And you'd unconsciously register the time it was taking to etch in each name, and the time somebody had lost. It was always *there.* It was ever-present. The actual work stopped sometime in my sophomore or junior year, but I think, like every other student passing through there, you could not help but be quiet as you walked through that hall. Also, you couldn't *not* touch the names. . . . The opportunity to touch the names is a little different from a lot of the WWI memorials where in many cases you cannot approach the names, even though you are reading them, because

they're much higher off the ground." Maya Lin, *Remarks*, in Grounds for Remembering: Monuments, Memorials, Texts 8–9, (C. Gillis, ed.) (Berkeley, Calif.: Occasional Paper of the Doreen B. Townsend Center for the Humanities, 1995).

42. In the written description accompanying her submission in the memorial competition, Lin had stated, "The memorial is composed not as an unchanging monument, but as a moving composition to be understood as we move into and out of it. . . . We the living are brought to a concrete realization of these deaths. Brought to a sharp awareness of such a loss, it is up to each individual to resolve or come to terms with this loss. For death is, in the end, a personal and private matter and the area contained within this memorial is a quiet place meant for personal reflection and private reckoning." Id., at 11–12.

43. Judith Ann Schiff, *Old Yale: Sacrifice in Stone* 88, Yale Alumni Magazine, May 1994.

44. Robert D. Putnam, *Bowling Alone: The Collapse and Revival of American Community* 47 (New York: Simon & Schuster, 1999).

45. Andrew Delbanco, *The Real American Dream: A Meditation on Hope* 1, 77, 79–80 (Cambridge, Mass.: Harvard Univ. Press, 1999).

4. Judges and Death

1. *In re Quinlan*, 348 A.2d 801, 818 (N.J. Super. Ch., 1975).

2. Joseph & Julia Quinlan, *Karen Ann: The Quinlans Tell Their Story* 214–15 (Garden City, N.Y.: Doubleday, 1977).

3. Id. at 115–22.

4. Id. at 116.

5. *Report of the Secretary's Commission on Medical Malpractice* 20, DHEW Publication No. (OS) 73–88, January 16, 1973.

6. Robert J. Blendon et al., *Public Opinion and Health Care: Bridging the Gap between Expert and Public Views on Health Care Reform*, 269 JAMA 2573, 2576 figure 4 (1993) (citing data derived from Louis Harris and Associates Poll, Roper Center for Public Opinion Research, January 22, 1993). Physicians had ranked ahead of every other occupational group in public opinion polls since the 1930s; see Paul Starr, *The Social Transformation of American Medicine* 143 (New York: Basic Books, 1982). See also Elliot Krause, *Death of the Guilds: Professions, States, and the Advance of Capitalism, 1930 to the Present* 36 (New Haven: Yale Univ. Press, 1996) ("[N]o profession in our sample has flown quite as high in guild power and control as American medicine, and few have fallen as fast").

7. Kristin Luker, *Abortion and the Politics of Motherhood* 46 (Berkeley: Univ. of California Press, 1984). Luker cites seventeen articles published in medical journals between 1907 and 1948 which, she says, are "illustrative (but hardly comprehensive) examples." 271–73 n.2.

8. Id. at 46–47.

9. This same attitude can be seen in the public status of contraception from the late nineteenth century into the mid-twentieth century—public condemnation as "sinful" and illegal coupled with virtually open disregard for the legal prohibitions, both among purveyors and law enforcement officials. See Andrea Tone, *Black Market Birth Control: Contraceptive Entrepreneurship and Criminality in the Gilded Age,* 87 J. Amer. History 435, 438–39 (2000) ("Paralleling Americans' response to other forms of regulated vice, a zone of tolerance was created in which birth control was routinely made, sold, bought, and used. Not openly endorsed, contraceptives were nonetheless accepted"— this notwithstanding the 1873 federal enactment of the Comstock Law prohibiting the "nefarious and diabolical traffic" of "vile and immoral goods" imported, sold or distributed "for the prevention of contraception.")

10. Luker, supra note 7, at 56.

11. Id.

12. Id. at 48.

13. See Luker's account of Sherri Finkbine's case, id. at 62–65. In 1962, Finkbine learned of the teratogenic risks of the drug thalidomide, which her husband had obtained for her in Europe and which she had taken during pregnancy. After arranging for an abortion with her regular physician, Finkbine contacted a local newspaper to warn other pregnant women of this risk; national news services relayed her story and a public furor suddenly erupted, which prompted Finkbine's physician to cancel the planned abortion and Finkbine to travel to Sweden for its performance. Finkbine was, as Luker observed, "abortion['s] own Karen Ann Quinlan." Id. at 62.

14. See Mary Ann Glendon, *Abortion and Divorce in Western Law* 48, 173 n.197 (Cambridge, Mass.: Harvard Univ. Press, 1987).

15. For advocacy of the parallel proposition that mental illness is a social construct fraudulently disguised as a biological reality, see Thomas Szasz, *The Manufacture of Madness* (New York: Harper & Row, 1970).

16. *Doe v. Bolton,* 410 U.S. 179, 208 (1973) (concurring opinion).

17. Id. at 221 (dissenting opinion of Justice White).

18. *Griswold v. Connecticut,* 381 U.S. 479 (1965).

19. *United States v. Vuitch,* 402 U.S. 62 (1971).

20. Id. at 96–97.

21. *Roe v. Wade,* 410 U.S. at 153.

22. Id. at 165.

23. Id. at 165–66 (emphasis added).

24. *Doe v. Bolton,* 410 U.S. at 199.

25. *Dent v. West Virginia,* 129 U.S. 122 (1889).

26. Starr, supra note 6, at 65.

27. Id. at 17, 140.

28. In *Planned Parenthood of Central Missouri v. Danforth,* 428 U.S. 52 (1976), the Court struck down a state statute requiring spousal consent to an abortion by focusing exclusively on the woman's right to choose for herself,

without any special role identified for her physician.

29. Evelyn Shuster, *Fifty Years Later: The Significance of the Nuremberg Code*, 337 New Eng. J. Med. 1436 (1997).

30. See David J. Rothman, *Other People's Bodies: Human Experimentation on the 50th Anniversary of the Nuremberg Code* 19–20 (Osler Society pamphlet).

31. The Holocaust itself was virtually ignored in public discourse until the 1960s; in the United States, it initially came into focus through the lens of the 1961 trial of Adolf Eichmann in Israel, but subsequently assumed a distinctive American meaning "in the fundamental tale of pluralism, tolerance, democracy, and human rights that America tells about itself." A. J. Wolf, *The Centrality of the Holocaust Is a Mistake,* in After Tragedy and Triumph: Essays in Modern Jewish Thought and the American Experience 40–41 (M. Berenbaum, ed.) (New York: Cambridge Univ. Press, 1990). Assessing the origins in the 1970s of "organised memorialisation" of the Holocaust in America, Raul Hilberg has suggested that "after the disorientation of Vietnam [American Jews and non-Jews alike] wanted to know the difference between good and evil. The Holocaust is the benchmark, the defining moment in the drama of good and evil [and] against this single occurrence, one would assess all other deeds. And so, memorialisation began in earnest, that is to say it became organised." (Quoted in E. T. Linenthal, *Preserving Memory: The Struggle to Create America's Holocaust Museum* 11 [New York: Viking, 1997].)

32. See Barron H. Lerner & David J. Rothman, *Medicine and the Holocaust: Learning More of the Lessons* 122 Annals of Int. Med. 321 (May 15, 1995); Robert N. Proctor, *Nazi Doctors, Racial Medicine, and Human Experimentation,* in The Nazi Doctors and the Nuremberg Code: Human Rights in Human Experimentation 18–31 (G. J. Annas & M. A. Grodin, eds.) (New York: Oxford Univ. Press, 1992); Christian Pross, *Nazi Doctors, German Medicine, and Historical Truth,* in id. at 32–52; Mario Biagioli, *Science, Modernity, and the "Final Solution,"* in Probing the Limits of Representation: Nazism and the "Final Solution," 185–205 (S. Friedlander, ed.) (Cambridge, Mass.: Harvard Univ. Press, 1992).

33. Jay Katz, *The Consent Principle of the Nuremberg Code: Its Significance Then and Now,* in The Nazi Doctors and the Nuremberg Code: Human Rights in Human Experimentation 228 (G. J. Annas & M. A. Grodin, eds.) (New York: Oxford Univ. Press, 1992).

34. This characterization has by now become the commonplace depiction for the treatment of dying patients in hospital intensive care units, not only in public discourse but among physicians. See Nicholas A. Christakis, *Managing Death: The Growing Acceptance of Euthanasia in Contemporary American Society,* in Must We Suffer Our Way To Death? Cultural and Theological Perspectives on Death by Choice 22–27 (R. P. Hamel & E. R. DuBose, eds.) (Dallas: SMU Press, 1996) ("In a setting where medical care is equated with 'excruciating pain,' 'imprisonment,' and 'torture,' . . . euthanasia in all its forms finds increasing acceptability.") Ironically enough, Karen Ann Quinlan's status as the icon for the contemporary expressions of revulsion toward medical care

was not affected by the widely reported fact that she was not actually kept alive by any high technologies, that she did not need the ventilator to sustain her continued life. This irony itself is one indication that public attitudes on these caretaking issues contain considerable internal contradictions which are publicly known but nonetheless unacknowledged.

35. On Tuskegee, see James Jones, *Bad Blood* (New York: Free Press, 1981); on Willowbrook, see David J. Rothman and Sheila M. Rothman, *The Willowbrook Wars* 271 (New York: Harper & Row, 1984).

36. See David J. Rothman, *Strangers at the Bedside* 182–89 (New York: Basic Books, 1991). In 1978 Congress broadened the mandate of this commission and changed its name accordingly to the President's Commission for the Study of Ethical Problems in Medicine.

37. See Shuster, supra note 29, at 1440.

5. Doctors and Death

1. Charles L. Bosk, *Forgive and Remember: Managing Medical Failure* 196, 201–2 (Chicago: Univ. Chicago Press, 1979). As to the ubiquity of death in elite surgeons' work, Bosk reports that one senior attending told him, "It would look suspicious if you are doing major surgery and, week after week, you have no deaths and complications. You're going to have these, especially deaths, if you do major surgery. You can lead a long and happy life without deaths and complications, but you have to give up major surgery." Id. at. 50.

2. Id. at 189.

3. Id. at 63.

4. See Judith P. Swazey & Renee C. Fox, *The Clinical Moratorium: A Case Study of Mitral Valve Surgery* (Cambridge, Mass.: Harvard Univ. Program in Technology & Society, 1970).

5. Frederic Hafferty, *Into the Valley: Death and the Socialization of Medical Students* 95 (New Haven: Yale Univ. Press, 1991).

6. Id. at 97, 110.

7. Id. at 95–96.

8. Id. at 123.

9. Id. at 122–23.

10. Id. at 124–25.

11. Anna Freud, *The Doctor-Patient Relationship*, unpublished address delivered at Western Reserve Medical School, October 29, 1964, reprinted in Jay Katz, *Experimentation with Human Beings* (New York: Russell Sage Foundation, 1972) at 643.

12. Id. at 642–43.

13. D. Hilfiker, *Healing the Wounds: A Physician Looks at His Work* 21 (Omaha, Neb.: Creighton Univ. Press, 1998).

14. In the film prepared for classroom teaching purposes, Milgram explicitly ascribed "malevolence" to the authority deployed in his experiment; his

subsequently published book was more neutral. Stanley Milgram, *Obedience to Authority: An Experimental View* (New York: Harper & Row, 1974).

15. Id. at 14–16.

16. Id. at 16–21.

17. Id. at 23, 55–57.

18. Id. at 21.

19. Id. at 41–42. In the initial design of the experiment, Milgram decided against the customary practice of using undergraduate psychology students as subjects because they were too likely to view the enterprise as fictitious. Id. at 14.

20. Id. at 76–77, 87–88 ("Mr. Gino [a teacher-subject] summarizes his reaction to his own performance. 'Well, I faithfully believed the man was dead until we opened the door. When I saw him, I said, 'Great, this is great.' But it didn't bother me even to find that he was dead. I did a job.'")

21. Id. at 35.

22. Id. at 54.

23. Id. at 135–52.

24. Stanley Milgram, *Some Conditions of Obedience and Disobedience to Authority* 18 Human Relations 68 (1965).

25. Milgram, supra n. 14, at 152.

26. David Luban, *Milgram Revisited*, 9 Researching Law 1 (1998).

27. Milgram, supra note 14, at 28–31.

28. SUPPORT Principal Investigators, *A Controlled Trial to Improve Care for Seriously Ill Hospitalized Patients: The Study to Understand Prognoses and Preferences for Outcomes and Risks of Treatments (SUPPORT)*, 274 JAMA 1591, 1595 (1995).

29. See Committee on Care at the End of Life, Institute of Medicine, *Approaching Death: Improving Care at the End of Life* 133 (C. Cassel & M. Field, eds.) (Washington, D.C.: National Academy Press, 1997).

30. Marguerite S. Lederberg, *Blaming the Victim: Can We Learn to Stop? Cancer as the Battleground*, 225, 226 in Celebrating Elie Weisel: Stories, Essays, Reflections (Alan Rosen, ed.) (South Bend, Ind.: Univ. of Notre Dame Press, 1998).

31. Id. at 227.

32. Milgram, supra note 14, at 21.

33. Compare Jonathan Lear's psychoanalytically informed "hypothesis [that] aggression emerges from a breakdown in the mind's effort to make meaning—that is, a breakdown which cannot be healed by subsequent efforts to make meaning." *Happiness, Death, and the Remainder of Life* 113 (Cambridge, Mass.: Harvard Univ. Press, 2000).

34. Sigmund Freud, *Criminals from a Sense of Guilt*, 14 Standard Edition of the Complete Psychological Works of Sigmund Freud 332 (James Strachey, ed.) (London: Hogarth Press, 1964).

6. Choosing Death

1. In his book *Aging and Old Age* 245–48 (Chicago: Univ. Chicago Press, 1995), Richard Posner asserts that legalized physician-assisted suicide is likely to reduce the numbers of suicides, especially of elderly people, because its availability would lead a rational calculator to forgo an earlier suicide to avoid the possibility of subsequent diminished physical capacity; Posner's reasoning ignores the possibility that the prospect of death unsettles the stable sense of "self" and ordinary reasoning capacity for assessing present versus future risk/benefit ratios, which is dependent on that sense of stability. His position is worth extended quotation because it lays bare the unrealistic psychology, the underlying hyperrationality, of contemporary reformist claims to exert rational control over death:

> [A]ssume that our hypothetical sufferer is not certain that [his] disease will progress to a point where he will prefer to be dead, though he is certain that if it does progress to that point he will be incapable of killing himself without assistance. . . . [Where] physician-assisted suicide is forbidden, . . . when the individual first learns his probable fate he must choose between two courses of action: one in which he commits suicide now, at a cost (in dread of death, pain, moral compunctions, whatever) of c; the other in which he postpones the decision to a time when, if he still wants to commit suicide, he will be unable to do so. The question is which course will confer greater utility on him. If he commits suicide now, he will have utility of $-c$. He will experience neither positive nor expected utility from living, because he will be dead, but he will incur the cost of getting from the state of being alive to the state of being dead. If he decides not to commit suicide now, he avoids incurring c and obtains whatever utility, positive or negative, continued life confers upon him. Because of uncertainty, that utility is an expected utility; it is equal to the weighted average of his negative utility in the doomed state,—Ud—the disutility that he will incur if it turns out that he really does have a terminal or otherwise horribly painful or disabling illness—and his positive utility in the healthy or at least relatively healthy state that he will be in if he recovers to the point of wanting to live after all: Uh.
>
> Each expected utility must be weighted by the probability (p or $1 - p$) that the individual will in fact find himself in the doomed or in the healthy state. He reasonably expects the former, but not with certainty: that is, $1 > pUd > (1 - p)Ud$. The sum of these utilities is $p(-Ud) + (1 - p)Uh$, and must be compared with the utility of committing suicide ($-c$). I assume that $Ud > c$, an important assumption that will be relaxed later. With these assumptions, our hypothetical individual will commit suicide if
>
> $$pUd > (1 - p)Uh + c \quad (10.1)$$
>
> —in words, if the expected utility of death now, which is to say the disutility averted by death now, exceeds the expected utility of life plus the cost of suicide. The loss of that expected utility, and the cost of suicide, are the costs that he incurs by committing suicide now. If $c = 0$, he will commit suicide if $pUd > (1 - p)Uh$, that is, if the expected (that is, probability-weighted) disutility of living in

what I am calling the doomed state exceeds the expected utility of living in the healthy state.

Since the doomed state is more likely—that is, $p > (1 - p)$—the anticipated disutility of that state need not be so great as the anticipated utility of the saved (healthy) state for suicide to be a rational decision; indeed, if p is high enough, the disutility of living in the doomed state could be considerably smaller than the utility of living in the saved state without making the decision to commit suicide an irrational one. This also depends on the size of c, however. If the cost of committing suicide is great enough, an individual will refrain from committing suicide even if he would consider himself much better off dead than alive. So c is a type of transaction cost, a one-way ticket to oblivion.

Contrast the situation in which the individual has a choice between committing suicide now, again at cost c and committing it later, at the same cost, with a physician's assistance. It is a real choice because, by virtue of the possibility of assistance (assumed to have been legalized), the individual can postpone the decision to commit suicide. If we assume for simplicity that the unbearable suffering that gives rise to $-Ud$, the disutility of the doomed state, will begin at some future time when the individual will know for certain that he will not recover into the relatively healthy state Uh, the assumption that suicide is possible later at a cost of c implies the substitution of c for Ud in inequality 10.1. That is, as soon as the doomed state sets in, the individual (with [a physician's] assistance . . .) will substitute for it a lesser disutility, the cost of committing suicide.

With this substitution into 10.1, our hypothetical individual will commit suicide now, rather than postpone the decision only if

$$pc > (1 - p)Uh + c \quad (10.2)$$

or equivalently if—$Uh > c$—which makes clear that he will not commit suicide now, since both Uh and c are positive. Even if discounting to present value is ignored, the cost of committing suicide with probability 1 must exceed that cost when multiplied by a probability of less than one and offset by some expectation of entering a state in which continued life will yield net utility. Indeed the cost of suicide now must exceed the *expected* cost of suicide later (since c is assumed constant and exceeds pc), even if the expected utility from living is ignored.

The analysis implies that if physician-assisted suicide in cases of physical incapacity is permitted, the number of suicides in the class of cases that I have modelled will be reduced by $1 - p$, the percentage of cases in which the individual contemplating suicide is mistaken about the future course of his disease or its effect on his desire to live. Moreover, in the fraction of cases in which suicide does occur (p), it will occur later than if physician-assisted suicide were prevented. Weeks, months, or even years of life will be gained, and with it net utility.

The intuition behind these results is straightforward. If the only choice is suicide now and suffering later, individuals will frequently choose suicide now. If the choice is suicide now or suicide at no great cost later, they will choose suicide later because there is always a chance that they are mistaken in believing that continued life will impose unbearable suffering or incapacity on them. They would give up that chance by committing suicide now. The possibility of physician-assisted suicide enables them to wait until they have more information before

deciding whether to live or die. Another way to put this is that the availability of physician-assisted suicide increases the option value of continued living.

2. See generally Sandra H. Johnson, *End-of-Life Decision Making: What We Don't Know, We Make Up; What We Do Know, We Ignore,* 31 Ind. L. Rev. 13 (1998).

3. The capstones of these interrelated reform claims came in 1990 with congressional enactment of the Patient Self-Determination Act, which required all federally funded medical facilities to facilitate patients' exercise of their choice-making rights, including the execution of advance directives, and the U.S. Supreme Court decision in *Cruzan v. Missouri Department of Health,* 497 U.S. 261, 269 (1990), which in effect recognized that mentally competent individuals have a constitutional right to refuse life-prolonging medical treatment.

4. Joanne Lynn, *Unexpected Returns: Insights from SUPPORT,* in To Improve Health and Health Care (S. Isaacs & J. Knickman, eds.) (San Francisco: Jossey-Bass, 1997) at 165.

5. Id. at 167.

6. Id. at 165–66.

7. Id. at 173. There was no difference in the proportion of patients in the intervention and the control groups who completed advance directives.

8. Id.

9. Id. at 175. ("The problem was not just that physicians were not asking patients their views. In addition, patients were not seeking to talk with physicians about such matters as resuscitation. Of those who had not talked with a physician about CPR [cardiopulmonary resuscitation], only 42 percent wanted to do so. Right after we asked patients their preferences concerning CPR, we asked them whether they wanted their preferences followed or would rather have their family and physicians make decisions for them. The vast majority wanted family and doctors to make the choice. Even for those who wanted no CPR and who had no family, most wanted just their doctors to make a choice later, rather than rely upon their own choice." Id. at 169.)

10. As Lynn observed regarding the close proximity of death and the typical entry of DNR orders, "Most were written as prognoses for survival dropped and within a few days of actual death. Mostly, there had not been explicit discussions with patients or families about how to plan for the likelihood of death until this discussion was undertaken. Until then, patients and families 'knew' that the illness was serious, but they still thought they could beat the odds." Id. at 178.

11. See generally Mildred Z. Solomon et al., *Decisions Near the End of Life: Professional Views on Life-Sustaining Treatments,* 83 Am. J. Pub. Health 14, 17 (1993), discussed in chapter 1 supra, at text accompanying notes 26–29. See also Miles J. Edwards & Susan W. Tolle, *Disconnecting a Ventilator at the Request of a Patient Who Knows He Will Then Die: The Doctor's Anguish,* 117 Ann. Int. Med. 254, 255–56 (1992). Describing their experience in disconnect-

ing respirator support at the request of a mentally competent post–polio syndrome patient, Drs. Edwards and Tolle reported, "We looked into the face of an alert man who we knew would soon die. Our more rational intellects told us that his disease, not us, would be the cause of his death. Deep feelings, on the other hand, were accusing us of causing death. From deep within us, feelings were speaking to us, making accusations, 'You are really killing him, practicing active euthanasia, deceptively rationalizing with your intellects that there is a difference.' "

12. On the ways that the exercise of self-determination has become not simply an option but a moral obligation for patients, see Carl Schneider, *The Practice of Autonomy: Patients, Doctors, and Medical Decisions* 137–180 (New York: Oxford Univ. Press, 1998).

13. *Washington v. Glucksberg,* 521 U.S. 702 (1997), *Vacco v. Quill,* 521 U.S. 793 (1997).

14. *Quill v. Vacco,* 80 F.3d 716, 730 (2nd Cir. 1996), rev'd sub nom. *Vacco v. Quill,* 521 U.S. 793 (1997).

15. See note 11, supra.

16. According to one early study regarding refusal of treatment, "physicians often seemed too ready to concede patients' 'right to refuse' rather than to recognize the clinical problems that lay at the bottom of the refusal (e. g., poor or inconsistent communication) and to take steps to remedy them. The disinclination of physicians to encourage patients over time to accept the treatment in question often left patients confused as to the validity of the original recommendation and, by implication, the competence of their physician." Paul S. Appelbaum & Loren H. Roth, *Patients Who Refuse Treatment in Medical Hospitals,* 250 JAMA 1296, 1301 (1983). A more recent study of the first operational year of the Oregon statute permitting physician-assisted suicide, conducted after Judge Miner's ruling, found that patients who sought assisted suicide did not report any undue psychological pressure; but these reports were based on their prescribing physicians' subsequent accounts and have no reliable probative worth for this proposition. Compare Arthur E. Chin et al., *Legalized Physician-Assisted Suicide in Oregon—The First Year's Experience,* 340 N. Eng. J. Med. 577 (1999) with Kathleen Foley & Herbert Hendin, *The Oregon Report: Don't Ask, Don't Tell,* 29 Hastings Center Report 37 (1999).

17. See Anne Scitovsky, *Medical Care in the Last Twelve Months of Life: The Relation between Age, Functional Status, and Medical Expenditures,* 66 Milbank Quarterly 640, 648 (1988); Helena Temkin-Greener et al., *The Use and Cost of Health Services Prior to Death: A Comparison of the Medicare-Only and the Medicare-Medicaid Elderly Population,* 70 Milbank Quarterly 679, 698–99 (1992).

18. *Compassion in Dying v. Washington,* 79 F.3d 790, 821–22 (9th Cir. 1996), rev'd sub nom. *Washington v. Glucksberg,* 521 U.S. 702 (1997) (emphasis in original).

19. See Timothy D. Quill et al., *Care of the Hopelessly Ill: Proposed Clinical Criteria for Physician-Assisted Suicide,* 327 N. Eng. J. Med. 1380, 1381 (1992):

In assisted suicide, the final act is solely the patient's, and the risk of subtle coercion from doctors, family members, institutions, or other social forces is greatly reduced. The balance of power between doctor and patient is more nearly equal in physician-assisted suicide than in euthanasia. . . . In voluntary euthanasia, the physician both provides the means and carries out the final act, with greatly amplified power over the patient and an increased risk of error, coercion, or abuse. . . . We recognize that this exclusion [of voluntary euthanasia] is made at a cost to competent, incurably ill patients who cannot swallow or move and who therefore cannot be helped to die by assisted suicide. . . . [T]his solution is less than ideal, but we also recognize that in the United States access to medical care is currently too inequitable, and many doctor-patient relationships too impersonal, for us to tolerate the risks of permitting active voluntary euthanasia.

See also Margaret P. Battin, *Euthanasia: The Way We Do It, The Way They Do It,* in Ethical Issues in Modern Medicine 286 (J. D. Arras & B. Steinbock, eds.) (Mountain View, Calif.: Mayfield Publ. Co., 5th ed., 1998):

The Netherlands . . . permits voluntary active euthanasia . . . [but a] 1995 policy statement of the Royal Dutch Medical Association expressed a careful preference for physician-assisted suicide in preference to euthanasia, urging that physicians encourage patients who request euthanasia to administer the lethal dose themselves as a further protective of voluntary choice.

20. Judge Guido Calabresi concurred in the invalidation of New York's law specifically on the ground that there had been no recent "affirmative statement forthcoming from the state of New York" signifying its continued commitment to prohibiting physician-assisted suicide. *Quill v. Vacco,* 80 F.3d at 741.

21. Opponents of the Oregon measure sought to block its implementation by litigation and by persuading the state legislature to require a second referendum vote. Both blocking efforts were ultimately unsuccessful; the litigative challenge was rejected by the Ninth Circuit, *Lee v. Oregon,* 107 F.3d 1382 (9th Cir.), cert. denied sub nom. *Lee v. Harcleroad,* 522 U.S. 927 (1997), and in 1996 the Oregon voters reiterated their approval by a much wider margin of 65 to 35 percent.

22. *Compassion in Dying v. Washington,* 79 F.3d at 831–32.

23. See Loes Pijnenborg et al., *Life-terminating Acts without Explicit Request of Patient,* 341 Lancet 1196, 1197 (1993) (Of all deaths in the Netherlands, 1.8 percent were voluntary euthanasia and 0.8 percent were involuntary); for a more expansive interpretation of these data, see Herbert Hendin, *Seduced by Death: Doctors, Patients, and the Dutch Cure* 75–76 (New York: W. W. Norton, 1997) ("The report revealed that in over one thousand cases, physicians admitted they actively caused or hastened death without any request from the patient. . . . [But] other forms of hastening death without the patients consent are common practice in the Netherlands as well. . . . In half of the 49,000 cases [of medical decisions at end of life], decisions that might [end] or were intended to end the life of the patient were made without consulting the patient. In nearly 20,000 cases (about 80 percent), physicians gave the patient's impaired ability to communicate as their justification for not seeking consent. This left

about 5,000 cases in which physicians made decisions that might [end] or were intended to end the lives of competent patients without consulting them.")

24. *Compassion in Dying v. Washington,* 79 F.3d at 832 n. 120 (emphasis in original).

25. See Committee on Care at the End of Life, Institute of Medicine, *Approaching Death: Improving Care at the End of Life* 202–3 (C. Cassel & M. Field, eds.) (Washington, D.C.: National Academy Press, 1997) ("[The 1990 Patient Self-Determination Act] appears to have had modest effects. . . . There are no national studies on the rates of persons completing advance directives, but studies of discrete populations (e.g., nursing home residents or hospital patients) conducted both before and after passage of the PSDA show rates between 5 percent and 29 percent. . . . [In the most recent study] investigators found a small increase of seriously ill patients having an advance directive since the PSDA went into effect (from one in five to one in four), but this increase did not translate into higher rates of documented resuscitation discussions or DNR orders for patients who seemed to want them.")

26. See Colleen M. O'Connor, *Statutory Surrogate Consent Provisions: An Overview and Analysis,* 20 Mental & Physical Disability Law Reporter 128, 133–38 (1996). See also section 5 of the Uniform Health-Care Decisions Act, approved by the National Conference of Commissions on Uniform State Laws in 1993 and the American Bar Association in 1994:

> (a) A surrogate may make a health-care decision for a patient who . . . has been determined by the primary physician to lack capacity . . .
>
> (b) An adult or emancipated minor may designate any individual to act as surrogate. . . . In the absence of a designation, or if the designee is not reasonably available, any member of the following classes of the patient's family who is reasonably available, in descending order of priority, may act as surrogate:
>
> (1) the spouse, unless legally separated;
> (2) an adult child;
> (3) a parent; or
> (4) an adult brother or sister.
>
> (c) If none of the individuals eligible to act as surrogate under subsection (b) is reasonably available, an adult who has exhibited special care and concern for the patient, who is familiar with the patient's personal values, and who is reasonably available may act as surrogate.

27. 1 Samuel 31:1–6 (translated in Robert Alter, *The David Story* 189–90 (New York: W. W. Norton, 1999).

28. 2 Samuel 1:1–16 (translated in id. at 195–98); ellipsis in original.

29. 1 Samuel 31:8–10 (translated in id. at 190–91).

30. 1 Samuel 24:6–7 (translated in id. at 148).

31. 1 Samuel 26:9 (translated in id. at 164).

32. Thus Freud speaks of suicide as "murderous impulses against others redirected upon [one]self" and the death of a loved one as a "shadow of the

object [falling] upon the ego . . . [in that] the loss of the object became transformed into a loss in the ego." This interweaving of self and others in the experience of death is the core linkage between mourning, depression, and "the fear that rises up at the menace of death." *Mourning and Melancholia*, 4 Collected Papers of Sigmund Freud (London: Hogarth Press, 1956) at 159, 162–63.

7. The Death Penalty

1. Though the death penalty is endorsed by some two-thirds of the American public, according to most recent opinion polls, this proportion has declined since the historic high point of 80 percent in 1994. See Jeffrey M. Jones, *Two-Thirds of Americans Support the Death Penalty,* Gallup Poll, Releases, March 2, 2001, www.gallup.com/poll/releases/pr010302.asp. Regarding the imposition of an execution moratorium in Illinois and similar movements elsewhere, see Death Penalty Information Center, Year End Report 2000, www.deathpenaltyinfo.org/yrendrptoo.html.

2. See Fox Butterfield, *Federal Study Finds Decline in Executions,* N. Y. Times, Dec. 11, 2000, A20 ("Of the 84 executions this year, 40, or almost half, have taken place in Texas, after review by Gov. George W. Bush. . . . That is the largest number of executions in one year in any state in the nation's history.") See also Neal Walpin, *Why Texas #1 in Executions,* Frontline, December 5, 2000, www.deathpenaltyinfo.org/Frontline-TX.html.

3. Sara Rimer & Raymond Bonner, *On the Record/Capital Punishment in Texas: Bush Candidacy Puts Focus on Executions,* N. Y. Times, May 14, 2000, A1.

4. *Furman v. Georgia,* 408 U.S. 238 (1972).

5. *Lockhart v. McCree,* 476 U.S. 162 (1986).

6. *McCleskey v. Kemp,* 481 U.S. 279 (1987).

7. See generally Robert A. Burt, *The Constitution in Conflict* 335–44 (Cambridge, Mass.: Harvard Univ. Press, 1992).

8. David Brion Davis, *From Homicide to Slavery: Studies in American Culture* 28 (New York: Oxford Univ. Press, 1986).

9. Id. at 36, 40.

10. Though most states had ended public executions by 1900, the last legalized public execution in the United States took place in Kentucky in 1936, attended by a crowd of "between ten and twenty thousand 'jeering' and 'festive' spectators." John D. Bessler, *Death in the Dark: Midnight Executions in America* 32, 59 (Boston: Northeastern Univ. Press, 1997).

11. See id. at 47–63.

12. See Davis, supra note 8, at 21–22.

13. Regarding the late-nineteenth-century expansion of open-ended discretionary criminal sentencing practices and the corresponding reduction of the jury's role, as the linkage was broken between determinations of guilt for specific substantive offenses and their penalties, see David J. Rothman, *Conscience and Convenience: The Asylum and Its Alternatives in Progressive America* (Boston: Little, Brown, 1980); Marvin Zalman, *The Rise and Fall of the Inde-*

terminate Sentence, 24 Wayne L. Rev. 45 (1977). The one outstanding persistence of this linkage was, in most states, the mandatory death penalty that would follow from jury determination of guilt for first-degree murder. See Lawrence M. Friedman, *Crime and Punishment in American History* (New York: Basic Books, 1993).

14. See Franklin E. Zimring & Gordon Hawkins, *Capital Punishment and the American Agenda* 29, table 2.1 (Cambridge: Cambridge Univ. Press, 1986).

15. Id. at 30 and table 2.2.

16. California's experience in 1967 seemed to forecast the future. In response to physicians' concerns about novel threats of criminal prosecution from a local prosecutor, the legislature enacted liberalized abortion criteria; this bill was signed by then-Governor Ronald Reagan, who did not yet conceive himself as a champion for pro-life protagonists—indeed, as a practical political matter, there were no pro-life protagonists around. See Kristin Luker, *Abortion and the Politics of Motherhood* 88 (Berkeley: Univ. of California Press, 1984). Within four years of this new enactment, the number of legal abortions in California increased from some 5,000 to more than 115,000—an increase of some 2000 percent; as Luker observes, "what had been proposed as a 'middle-way' solution had in fact become 'abortion on demand.' . . . [B]y late 1970, of all women who applied for an abortion, 99.2 percent were granted one." Id. at 94.

17. *Brown v. Board of Education,* 347 U.S. 483 (1954).

18. *Furman v. Georgia,* 408 U.S. 238 (1972).

19. *Planned Parenthood of Central Missouri v. Danforth,* 428 U.S. 52 (1976); see chapter 4, supra, at text accompanying note 24.

20. *Gregg v. Georgia,* 428 U.S. 153, 196 (1976).

21. *Woodson v. North Carolina,* 428 U.S. 280, 302–3 (1976).

22. Robert Weisberg, *Deregulating Death,* 1983 Sup. Ct. Rev. 305, 305 n. 1.

23. *Coker v. Georgia,* 433 U.S. 584 (1977).

24. *Enmund v. Florida,* 458 U.S. 782 (1982).

25. *Lockett v. Ohio,* 438 U.S. 586 (1978).

26. *Gardner v. Florida,* 430 U.S. 349 (1977).

27. Utah had executed Gary Gilmore on January 17, 1977, but Gilmore had waived any appeal from his sentence. The Supreme Court, in permitting his execution, invoked the same rationalist principles that have guided the contemporary reformist agenda in the administration of death for terminally ill people and abortion—that Gilmore's decision was "voluntary," that he had been certified as "mentally competent" by a psychiatrist, and that no one but he, as a free-standing self-determining individual, had any socially cognizable stake in his decision—not even his mother, who petitioned for a hearing regarding the constitutionality of the Utah statute under which her son was to be executed. *Gilmore v. Utah,* 429 U.S. 1012 (1976); on Gilmore's execution, see *New York Times,* Jan. 18, 1977, 1, col. 4.

28. *Spinkellink v. State,* 313 So. 2d 666, 668 (Fla. 1975). Spenkelink's name was repeatedly and variously misspelled in the case reports, see *Spinkellink v. Wainwright,* 578 F.2d 582, 582 n. 1 (5th Cir. 1978).

29. *Spenkelink v. State,* 350 So. 2d 85 (Fla.), cert. denied, 434 U.S. 960 (1977).

30. Id; *Spenkelink v. State,* 372 So. Ed 65 (Fla. 1979).

31. *Spinkellink v. Wainwright,* 578 F.2d 582 (5th Cir. 1978), cert. denied, 440 U.S. 976 (1979); *Spinkellink v. Wainwright,* 596 F.2d 637 (5th Cir. 1979).

32. *Spenkelink v. State,* 350 So. 2d 85, 86 (Fla. 1977) (England, C.J., concurring); *Spenkelink v. Wainright,* 372 So. 927, 927 (Fla. 1979) (England, C.J., concurring).

33. Transcript of student tape recording of seminar with Arthur England, Yale Law School, April 18, 1985. Used by permission.

34. Ramsey Clark, *Spenkelink's Last Appeal,* The Nation, Oct. 27, 1979, at 385.

35. Id. at 400–401.

36. Id. at 401–2.

37. 28 U.S.C. sec. 2254 (1982).

38. *Spenkelink v. Wainright,* 442 U.S. 901, 905–6 (1979) (dissenting opinion, quoting *Sanders v. United States,* 373 U.S. 1, 18 [1963]).

39. 442 U.S. at 902–3.

40. Id. at 904.

41. Clark, supra note 34, at 403.

42. *Spinkellink v. Wainright,* No. 79–8215 (5th Cir., May 24, 1979) (unpublished memorandum).

43. Clark, supra note 34, at 403–4.

44. *Furman v. Georgia,* 408 U.S. 238, 405–12 (1972) (dissenting opinion).

45. *Callins v. Collins,* 510 U.S. 1141, 1144 (1994) (dissenting opinion).

46. Blackmun advanced this more limited proposition essentially as an alternative argument: "But even if the constitutional requirements of consistency and fairness are theoretically reconcilable in the context of capital punishment, it is clear that this Court is not prepared to meet the challenge." Id. at 1150.

47. Id. at 1149.

48. Id. at 1145.

49. Id. at 1146, citing *Woodson v. North Carolina,* 428 U.S. 280, 304 (1976).

50. Id. at 1147, citing *Lockett v. Ohio,* 438 U.S. 586, 604 (1978).

51. Id.

52. *McGautha v. California,* 402 U.S. 183 (1971).

53. The attempt, Harlan said, to provide rationalized standards to control or even to influence jury discretion "was an intractable problem . . . which the history of capital punishment has from the beginning reflected. . . . [T]o identify before the fact those characteristics of criminal homicides and their perpetrators which call for the death penalty, and to express these characteristics in language which can be fairly understood and applied by the sentencing authority, appear to be tasks which are beyond present human ability." 402 U.S. at 207–8. Harlan invoked Justice Benjamin Cardozo's observation, forty years earlier, that legislative efforts to limit imposition of the death penalty by speci-

fying various degrees of murder were nothing more than "a privilege offered to the jury . . . for the exercise of mercy [but] given to them . . . in a mystifying cloud of words." Id. at 198, citing Benjamin Cardozo, *What Medicine Can Do for Law*, in Law and Literature (1931).

54. *Walton v. Arizona*, 497 U.S. 639, 656 (1990) (concurring opinion); *Callins v. Collins*, 510 U.S. 1141 (1994) (concurring opinion).

55. *Graham v. Collins*, 506 U.S. 461 (1993) (concurring opinion).

56. *Callins v. Collins*, 510 U.S. at 1148.

57. Id. at 1142.

58. Sigmund Freud, *Thoughts for the Times on War and Death* (1915), in 14 Standard Edition of the Complete Psychological Works of Sigmund Freud 289 (James Strachey, ed.) (London: Hogarth Press, 1964).

59. Id. at 291.

60. Arthur Koestler, *Reflections on Hanging*, cited in *Witherspoon v. Illinois*, 391 U.S. 510, 520 and n. 17 (1968).

61. *Callins v. Collins*, 510 U.S. 1141, 1142 (1994) (dissenting opinion).

62. *Lockhart v. McCree*, 476 U.S. 162 (1986). For detailed evaluation of the Court's reasoning, see Robert A. Burt, *Disorder in the Court: The Death Penalty and the Constitution*, 85 Mich. L. Rev. 1741, 1786–91 (1987).

63. *Lockhart v. McCree*, 476 U.S. at 185.

64. For an extensive recitation of the data, see Samuel Gross, *Race and Death: The Judicial Evaluation of Discrimination in Capital Sentencing*, 18 U.C. Davis L. Rev. 1275 (1985).

65. *McCleskey v. Kemp*, 481 U.S. 279, 292 n. 7 (1987).

66. See Burt, supra note 62, at 1795–1800.

67. In *McCleskey v. Zant*, 499 U.S. 467 (1991), the Court essentially eliminated the possibility of more than one federal habeas review; in *Coleman v. Thompson*, 501 U.S. 722 (1991), the Court overturned a 1963 ruling that permitted federal habeas review of claims barred by state procedural rules so long as the petitioner did not deliberately intend to bypass the state tribunals; in *Pulley v. Harris*, 465 U.S. 37 (1984), the Court ruled that states were not required to systematically monitor the consistency and proportionality of their general death penalty sentencing practices. According to recently compiled data, between 1983 and 1995 the proportion of federal habeas relief granted in capital cases was 35 percent (of 531 decisions rendered in all federal courts), dropping from an average of 72 percent (of 32 decisions) between 1978 and 1982. James S. Liebman, *Life after Death: The Fate of Capital Sentences after Imposition at Trial*, unpublished memorandum, June 16, 1999 (cited with permission).

68. *Coleman v. Balkcom*, 451 U.S. 949, 963–64 (dissenting from denial of certiorari).

69. This was Justice John Paul Stevens's estimate, based on the certiorari petitions filed in capital cases during the preceding ten months; id. at 950 (Stevens, J., concurring in denial of certiorari).

70. Id. at 958–59, 962 (dissenting from denial of certiorari).

71. Jack Greenberg, *Capital Punishment as a System,* 91 Yale L. J. 908, 917–18 (1982). In 1983, Justice Marshall reported that federal courts of appeals had overruled lower court rulings to grant relief to death-sentenced prisoners, in some 70 percent of the cases decided since 1976. *Barefoot v. Estelle,* 463 U.S. 880, 915 (1983). At the same time, state appellate courts were also reversing death sentences at a high rate. For example, between 1972 and 1984, the Florida Supreme Court reviewed 247 capital cases and set aside 116 or 47 percent. M. Vandiver & M. Radelet, *Post*-Furman *Death Sentences in Florida* (September 20, 1984) (unpublished manuscript, Capital Punishment Project, Sociology Dep't, Univ. of Florida). A 1985 study found a similar proportion of death sentence reversals in state courts generally. NAACP Legal Defense Fund, Inc., *Death Row, U.S.A.* (October 1985) (unpublished manuscript).

72. *Vasquez v. Harris,* 503 U.S. 1000 (1992).

73. See John T. Noonan, Jr., *Horses of the Night: Harris v. Vasquez,* 45 Stan. L. Rev. 1011, 1020 (1993).

74. This indictment was made explicit by former Judge Robert Bork in a newspaper commentary: "Perhaps the most dismaying thing is the display of civil disobedience within the federal judiciary. . . . What is new, and exemplified by the legal disaster of the Harris case, is the resistance of lower-court judges both to the law and to the Supreme Court. Those judges who, after years of examination and re-examination of the conviction, repeatedly issued last-minute stays of execution evidently thought their personal opposition to capital punishment was reason enough to defy what law and their judicial superiors demanded." *An Outbreak of Judicial Civil Disobedience,* Wall Street Journal, April 29, 1992, A19.

75. Noonan, supra note 73, at 1020 ("Whether the Court had jurisdiction to issue such a blanket anticipatory order is doubtful. Who determines the jurisdiction of the Supreme Court but the Supreme Court? Yet the Supreme Court must abide [by] rules. In any event, the order was effective and final. The horses of the night had galloped. Harris was put to death at 6:30 in the morning.") Judge Noonan—a Reagan appointee to the Ninth Circuit Court of Appeals who had not concurred in any of the stays issued in *Harris*—elaborated his suggestion of Supreme Court lawlessness by revealing that the Court had issued its final order in the *Harris* case without consulting those members of the Court who had dissented from its previous dispositions. Judge Noonan stated, "So the author was informed by one of the dissenters." Id. at 1020 n. 50.

76. In a 1981 case, Justice John Paul Stevens somewhat acidly observed that capital punishment "questions have not been difficult for three members of the Court," noting that "Justices Brennan and Marshall have invariably voted to set aside the death penalty and, if my memory serves me correctly, Justice Rehnquist has invariably voted to uphold the death penalty." *Coleman v. Balkcom,* 451 U.S. 949, 951 and n. 2 (concurring in denial of certiorari).

77. *Gregg v. Georgia,* 428 U.S. 153, 225–26 (1976) (concurring opinion).

78. *McCleskey v. Kemp,* 481 U.S. 279, 314–15, 319 (1987).

79. *McCleskey v. Kemp,* 481 U.S. at 339 (dissenting opinion).

80. Id. at 339, 342.

81. Regarding the different sequence in public attitudes toward the death penalty in the United States and western Europe, see Franklin E. Zimring & Gordon Hawkins, *Capital Punishment and the American Agenda* (Cambridge: Cambridge Univ. Press, 1986), chapter 2. Attitudes toward abortion have also sharply diverged between us and them since the 1970s; see Margaret Talbot, *The Little White Bombshell,* N. Y. Times Magazine, July 11, 1999, 40 ("In the United States . . . abortion is a far more volatile issue [than in western Europe.]")

82. Zimring & Hawkins, supra note 81, at 26–33.

83. See Butterfield, supra note 2 ("Eighty-four prisoners have been executed in the United States this year, a 14 percent decline from the 98 put to death in 1999, in what some experts believe is one sign of a new sense of caution and skepticism about the death penalty among both politicians and the public. . . . [T]hough a majority of Americans continue to favor the death penalty, support for it has declined. For example, a Gallup Poll last February showed that support for the death penalty had dropped to 66 percent from 80 percent in 1984.")

84. See Stephen Bright & Patrick Keenan, *Judges and the Politics of Death: Deciding between the Bill of Rights and the Next Election in Capital Cases,* 75 Boston Univ. L. Rev. 759 (1995); Stephen Bright et al., *Breaking the Most Vulnerable Branch: Do Rising Threats to Judicial Independence Preclude Due Process in Capital Cases?* 31 Colum. Human Rights L. Rev. 123 (1999).

85. Notwithstanding the Supreme Court's intense suppressive efforts, abetted by congressional enactments (see, especially, the Antiterrorism and Effective Death Penalty Act of 1996, Pub. L. No. 104–132, 110 Stat. 1214), many lower courts in both the state and federal system continue to chafe at the individual instances of systemic injustice that they see. According to recent research, the reversal rates of death penalty impositions in these courts persist at the high levels of the early 1980s—68 percent of the cases adjudicated through 1995, as compared to a reversal rate of less than 10 percent in noncapital criminal cases. *Death Sentences Being Overturned in 2 of 3 Appeals,* N.Y. Times, June 12, 2000, 1, col. 6. This divergence between the Supreme Court's adamant turning away and lower courts' misgivings only occasionally explodes into high visibility, as in the imbroglio with the Ninth Circuit in the *Harris* case; but, as with *Harris,* these divergent perspectives fuel a persistent sense of systemic wrongdoing on all sides in the administration of the death penalty.

8. All the Days of My Life

1. *Superintendent of Belchertown State School v. Saikewicz,* 370 N.E.2d 417 (1977). See Robert A. Burt, *Taking Care of Strangers: The Rule of Law in Doctor-Patient Relations* 148–49, 155–58 (New York: Free Press, 1979).

2. Raymond S. Duff & A. G. M. Campbell, *Moral and Ethical Dilemmas in the Special-Care Nursery,* 289 New Eng. J. Med. 890, 891, 894 (1973).

3. See *Declaratory Judgment in the Infant Doe Case,* reprinted in 2 Issues in Law & Medicine 77 (1986).

4. See U.S. Commission on Civil Rights, *Medical Discrimination against Children with Disabilities* (Washington, D.C.: Government Printing Office, 1989).

5. See Rene Anspach, *Deciding Who Lives: Fateful Choices in the Intensive-Care Nursery* 58–108 (Berkeley: Univ. California Press, 1993).

6. See *In the Matter of Baby K,* 16 F.3d 590 (4th Cir. 1994) (upholding parent's authority to direct treatment for a seriously ill infant, notwithstanding physicians' determination of futility).

7. See Dan W. Brock, *Physician-Assisted Suicide Is Sometimes Morally Justified* in Physician-Assisted Suicide 91–95 (R. F. Weir, ed.) (Bloomington: Indiana Univ. Press, 1997); David Orentlicher, *The Alleged Distinction between Euthanasia and the Withdrawal of Life-Sustaining Treatment: Conceptually Incoherent and Impossible to Maintain,* 1998 Univ. Ill. L. Rev. 837; Richard Epstein, *Mortal Peril: Our Inalienable Right to Health Care?* 290–92 (Reading, Mass.: Addison-Wesley Pub. Co., 1997).

8. Oregon Death with Dignity Act, OR. Rev. Stat. secs. 127.800–897 (1996).

9. National Conference of Commissioners on Uniform State Laws, Uniform Health-Care Decisions Act (1993), section 5(e).

10. See J. Andrew Billings & Susan D. Block, *Slow Euthanasia,* 12 J. Palliative Care 21 (1996); David Orentlicher, *The Supreme Court and Physician-Assisted Suicide: Rejecting Assisted Suicide but Embracing Euthanasia,* 337 N. Eng. J. Med. 1236 (1997).

11. See Susan Anderson Fohr, *The Double Effect of Pain Medication: Separating Myth from Reality,* 1 J. Palliative Medicine 315, 320 (1998) ("The literature contains little data to support the belief that appropriate use of opioids hastens death in patients dying from cancer and other chronic diseases"); but compare Howard Brody, *Double Effect: Does It Have a Proper Use in Palliative Care?,* 1 J. Palliative Medicine 329, 330 (1998) ("Fohr has dealt only with the appropriate use of opioids for analgesia, and . . . has omitted mention of terminal sedation, especially in the particular form of barbiturate coma [where] the picture is far less neat. . . . [I]t is hard to question the empirical generalization that barbiturate coma shortens life . . . especially if one does not offer artificial support of ventilation or hydration, which one generally would not do (for excellent reasons) within a palliative care environment.")

12. See generally Timothy E. Quill et al., *The Rule of Double Effect—A Critique of Its Role in End-of-Life Decision Making,* 337 N. Eng. J. Med. 1768 (1997); Daniel Sulmasy, *The Use and Abuse of the Principle of Double Effect,* 3 Clinical Pulmonary Med. 86 (1996).

13. See Kathleen M. Foley, *Competent Care for the Dying instead of Physician-Assisted Suicide,* 336 N. Eng. J. Med. 54, 55–6 (1997) ("Physicians

do struggle with doubts about their own intentions. The courts' arguments [equating a lethal prescription with withdrawing life-sustaining treatment and with aggressive treatment of pain] fuel their ambivalence about withdrawing life-sustaining treatments or using opioid or sedative infusions to treat intractable symptoms in dying patients. . . . Yet saying that physicians struggle with doubts about their intentions is not the same as saying that their intention is to kill. . . . Specialists in palliative care do not believe they practice physician-assisted suicide or euthanasia.")

14. *Washington v. Glucksberg*, 521 U.S. 702, 736–37 (1997). Justices Ruth Bader Ginsburg and Steven Breyer joined this concurrence; in his own concurring opinion, Justice Breyer stated, "The laws of New York and of Washington do not prohibit doctors from providing patients with drugs sufficient to control pain despite the risk that those drugs themselves will kill. . . . Medical technology . . . makes the administration of pain-relieving drugs sufficient, except for a very few individuals for whom the ineffectiveness of pain control medicines can mean, not pain, but the need for sedation. . . . This legal circumstance means that the state laws before us do not infringe directly upon the (assumed) central interest [put forward by the plaintiffs] in dying with dignity." Id. at 791–92.

15. See Holcomb B. Noble, *Doctors Increasingly Shielded in Prescribing Powerful Painkillers*, N.Y. Times, Aug. 9, 1999. See also *Oregon Board Disciplines Doctor for Not Treating Patients' Pain*, N.Y. Times, Sept. 4, 1999, A26.

16. *Compassion in Dying v. Washington*, 79 F.3d 790, 801–2 (9th Cir. 1996), citing *Planned Parenthood v. Casey*, 505 U.S. 833, 851 (1992).

17. See generally Jay Katz, *The Silent World of Doctor and Patient* (New York: Free Press, 1984).

18. See Ezekiel J. Emanuel & Linda L. Emanuel, *Four Modes of the Physician-Patient Relationship*, 267 JAMA 2221 (1992).

19. See Nancy Dubler, *Limiting Technology in the Process of Negotiating Death*, 1 Yale J. Health Policy, Law & Ethics 297–98 (2001) ("[D]eath has re-emerged as an acceptable outcome of medical practice . . . for patients whose prognosis is hopeless. [But] financial disincentives for long-term hospital stays must make us wary of determining the prognosis of hopelessness too easily. Capitated systems and prospective payment mechanisms provide incentives for shortened lengths of stay. This financial fact of life must not be permitted to contaminate decisions about death. . . . [H]ealth care organizations and institutions [have recently] reevaluate[d] their practices and protocols for managing patients at the end of life and especially in expensive intensive care units. In the aggregate, the results may be beneficial to patients and families as new perceptions and practices limit the endless process of dying that had become the norm in many health care centers. But not surprisingly, dangers of discrimination, creation of levels of care linked to layered reimbursement, and unnecessarily hastened deaths lurk in newly found perceptions of palliative and hospice care.")

20. Many advocates for legal recognition of physician-assisted suicide insist

that the moral integrity of the "self-determination principle" would be inappropriately compromised by any consideration of adverse social consequences that might follow from this legalization. These advocates insist, that is, that the only proper framework for moral analysis is "deontological" rather than "consequentialist" or pragmatically utilitarian. See, e.g., Brody, supra note 11, at 329–30. But the conceptual incoherences of the self-determination principle moot its application in death-dispensing decisions, even when viewed exclusively within a deontological framework.

21. See Robert A. Burt, *The Constitution in Conflict* 349–51 (Cambridge, Mass.: Harvard Univ. Press, 1992).

22. See id. at 347–51; Kristin Luker, *Abortion and the Politics of Motherhood* 94 (Berkeley: Univ. California Press, 1984) ("[Between 1968 and 1972] the number of abortions sought and performed in California increased by *2000 percent.* Moreover, by 1970 it was becoming apparent that what had been proposed as a 'middle-way' solution had in fact become 'abortion on demand.' . . . By 1971, women in California had abortions because they wanted them, not because physicians agreed that they could have them.")

23. See *Planned Parenthood of Southeastern Pennsylvania v. Casey,* 505 U.S. 833 (1992).

24. In *Maher v. Roe,* 432 U.S. 464 (1977) and *Harris v. McRae,* 448 U.S. 297 (1980), the Supreme Court upheld congressional and state legislation specifically denying financial assistance for abortions; on the practical obstacles to obtaining abortions, see Jack Hitt, *Who Will Do Abortions Here?* N.Y. Times Magazine, Jan. 18, 1998, 20.

25. See text accompanying note 7, chapter 4, supra.

26. On the likely shortcomings of screening mechanisms, see Robert A. Burt, *Misguided Guidelines,* 6 Psychology, Public Policy & Law 382 (2000); Daniel Callahan & Margot White, *The Legalization of Physician-Assisted Suicide: Creating a Regulatory Potemkin Village,* 30 Univ. Richmond L. Rev. 1 (1996).

27. See generally Burt, supra note 21, at 265–310.

28. Orlando Patterson, *Slavery and Social Death: A Comparative Study* (Cambridge, Mass.: Harvard Univ. Press, 1982).

29. Mary Douglas, *Purity and Danger: An Analysis of the Concepts of Pollution and Taboo* 174 (London: Routledge & Kegan Paul, 1966).

30. Id. at 167–71.

31. Id. at 170–71.

32. Genesis 2:17.

33. Letter of 21 December 1817, in *Selected Letters of John Keats* 92 (Lionel Trilling, ed.) (New York: Farrar, Strauss and Young, 1951).

34. Speech at naturalization ceremony, 1944, quoted in Gerald Gunther, *Learned Hand: The Man and the Judge* 548–49 (New York: Knopf, 1994); *Repouille v. United States,* 165 F.2d 152 (2d Cir. 1947) at 153.

35. W. H. Auden, *We're Late,* in The Collected Poetry of W. H. Auden 26–27 (New York: Random House, 1945).

INDEX

Text:	10/13 Galliard
Display:	Akzidenz Grotesk
Compositor:	G&S Typesetters, Inc.
Printer and binder:	Sheridan Books, Inc.